Animal Cruelty Investigations: A Collaborative
Approach from Victim to Verdict™

Cover photo:

Abraham was one of 149 dogs seized in a large-scale animal neglect case in Oregon requiring strong inter-disciplinary collaboration. After gaining 20 pounds (25% of his body weight), Abe, as he came to be known, found his forever home in Oregon. The plight of the animal victims in that case prompted significant strengthening of Oregon's animal protection laws.

Animal Cruelty Investigations: A Collaborative Approach from Victim to Verdict™

Edited by

Kris Otteman
DVM, Diplomate ABVP Shelter Medicine Practice, CAWA
Courtesy Faculty Carlson College of Veterinary Medicine, Oregon State University, USA

Linda Fielder
CAWA
Animal Legal Defense Fund, Cotati, CA, USA

Emily Lewis
JD, MSEL
Animal Legal Defense Fund, Cotati, CA, USA

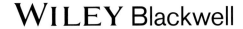

Registered Office
John Wiley & Sons, Inc., 111 River Street, Hoboken, NJ 07030, USA

Editorial Office
111 River Street, Hoboken, NJ 07030, USA

For details of our global editorial offices, customer services, and more information about Wiley products visit us at www.wiley.com.

Wiley also publishes its books in a variety of electronic formats and by print-on-demand. Some content that appears in standard print versions of this book may not be available in other formats.

Library of Congress Cataloging-in-Publication Data Applied for

PB: 9781119764885

Cover Design: Wiley
Cover Image: Courtesy of John Valls

Set in 9.5/12.5pt STIXTwoText by Straive, Pondicherry, India

Printed in Singapore
M113138_070122

Contents

List of Contributors

Editors

Linda Fielder, CAWA
Animal Legal Defense Fund
Cotati, CA
USA

Emily Lewis, JD, MSEL
Animal Legal Defense Fund
Cotati, CA
USA

Dr. Kris Otteman, DVM, Diplomate ABVP Shelter Medicine Practice, CAWA
Courtesy Faculty Carlson College of Veterinary Medicine,
Oregon State University
USA

Contributors

Dr. Zarah Hedge, DVM, MHP, DACVPM, DABVP
Shelter Medicine Practice
San Diego, CA
USA

Jake Kamins, JD
State of Oregon Animal Cruelty Deputy
District Attorney
Corvallis, OR
USA

David B. Rosengard, JD, LLM
Managing Attorney, Animal Legal
Defense Fund
Adjunct Professor of Animal Law, Lewis &
Clark Law School
Cotati, CA
USA

Preface

The authors have worked together to promote the investigation and prosecution of crimes against animals for over a decade. We have put our best efforts forward in hoarding cases that made the national news and cases of anonymous animal victims with no known owner, witnesses, or suspect. Despite our fierce dedication to the cause, there were moments, months, even years, that led to frustration, tested our fortitude, and pushed the boundaries of our tolerance for impediments. It is in those moments that we garnered the information and experience that we share with you in this book. We have faced many challenges in working on these cases and realized over time that our most successful responses were born out of a collaboration of disciplines and expertise. Not one of us could have approached our work in this field alone and we do not expect that from our readers.

Use the information in this book to empower you and your agency to respond to animal cruelty with confidence and integrity. Animal cruelty casework is difficult, particularly if you do not have the resources, support, and expertise you need. Let this book help identify those gaps in your jurisdiction and guide a solution regardless of the magnitude of the perceived roadblocks.

Confronting and addressing animal cruelty is important. If for no other reason than it is against the law in every state. That aside, animal abuse is a violent crime and to think the cycle of violence begins or ends with animals would be naive. The safety of your community is directly related to how seriously you take animal cruelty allegations. In our years of work on these cases, the frequency with which mental illness correlated to maltreatment of animals became glaringly evident. More often than not, the owner of a neglected animal needed community resources as much as the victim animal. Failing to adequately respond to neglected animals in your jurisdiction simultaneously ignores individuals who are struggling with mental health issues. Finally, animals are sentient beings, made vulnerable by their inability to put words to their experiences. They rely on veterinarians, field officers, and prosecutors to speak on their behalf with equal advocacy as any victim would receive.

After years in the field, each of us can recall a case that we wish had turned out differently for the animal or humans involved. For any one of you who can name *that* animal cruelty case, the one that keeps you up at night, the one you wish had turned out differently, the one you learned from, the one that simply did not seem fair, this book was born out of that indignation and the drive to facilitate justice in honor of those victims who never found it and future victims who deserve it.

Acknowledgments

General Acknowledgments

Writing this book was an exercise in perseverance and teamwork. Having worked together closely for many years, we consider ourselves masters of teamwork. As for perseverance, we've learned that a bend in the road is not the end of the road, and we are grateful to be continuing this journey together. We relied on each other throughout this process, but our thanks goes out to the people who kept us organized, contributed their expertise, and offered genuine feedback. Thank you to contributing authors Dr. Zarah Hedge, Jake Kamins, Esq., and David Rosengard, Esq. Each of you brings a deep well of experience and insight to this text. Thank you to Anika Moje for reviewing our work with a keen eye for detail, keeping us on task, and providing support and constant encouragement. Thank you to Kathleen Wood, Esq., for repeatedly lending your vast expertise on state law nuances and Conor Lamkin for your extensive legal research assistance. Our appreciation goes out to Scott Heiser, Esq. and Michelle Welch, Esq., for their contributions to the Specific Case Protocols. Thank you to Nichole Waldner for editing and formatting our manuscript, Jacqui Monahan for designing our graphics and templates, and to Merryl Le Roux, Erica Judisch, and Wiley Publishing for guiding us through the submission and publishing process. Thank you to the Oregon Humane Society for the use of case materials and photographs throughout this text.

Linda Fielder's Acknowledgments

This book was created not only by the authors and contributors, but by every individual who worked alongside us responding to animal cruelty cases. The members of the Humane Investigations and Medical teams at the Oregon Humane Society were a committed, talented, compassionate group I considered family. We sweated inside Tyvek suits and maneuvered through crime scenes stacked with garbage, mircd in mud, and filled with treacherous hazards both living and inanimate. We worked together through long days and beyond exhaustion. Never satisfied with doing just enough, my colleagues helped support the mindset of constant learning and always finding ways to do better, always for the animals.

In the field of animal cruelty investigations, having a support network outside the organization or agency is critical to one's mental health and stamina. I am fortunate to have a chosen family of friends who made sure to check in when the work became heavy, both in the field and during the challenges of writing this manuscript. Finally, I owe a debt of gratitude to the experts who have contributed to the field of veterinary forensic medicine and whose texts I carried with me to the exam room, kept on the bedside table, and recommended to anyone who wanted to learn more about the science behind animal cruelty investigations. This book is intended to support those excellent works that came before it.

Emily Lewis' Acknowledgments

Many years ago, the Criminal Justice Program at the Animal Legal Defense Fund graciously allowed me to volunteer as a recent college graduate, adrift in the world with a degree but no specific direction, save my compassion for animals. That position opened my eyes both to the horrific crimes perpetrated against animals and the network of remarkable professionals committed to seeking justice on their behalf. I had found my path.

In the years that followed, lawyers, professors, veterinarians, and animal welfare professionals whom I held in the highest esteem became mentors and eventually colleagues. I will never be able to adequately convey the level of gratitude I have for the individuals who created opportunities and then mentored me on the path of this career that has enriched my life in so many ways. This book is a testament to your leadership, guidance, and inspiration. Thank you for constantly raising the bar and never doubting my ability to meet it.

To my most wonderful, supportive family and amazing loyal friends, thank you for being the counterbalance to the heaviness of this work and shining a light on those days when the world can seem full of shadows. You are the constant reminder that there is good in the world and have always fueled my sustained optimism that it is worth fighting for that good.

Sentiments of gratitude cannot come without also acknowledging the motivation behind this work. To the individuals involved in animal cruelty cases – once or every day – who are open to unique partnerships and willing to rely on them, who value the insight of experts, and who use their experiences to teach others: you are inspiring, you make a difference, you are both the reason for this book and the answer for the animals.

Dr. Kris Otteman's Acknowledgments

Working in a local veterinary practice in the early years of my career, I encountered animals who had suffered cruelty, however during this time, laws were not in place that recognized these crimes or offered any legal consequences on behalf of the animal victim. As the fields of veterinary medicine, animal welfare, and animal protection laws have grown and aligned in recent years, the resulting synergy has been incredible to witness. The tangible benefits to the animals and the people in our communities through teamwork, compassion, education, and emerging science have profoundly changed the world for the better.

The Oregon Humane Society provided the mission and the resources necessary for us to contribute to the incredible evolution of humane investigations in the United States through practical example and teaching others. I am eternally grateful to all the amazing people who made this possible. Every action certainly influences others and I am grateful for the opportunity to be a positive force and example that propels this field forward.

Thank you to my father, Dr. Richard H. Otteman, for inspiring me to never stop learning and to have the courage to make a difference even in the face of fear or uncertainty.

To my ever encouraging and best critic, my husband Jeff, thank you for supporting this effort to put into writing the passion and energy my co-authors and I have for collaboration in the fight against animal cruelty. Your sage advice and wisdom sustain me.

To the social workers, law enforcement, prosecutors, animal control and animal welfare workers, veterinarians, and veterinary staff who give of their time, talents, and treasure to act and continue this momentum – thank you and *do not tire*. It is my hope that this book is a thank you to all my colleagues who have paved the way and an encouragement to all who may begin or choose to continue this journey of truly making reverence for life a reality for all creatures great and small.

About the Companion Website

This book is accompanied by a companion website:

www.wiley.com/go/otteman/victimtoverdict

The website includes:

- Introduction to the Appendix
- Appendix A–Specific Case Protocols
- Appendix B–Forms and Checklists
- Appendix C–Templates and Agreements
- Appendix D–Resources

1

Introduction
Emily Lewis

All 50 states now criminalize cruelty to animals in one way or another. With animals as live evidence unable to put words to their suffering or the criminal act perpetrated upon them, attaining justice for victim animals is conditional on the successful collaboration of veterinarians, law enforcement, and prosecutors. Not only do these cases require each of these disciplines to understand and execute their role with precision in order to be successful, but they must also understand the duty, constraints, and capabilities of each other in the context of an animal cruelty case. The laws may differ between states in nuanced ways, but the foundation of a thorough and fair animal cruelty investigation remains relatively static across state lines. This book provides a multidisciplinary guide to building that foundation in every case.

1.1 Making the Most of This Resource

1.1.1 How to Use This Book

Whether you are working in the field or training members of your community, this book can be a valuable resource. It is written to be equally comprehensible across disciplines and experience levels. It can function as a guide for field officers to use when actively responding to reports of animal cruelty, while also providing forms and templates ready for use in the field. It can provide clarity to veterinary staff at a community clinic on what to do when they are presented with a suspected victim of animal cruelty. Seasoned and novice prosecutors can reference this book upon assignment of an animal cruelty case to understand the players and nuances of such cases.

The book is written and organized in a way that facilitates its use as a quick, situational reference source or as a comprehensive manual suited for field work or a classroom setting.

1.1.2 Roadmap

The chapters are ordered to follow the typical trajectory of an escalating criminal animal cruelty case. Before addressing the investigation aspect of these cases, the book first emphasizes the importance of a preliminary understanding of the subject matter of the investigation, found in Chapter 2. From there, the chapters discuss the various phases and components of a thorough investigation, starting

Animal Cruelty Investigations: A Collaborative Approach from Victim to Verdict™, First Edition.
Edited by Kris Otteman, Linda Fielder, and Emily Lewis.
© 2022 John Wiley & Sons, Inc. Published 2022 by John Wiley & Sons, Inc.
Companion website: www.wiley.com/go/otteman/victimtoverdict

with the baseline expectations for each case assessment (Chapter 3) through execution of a search warrant and evidence collection (Chapters 9 and 10). The final third of the book discusses the phases of a case that typically occur after the initial investigation and/or search warrant execution (Chapter 11, 12, and 13), concluding with remedies for animal ownership and trial (Chapters 15 and 16).

Acknowledging that differing animal cruelty offenses present unique hallmarks or challenges, Appendix A: Specific Case Protocols is included as a quick reference source. This appendix is organized by the nature of the crime or injury and provides in-the-moment advice and reminders specific to that type of animal cruelty case, while cross-referencing recommended forms, checklists, agreements, templates, and resources provided in Appendices B–D.

1.2 Why Definitions Are Important

Endeavoring to impart knowledge of the expectations and challenges posed to multiple professional disciplines involved in animal cruelty investigations begins with a foundation in relevant terminology. The words used by veterinarians, field officers, and prosecutors alike can have far-reaching implications in an animal cruelty case. This in and of itself is a compelling reason to discuss verbiage. Beyond that motivation, we acknowledge that states, agencies, and individuals are going to have their own nuanced definition of words and concepts frequently referenced in this book. There are venues to delve into those nuances and make the case as to why one definition may be better than another, but this book is not that venue. The overarching concepts behind these terms and phrases should be relatively consistent across states and disciplines and the way this book uses them should be easily adapted to the way you, your organization, or your state uses those words. Do not let semantics detract from the fundamentals imparted in the chapters that follow.

1.3 Terms and Phrases: Animal Cruelty Cases

Each state uses different verbiage to craft its cruelty laws, but across the board there are certain concepts found in every state's animal protection laws. These are important concepts and definitions to understand and will be continually referenced throughout this book.

1.3.1 Animal

At first impression, it would seem that "animal" could be easily defined, but in reality, states struggle with how to categorize this noun in the context of their criminal code. Some states list what *are* considered "animals" in that state [1, 2]. Other states define the term by saying what it is *not* [3, 4]. Other states choose a more succinct definition and simply say an animal is defined as a nonhuman animal [5]. And some states choose to take the opportunity to narrow the definition beyond what one would typically interpret to be an "animal" [6, 7]. For the purposes of this book, we are discussing animal species who are subject to your state's animal cruelty laws.

1.3.2 Active Animal Cruelty

An individual (or corporation) can commit what has been identified as "active animal cruelty." These are acts that are decisive, acute, and done with intention. The mental states typically associated with this type of animal cruelty are malicious, intentional, purposeful, and knowing. Examples of statutes that would fit under this category are aggravated animal abuse, aggravated cruelty to animals, torture, and sexual assault of an animal. Throughout this book, unless a specific crime is being referenced, the phrase "animal abuse" will be used to indicate active animal cruelty.

1.3.3 Passive Animal Cruelty

All states criminalize certain types of "passive animal cruelty." This can be identified when the *inaction* of an individual (or corporation) causes undue suffering to an animal. Reckless and criminally negligent are the mental states often connected with these types of crimes, though inaction of an individual can also be intentional or knowingly done. Examples of statutes that would fit under this category are those that require the provision of minimum care (food, water, shelter, veterinary care) to animals. Throughout this book, unless a specific crime is being referenced, the phrase "animal neglect" will be used to indicate passive animal cruelty.

1.3.4 Good Animal Husbandry

In the context of animal cruelty work, the phrase "good animal husbandry" needs to be distinguished from the phrase "accepted animal husbandry practices." The latter is a phrase frequently used when exempting certain agricultural and food production practices from the animal cruelty laws in a state. The former colloquially refers to providing species-appropriate care to an animal in one's custody and can provide the basis for minimum care standards in a state.

1.3.5 Mandatory Reporting

Across many professional disciplines, particularly those likely to encounter vulnerable populations, there exists a duty to report certain actions, statements, observations, or suspicions to law enforcement. The field of animal welfare is no different. Lawyers and police officers working in this field are mandatory reporters of child and elder abuse. Social workers and human services employees are also mandatory reporters of child abuse. Veterinarians in many states[1] are mandatory reporters of animal cruelty. Being a mandatory reporter means you *must* report, it is not optional, and it is not transferable; not reporting could result in disciplinary action.

By passing laws requiring animal control officers to report suspected child abuse or permitting social service employees to report suspected animal cruelty, states are promoting cross-reporting. If there is one vulnerable entity being victimized, other vulnerable populations in the situation are at risk of also being victimized; cross-reporting ensures that this likelihood is not overlooked.

1.4 Terms and Phrases: Veterinary Medicine

1.4.1 Acute

Refers to a condition or situation that has occurred very recently. Acute conditions may become chronic health concerns.

---

1 As of January 2021, veterinarians are mandatory reporters of animal cruelty in 19 states. Animal Legal Defense Fund (2020). Laws in favor of veterinary reporting of animal cruelty. https://aldf.org/project/veterinary-reporting (accessed 4 August 2021).

1.4.2 Bright, Alert, and Responsive (BAR)

"Bright, Alert, and Responsive" is an acronym veterinarians use to indicate an animal's presentation is normal.

1.4.3 Blunt Force Trauma

An injury or group of injuries caused by tissue impacting or colliding with a blunt object.

1.4.4 Body Condition Score (BCS)

A quantitative, yet subjective, method for evaluating body fat and overall condition using a standardized numbering system. There are various BCS scoring charts available for reference that are species specific. When you are assigning an animal a BCS using a chart for reference, be sure to include the name of the chart you are referencing and words from the description associated with the BCS you are assigning to the animal.

1.4.5 CBC/Chemistry

Stands for complete blood count and blood chemistry panel. These are blood tests veterinarians may order in furtherance of the diagnostic phase of an exam or to evaluate the overall health status and well-being of an animal.

1.4.6 Chronic

Refers to a condition or situation that is persistent or reoccurring having not occurred very recently (hours or days).

1.4.7 Easy Keeper

A term used to refer to a livestock animal who maintains a normal body weight on a relatively modest or average amount of feed.

1.4.8 Lividity

An unnatural coloration of the skin, caused by fluid leakage within the tissues; can be useful in determining the positioning of a body at the time of death and whether a body was moved after death.

1.4.9 Necropsy

An autopsy performed on a deceased animal.

1.4.10 Nonaccidental Injury or Death

Injury or death that has been deliberately inflicted.

1.4.11 PE

An acronym for "physical exam."

1.4.12 Predation

The hunting or scavenging of an animal or animal remains by another animal for food. Victims of predation are often mistaken for victims of animal cruelty perpetrated by humans. There are certain hallmarks of predation that veterinarians can use to distinguish between those scenarios (see Chapter 11).

1.4.13 Radiographs

Radiograph means X-ray.

1.4.14 Rigor

The result of chemical changes in the body that cause stiffening and contraction of the joints and muscles; occurs one to six hours after death.

1.4.15 Subjective, Objective, Assessment, and Plan (SOAP) Note

SOAP is a standardized method of documentation within an animal's medical record.

1.4.16 Stereotypic Behavior

Abnormal behaviors seen in animals confined and deprived of environmental enrichment (i.e. circling, pacing, self-mutilation).

1.4.17 Unremarkable

Used when describing results that are normal or where nothing out of the ordinary has been found.

1.4.18 Veterinary Forensics

The collection of data from an animal and related materials that can be used for the investigation of animal abuse, neglect, or nonaccidental death.

1.5 Terms and Phrases: Law Enforcement and Field Services

1.5.1 Affidavit

Generally speaking, a sworn statement. Also, the supporting document of a search warrant request that outlines the probable cause motivating the warrant request.

1.5.2 Chain of Custody

The documentation that tracks a piece of evidence and who it comes into contact with, from where it was found at the scene of a crime to the point it is being offered as evidence of that crime.

1.5.3 Citation

An official notice of a violation of state law generated by someone with authority to enforce those laws (i.e. law enforcement).

1.5.4 Civilian

Any individual who is not a sworn peace officer.

1.5.5 Custodial

In the criminal context, when a person is in the custody of a state agency and cannot leave of their own free will. Custody can be defined as literal physical custody (i.e. in handcuffs or in prison) or constructive custody, which occurs when the circumstances of an interaction with a representative from a state agency are such that the individual does not feel they are free to leave.

1.5.6 Evidence

Statements, objects, or information that indicates an alleged fact is more likely or less likely to be true [8].

1.5.7 Interview

The questioning of a witness or a suspect in furtherance of an investigation.

1.5.8 Miranda

A series of warnings/rights that must be stated verbally and/or in writing to a person who is in the custody of an individual acting on behalf of the state or the federal government before the person is asked any questions about their involvement in a situation under criminal investigation [9].

1.5.9 Officer Safety

A term used to refer to the topics of policies, procedures, and trainings employed by law enforcement agencies in order to best protect their agents in the field from harm.

1.5.10 Probable Cause

There is information available to indicate that a crime more likely than not has occurred or is occurring.

1.5.11 Protective Custody

In the context of animal cruelty cases, the retention of a victim animal for inspection, preservation, and security from abuse, neglect, or danger during which chain of custody is maintained.

1.5.12 Public Information Officer (PIO)

A peace officer designated by a law enforcement agency to be the liaison between the department and representatives of the media.

1.5.13 Reasonable Suspicion

There is some reason beyond a "hunch" that creates the belief that a crime has or is occurring.

1.5.14   Reporting Party

A person who reports a concern about a situation to an entity with authority to act.

1.5.15   Risk Assessment

A standardized procedure in which law enforcement evaluates the risks associated with locations and individuals they are likely to encounter when pursuing a particular tactical move in an investigation. Routinely done prior to search warrant executions.

1.5.16   Search Warrant

An order from a judge that commands a peace officer to search a specified location and seize specific evidence of a particular crime(s).

1.5.17   Seizure

In the context of criminal cases, taking custody of an individual's property or the individual themselves, within the bounds and under the authority of a warrant.

1.5.18   Suspect

An individual who is believed to have committed a crime but against whom no criminal charges have been filed yet.

1.5.19   Third-Party Owner

An individual, not the suspect, who has an ownership interest in an item of property.

1.5.20   Witness

An individual who has knowledge pertaining to or has personally experienced (with any one of their senses) anything relevant to a criminal investigation.

1.6   Terms and Phrases: Criminal Law

1.6.1   Alford Plea

A plea that maintains innocence but acknowledges that the prosecution could meet its burden of proof with the evidence available.

1.6.2   Arraignment

The proceeding in which charges are officially filed and the defendant enters a plea of guilty or not guilty.

1.6.3   Authentication

A process that seeks to admit items into evidence by proving they are true or genuine [10].

1.6.4   Brady Material

Any information or evidence that is favorable to the defendant. Nondisclosure by the prosecution is a violation of the defendant's constitutional rights [11].

1.6.5   Brief

A persuasive document written for submission to a judge or court about an issue in a case.

1.6.6   Charging Enhancement

Statutory provision that allows for more serious charges, when particular conditions are met, either by the defendant or by the circumstances of the crime. For example, in Nevada the crime of torturing a companion animal is a Class D felony but rises to a Class C felony if done to intimidate another person. In Idaho, the misdemeanor crime of torturing a companion animal rises to a felony if the perpetrator has a prior conviction involving voluntary infliction of bodily injury upon a human within 10 years [12, 13].

1.6.7   Charging Information

This is the document the prosecuting attorney files with the court to initiate criminal charges that are supported by probable cause.

1.6.8   Defendant

A criminal defendant is someone who has been charged with a crime.

1.6.9   Diversion

An arrangement that results in dismissal of the charges if a defendant complies with the terms of a plea agreement (see below) for a specified length of time without any violations.

1.6.10   Expert Witness

An expert witness is "[a] witness qualified by knowledge, skill, experience, training, or education to provide a scientific, technical, or other specialized opinion about the evidence or a fact issue" [14]. A veterinarian will almost always be considered an expert witness. Expert witnesses are treated differently than other witnesses in a trial (see Chapter 16 on trials for more information).

1.6.11   Forfeiture

A legal divestment of property that is ordered by a court.

1.6.11.1   Preconviction Forfeiture

A legal proceeding that is utilized in animal cruelty cases to address the cost of caring for victim animals until a criminal trial takes place. Once a preconviction forfeiture petition is filed, a defendant animal owner has a certain amount of time to pay a bond amount that will be used to provide care for their animals while they await trial. If the defendant animal owner cannot pay the bond amount, then ownership of the animals is transferred by an order of the court to a designated entity.

1.6.11.2 Postconviction Forfeiture

A divestment of property that occurs as a result of a criminal conviction.

1.6.12 Foreclosure

The process of terminating an ownership interest in property in order to gain title to the property or satisfy an unpaid debt connected to the property. In an animal cruelty case, the property consists of the animal/animals seized in the case. The unpaid debt is the costs of care that have accrued since the animal(s) was taken into custody.

1.6.13 Grand Jury

A body of citizens that reviews evidence presented by the prosecutor to determine if the prosecutor has probable cause to charge the suspect with a crime.

1.6.14 Hearing

A proceeding that takes place in front of a judicial officer to determine issues related to a case.

1.6.15 Judgment

A ruling in a case by a court containing its final determination in the case. Depending on the determination and the court, the judgment may be subject to appeal.

1.6.16 Lay Witness

A lay witness is "[a] witness who does not testify as an expert and who is therefore restricted to giving an opinion or making an inference that (1) is based on firsthand knowledge, and (2) is helpful in clarifying the testimony or in determining facts" [14].

1.6.17 Lien

"A legal right or interest that a creditor has in another's property, lasting usually until the debt or duty that it secures is satisfied" [15]. In an animal cruelty case, several states have laws that specifically create a lien for the costs of care that an agency or individual provides to the animals connected to a criminal animal cruelty case. The agency or individual can foreclose on those liens, the result of which is repayment of the costs or transfer of ownership of the property to satisfy the debt (see Chapter 15 for more information about liens and foreclosure).

1.6.18 Mental State

Mental state refers to an element of every animal cruelty offense: the state of mind of the perpetrator of the cruelty. Wording can vary slightly between states, but generally the mental state the prosecution is required to prove falls into one of these four areas [16].

1.6.18.1 Criminal Negligence

The perpetrator should have been aware of a risk and a reasonable person in their situation would have been aware of the risk.

1.6.18.2 Recklessly

The perpetrator disregards substantial and unjustifiable risk that a particular result will occur and engages in conduct that causes that result. This disregard for the risk deviates from that of an average law-abiding citizen.

1.6.18.3 Knowingly

The perpetrator consciously engages in conduct knowing that a particular result is likely if not certain.

1.6.18.4 Purposefully or Intentionally

The perpetrator has the conscious objective to engage in the conduct and cause the result of the conduct.

1.6.19 Motion

A document filed in a case requesting the court/judge to take a particular action.

1.6.20 No Contest

A plea that does not admit guilt but does not challenge the charges.

1.6.21 Plea Bargain/Agreement

An agreement the defendant makes to negotiated charges and sentencing provisions, and results in a conviction [17].

1.6.22 Pretrial Hearing

A court proceeding that takes place prior to a trial to assess trial readiness, or to address and sometimes narrow, the issues in a case [18].

1.6.23 Possession Ban

A sentencing provision that prevents a defendant from possessing animals, a certain species of animal, or a particular animal for a period of time.[2]

---

2 As of January 2021, 17 states have mandatory possession bans for convicted animal cruelty offenders. Animal Legal Defense Fund (2020). Laws supporting post-conviction possession bans. Animal Legal Defense Fund. https://aldf.org/project/post-conviction-possession-ban (accessed 4 August 2021).

1.6.24   Probation

A sentence that a defendant can receive that involves certain stipulations a defendant must meet after being released postconviction. Probation can be included with incarceration as part of a sentence, or in lieu of incarceration.

1.6.24.1   Bench Probation

Bench probation means the defendant will not have to check in with a probation officer but would have to appear before the trial judge if they are found to be in violation of one of the stipulations.

1.6.24.2   Supervised Probation

Supervised probation means the defendant will have to routinely check in with a probation officer to confirm they are adhering to their stipulations.

1.6.25   Release Order

An order by the court allowing a defendant to be released into the community pending trial, with restrictions that must be adhered to by the defendant.

1.6.26   Restitution

A monetary amount determined to redress a crime victim's injuries or losses that a defendant can be ordered to pay as part of sentencing.

1.6.27   Sentencing

The phase of the criminal justice process that determines how the defendant will be held accountable if they are convicted of a crime(s). This can include but is not limited to jail time, probation, fines, restitution, and mandatory counseling.

1.6.28   Stipulate

When two lawyers (generally adverse parties) agree to something relevant to their case. For example, to agree that a piece of evidence (lab results, photograph, video, etc.) can be admitted without authentication by a witness [19].

1.6.29   Testimony

Statements made by an individual under oath.

1.6.30   Trial

"A formal judicial examination of evidence and determination of legal claims in an adversary proceeding" [20]. In a criminal trial the defendant has the right to choose between a bench trial and a jury trial.

1.6.30.1   Bench Trial

A trial that takes place without a jury and the judge determines both questions of fact and law.

1.6.30.2 Jury Trial

A trial where a jury is convened to determine questions of fact that equate to elements of the charged offenses.

1.6.31 Victim

A being who has been injured through the commission of a crime.

1.6.32 Voir Dire

The process of selecting a jury for a trial. A judge and all attorneys representing a party in the case are permitted to ask questions of jury members and are permitted to eliminate a specified number of jurors.

1.7 Looking Ahead

Armed with this foundation of vocabulary relevant to animal cruelty case work, the next building block to a strong investigation is an understanding across disciplines of what basic care animals need in order to maintain their health and well-being.

References

1 Arizona – "[M]ammal, bird, reptile or amphibian." Arizona Revised Statutes Annotated, title 13, chapter 29, s 13-2910(H) (1) 2019 (AZ).

2 Oklahoma – "[A]ny mammal, bird, fish, reptile or invertebrate, including wild and domesticated species, other than a human being." Oklahoma Statutes Annotated, title 21, Pt VII, chapter 67, s 1680.1 1991 (OK).

3 Delaware – "'Animal' does not include fish, crustacea, or molluska." Delaware Code Annotated, title 11, Pt I, chapter 5, subchapter VII, subpart A, s 1325(a) (11) 1972 (DE).

4 Georgia – "'Animal' shall not include any fish nor shall such term include any pest that might be exterminated or removed from a business, residence, or other structure." Code of Georgia Annotated, title 16, chapter 12, article 1, s 16-12-4(a) (1) 2014 (GA).

5 Kansas – "[E]very living vertebrate except a human being." Kansas Statutes Annotated, chapter 21, article 64, s 717B.1(1) 2011 (KS).

6 Iowa – "Nonhuman vertebrates, but not including: Livestock; Game, fur-bearing animals, fish, reptiles, and amphibians, unless owned, confined or controlled by a person; Nuisance non-game species." Iowa Code Annotated, title XVI, subtitle 1, chapter 717B, s 1 1994 (IA).

7 Nebraska – "Any vertebrate member of the animal kingdom [except an] uncaptured wild creature or a livestock animal." Revised Statutes of Nebraska Annotated, chapter 28, article 10, s 2 1990 (NE).

8 Garner, B.A. (ed.) (2019). *Black's Law Dictionary Standard*, 11e, 697–698. St. Paul, MN: Thomson Reuters.

9 *Miranda vs. Arizona*, 86 St. Ct. 1602, (1966).

10 Garner, B.A. (2019). *Black's Law Dictionary Standard*, 11e, 163. St. Paul, MN: Thomson Reuters.

11 Garner, B.A. (2019). *Black's Law Dictionary Standard*, 11e, 231. St. Paul, MN: Thomson Reuters.

12 Nevada Revised Statutes Annotated, title 50, chapter 574, Cruelty to Animals, s 574.100(1) (a) 2017 (NV).

13 Idaho Code Annotated, title 25, chapter 35, ss 25-3504A; 25-3520A(3) (b) 2016 (ID).

14 Garner, B.A. (2019). *Black's Law Dictionary Standard*, 11e, 1920. St. Paul, MN: Thomson Reuters.

15 Garner, B.A. (2019). *Black's Law Dictionary Standard*, 11e, 1107. St. Paul, MN: Thomson Reuters.

16 Uniform Laws Annotated, Model Penal Code, P I, article 2, s 2.02 2020 (USA).

17 Garner, B.A. (2019). *Black's Law Dictionary Standard*, 11e, 1394. St. Paul, MN: Thomson Reuters.

18 Garner, B.A. (2019). *Black's Law Dictionary Standard*, 11e, 1438. St. Paul, MN: Thomson Reuters.

19 Garner, B.A. (2019). *Black's Law Dictionary Standard*, 11e, 1712. St. Paul, MN: Thomson Reuters.

20 Garner, B.A. (2019). *Black's Law Dictionary Standard*, 11e, 1812. St. Paul, MN: Thomson Reuters.

2

Animal Basics

Kris Otteman, Zarah Hedge, and Linda Fielder

While laws require that animals must receive basic minimum care, the legal definition of what constitutes basic care varies by species. The husbandry needs of a horse look wildly different from those of a guinea pig. In providing accurate and thorough investigations of animal cruelty cases, it is important for each of the experts involved to have the appropriate level of baseline or deep expertise pertaining to the specific species they will be involved with. This knowledge of animal basics provides guidance and analysis when answering the most common questions facing investigators, law enforcement, prosecutors, animal control officers, and veterinarians responding to concerns regarding abuse or neglect of an animal. When approaching these cases, it is important to ask: "Is the appearance of the animal within normal limits? Is the diet appropriate for the age, condition, and species involved? Is the care provided meeting the basic husbandry needs of the animals and the standards set forth in the county or state code, rules, or laws?" A foundation in animal basics will guard against failures in addressing animal cruelty. This chapter will offer an introduction to animal husbandry, which is the management and care of animals and includes the areas of nutrition, sanitation, housing, and environmental requirements for some common species. We will also introduce the Five Freedoms and examine how they helped shape animal protection laws and establish the field of animal cruelty investigations.

Veterinarians possess expert knowledge about the basic needs of animals and are trained and qualified to diagnose and treat animal diseases and illnesses. Law enforcement and investigators will benefit from trainings and resources that provide basic animal knowledge to increase the effectiveness of their work and are encouraged to enlist the aid of a veterinarian who is comfortable with the species in question when working animal cruelty cases and assessing animal welfare deficiencies.

States define the word "animal" differently. In your state, companion animals may have statutory requirements from which livestock are exempt. The same is true for other species such as birds, insects, and aquatics. Know how your state defines animals and what statutes apply to them [1].

Animal Cruelty Investigations: A Collaborative Approach from Victim to Verdict^{TM}, First Edition.
Edited by Kris Otteman, Linda Fielder, and Emily Lewis.
© 2022 John Wiley & Sons, Inc. Published 2022 by John Wiley & Sons, Inc.
Companion website: www.wiley.com/go/otteman/victimtoverdict

2.1   The History of the Five Freedoms and Their Impact on Animal Welfare Laws

The Five Freedoms were developed in the 1960s to establish standards of minimum care for animals, particularly those raised for food, and have since been accepted in the United States and across the world [2]. They are the basis from which laws concerning the care and treatment of captive animals developed. An understanding of the Five Freedoms acts as a foundation for animal cruelty investigations, when determining if an animal's basic needs are being adequately met. The Five Freedoms are uniformly applicable to animals in livestock and farming operations, breeding and shelter facilities, and any environment where an animal is confined or enclosed in any manner, including animals kept as pets. They are as follows [3]:

Freedom from Hunger and Thirst: by ready access to fresh water and a diet to maintain health and vigor.
Freedom from Discomfort: by providing an appropriate environment including shelter and a comfortable resting area.
Freedom from Pain, Injury, or Disease: by prevention or rapid diagnosis and treatment.
Freedom to Express Normal Behavior: by providing sufficient space, proper facilities, and company of the animal's own kind.
Freedom from Fear and Distress: by ensuring conditions and treatment which avoid mental suffering.

The Five Freedoms, along with the Animal Welfare Act [4], a federal law that sets minimum standards of care for animals in breeding and laboratory environments, serve to memorialize the fact that a failure to provide for an animal's basic needs is both inhumane and unlawful, and that animals deprived of these provisions suffer pain and mental anguish.

2.2   Veterinarians as Experts in the Field

When working on any case, but especially those with less common species, involving an experienced veterinarian or other expert can be essential to the proper understanding and workup of the case. For example, when investigating neglect within a large avian breeding facility, a zoo veterinarian may be able to accompany investigators on scene and help with assessment of the environment and basic animal needs. Such an expert may also provide expertise in identifying and gathering evidence and the humane removal and housing of multiple species, if necessary. Veterinarians and other animal experts may also play a vital role in planning the logistics and resource needs of complex cases or those involving multiple animals or a variety of species. While a veterinarian is not needed in all cases, most situations will benefit significantly from a doctor's involvement.

Involving a veterinarian to assess and report on animal cruelty investigations improves efficiency and accuracy when situations may seem complex or impossible. Calling on help early in an investigation can prevent missteps or loss of valuable evidence. Proactively finding community resources to supplement an officer or prosecutor's basic animal knowledge further supports the quality of the investigation. Consider reaching out to experts from government agencies such as the Department of Agriculture, veterinary colleges, or reputable organizations with expertise in specialized areas of nutrition or husbandry, such as marine mammal or exotic species experts. Seek out veterinarians who work in shelter medicine and may be available or can offer a referral to a veterinarian who can assist. When possible, build a network of contacts and experts that you can rely on in the event an urgent case arises. Help can be challenging to find once an emergency is underway.

2.3   With So Many Species, Where to Begin?

Animal cruelty cases most commonly involve species with close relationships to humans, mainly dogs, cats, rabbits, and horses. However, livestock such as pigs, cattle, goats, llamas, and exotic species, including reptiles, birds, marsupials, aquatics, captive wild animals, and all others may be victims of neglect or abuse.

The animal basics covered in this chapter focus on the most common domestic species, including dogs, cats, small mammals, captive avian species, small ruminants, cattle, and horses. This information is intended as a baseline and stepping-off point that you can build upon as time goes on. Websites that provide information written or reviewed by verified experts are good sources of information, and continuing education offered by colleges and professional veterinary and animal welfare organizations also offer high-quality information and training.

2.4   Defining Animals by Category

As a reminder, state statutes often have very specific definitions of animals and which statutes apply to them, but below are some general definitions of common terms used when describing categories or types of animals:

Livestock: animals raised in an agricultural setting, including hoofstock and equines.
Domestic animals: animals that have been adapted over generations to live alongside humans.
Pets or companion animals: a domesticated animal kept for companionship or pleasure.
Small mammals: rodents or other small mammals kept as pets, such as rats, guinea pigs, ferrets, and hedgehogs.
Avian: any bird.
Poultry: domestic fowl such as chickens, ducks, geese, and turkeys.
Reptiles: scaled animals such as snakes, lizards, turtles, and tortoises.
Amphibians: cold-blooded animals such as frogs, toads, newts, and salamanders.
Aquatics: an animal that lives exclusively in water.

Some state statutes also categorize particular animals further as "wildlife" or classify certain species such as large cats or monkeys as "exotics."

2.5   Animal Basics by Species

It is impossible to cover every animal species' specific care needs in this book, but below are some general environmental, health, and nutritional considerations for species frequently encountered in animal cruelty investigations.

2.5.1   Hoofstock

Cattle, including beef and dairy breeds, llamas, alpacas, and sheep, including meat and wool breeds, and a variety of goats fall into the category that is referred to as hoofstock. These animals are all grazing and foraging animals that may have access to a range and can seek food freely or may be confined

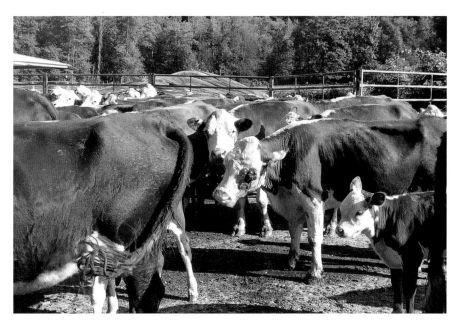

Figure 2.1 Feed requirements for cattle and other hoofstock can be calculated based on the animals' average or estimated ideal weight. *Source:* Oregon Humane Society.

and (Figure 2.1) fed in a pasture, feedlot, or dairy environment. Food consumption can be estimated based on body weight and ranges from 1% to 4%, depending on the species, life stage, and productivity. High-producing dairy cattle will consume 4% of their body weight (50 lb dry feed for a 1200 lb cow) per day, while a pet pygmy goat that spends her day resting and playing will consume 1 lb of food a day. Water consumption can also be calculated based on the same concepts of weight, species, utilization, and environment. With access to clean water, these animals will drink what they need. Hoofstock have a natural tendency to wear hooves down to a healthy length and shape, but in some cases require hoof care such as shaping and trimming. Regular deworming for intestinal and external parasites is required on a routine basis and is dependent upon the region and environment the animals live in. Some breeds of cattle and goats are dehorned early in life and certain breeds of sheep are tail docked as lambs to prevent fly attraction and damage during warm periods. Many of these breeds are ear tagged or microchipped for identification purposes and for registration with breed affiliates and government agencies as required. Breeding progress in sheep and cattle is monitored in some herds by use of paint markers that apply a color blot to the female's back when she is bred. All these species give birth in a pasture or barn setting unaided in most situations, but emergency procedures and veterinary intervention may be necessary when dystocia (difficulty birthing) arises. Breeds of goats, sheep, alpacas, and llamas grow long thick coats that may require shearing. Body condition can be difficult to evaluate in these species without a hands-on opportunity as the coat obscures their body, while visual evaluation is fairly straightforward for cattle breeds or short-coated goats.

2.5.2 Equine

Horses, donkeys, and mules are foraging animals eating grass and hay throughout the day. They require access to hay and/or pasture equal to 1–2% of their body weight (10–20 lb for a 1000 lb horse) per day. They drink 5–10 gal of water per day. Equine species require regular hoof trimming to allow them to walk and stand comfortably. Without regular maintenance, equine hooves are prone to painful splitting and curling. Equine teeth have evolved to grind grasses and grains. They develop sharp points and caps that must be filed away or removed by a veterinarian (a procedure known as floating) in order for the horse to efficiently chew its food. All equines are prone to parasites and require periodic deworming to avoid infestations, which can lead to illness and even death in some cases. Pregnant, nursing, and senior equines may require specialized diets and more frequent veterinary care to maintain their health and comfort.

2.5.3   Feline (Domestic Cats)

Cats are often kept as indoor pets but can also be found living exclusively outdoors as community cats (which can consist of tame or unsocialized felines living singly, in small groups, or in larger colonies [Figure 2.2]). Cats are carnivores and have a higher protein requirement than other mammals. They require access to potable water and an area free from their feces and urine. Cats kept in crowded or confined conditions frequently develop upper respiratory and eye infections characterized by congestion, nasal and eye discharge, sneezing, and wheezing. They are also at a higher risk of developing skin conditions such as ringworm or scabies, and viral diseases including feline immunodeficiency virus (FIV) and feline leukemia virus (FeLV) [5]. Unaltered cats breed prolifically, and unneutered male cats are known to fight each other, which can cause wounds that may develop into painful abscesses. Outdoor cats need access to shelter from extreme hot and cold temperatures.

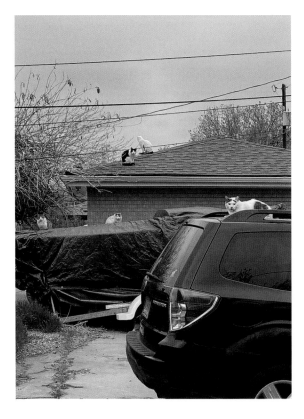

Figure 2.2   Community cats may be tame or unsocialized and often live in colonies. *Source:* Kayte Wolf.

2.5.4   Canine (Domestic Dogs)

Dogs' relationships with people vary tremendously from being kept as indoor companions, as outdoor guardians protecting livestock or property, or kept strictly outdoors, sometimes chained or fenced in, with little human contact. Some states prohibit chaining dogs (often with certain exceptions), while chaining is allowed in others. Chains and collars must fit appropriately and not cause wounds or be so tight as to damage or become embedded in the skin (Figure 2.3). Dogs require an area clear of environmental hazards, access to potable water, and shelter that provides protection from extreme temperatures and allows them to stay dry and away from their feces and urine. Dogs are omnivores whose nutritional requirements are based on size, age, and activity level. They can develop viral diseases and parasite infections, some of which are zoonotic (contagious to humans), such as rabies and hookworms. Vaccination and deworming prevent these conditions from debilitating or killing dogs and protects humans from infection. Breeds with particular hair coats require grooming to prevent matting, which can become painful, interfere with mobility, and contribute to skin infection and disease. Dogs, especially seniors, require regular nail trimming to keep their nails from curling and becoming embedded in their paw pads. Routine dental care is required for most dogs, especially as they age. Painful dental disease later in life, requiring veterinary care, can become a serious health concern in the canine.

2.5.5   Small Mammals (Rabbits, Guinea Pigs, Mice, Rats, Ferrets)

Inappropriate husbandry and diet are common causes of disease in small mammals. Rabbits and guinea pigs are herbivores and require a high-fiber diet, while rats and mice are omnivores. Ferrets, weasels, and mink are omnivores and require meat protein as well. Their nutritional requirements in captivity are best met by commercial diets developed for their species, supplemented with appropriate fresh foods. Guinea pigs require vitamin C in their diet as they are unable to produce this in their body like other mammals. Small mammals require constant access to potable water. Small mammals are intelligent and social animals. Providing appropriate housing will ensure they are able to display their normal behaviors. These species benefit from living in pairs or groups, but they can cause severe injuries and even death if fighting occurs. Adequately sized enclosures allow for the animals to eat, sleep, and exercise and allow them to be free from their waste. Some rodents

(a)

(b)

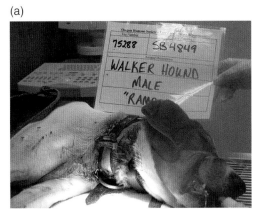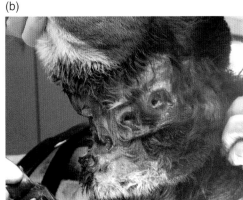

Figure 2.3   Tight collars may become embedded in an animal's skin causing painful wounds and infection. *Source:* Oregon Humane Society.

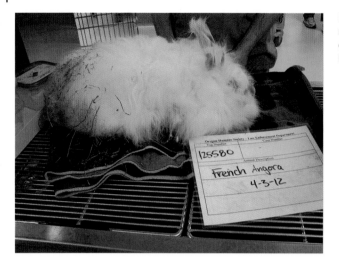

Figure 2.4 Angora rabbits require regular grooming to prevent matting of their long coats. *Source:* Oregon Humane Society.

require substrate or bedding for burrowing and sleeping. Enclosures should be free from hazards and cages with wire floors should be kept in good repair so as not to injure the animal's feet or entrap them. Cages with wire bottoms should always include a solid bed or resting platform where the animal can relieve itself from the constant pressure of standing on wire, which coupled with contact with feces and urine, leads to painful ulcerations and infection of the feet and hocks. Rabbit enclosures ideally have a thick and soft flooring, and wire or mesh flooring throughout the enclosure should be avoided. Rabbits do not have footpads, but have coarse fur covering the toes and paws. Rabbits kept in wire housing without access to soft, solid flooring commonly develop a condition called pododermatitis, which is an infection of the paw, and can be a serious and life-threatening condition. Most small mammals do not do well in extreme heat or cold and some, like rabbits, are prone to heat stroke and must have access to a shaded area if housed outdoors. Overcrowding is stressful to small mammals and can cause them to fight with and cannibalize their cage mates and offspring. Dental health is very important in small mammals and is a common cause of medical concern in these species. All teeth in rabbits and guinea pigs are continuously growing, throughout the life of the animal, and they require oral examination at veterinary visits. Rabbits may suffer from malocclusion, a condition in which their teeth are misaligned causing them to become overgrown and curled, which can prohibit them from chewing their food. This condition is sometimes visible, but the teeth may grow backward into the cheek and so a visual inspection of the mouth is advised when malocclusion is suspected. Some species of rabbit (Figure 2.4) and guinea pig have long hair coats that require consistent grooming. Severe matting can lead to pain and skin infections.

2.5.6 Avian

Birds kept as pets range from finches and pigeons to large parrots. They have adapted genetically over centuries so that their beaks are specially shaped to collect, open, and ingest the fruits and seeds native to their region of origin. Parrots have large, hooked bills for cracking open hard palm nuts, while finches have small triangular beaks designed to pluck tiny grass seeds from their stems. For this reason, birds in captivity must be provided with a diet modeled after what they were designed to eat in nature. There are hundreds of commercially available diets for every type of bird

Figure 2.5 Captive birds may develop feather picking behaviors owing to stress, diet, or underlying health concerns. *Source:* Oregon Humane Society.

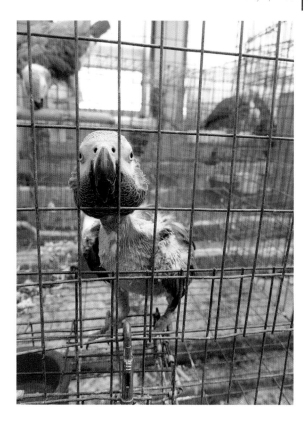

kept as a pet. Birds have high metabolisms and must eat frequently throughout the day, so food should always be available. When assessing feed, keep in mind that birds tend to drop spent seed hulls back into feed cups and hoppers, so what might appear as a full seed dispenser may actually be filled with empty seed hulls. Birds always require access to clean, potable water. Some birds, like pigeons and doves, may be suited to living in outdoor aviaries, but most pet birds are quite sensitive to cold temperatures. Cages should be large enough for the bird to move around, extend its wings, access its food and water, and be free from its waste. Birds require perches to rest and sleep on. They may be housed in pairs, groups, or singly. Breeding pairs require a nest or nest box in which to lay their eggs and tend their young. Health considerations for birds include monitoring for any changes in respiration or difficulty breathing, distress related to difficulty laying or retained eggs, and attention to overgrown beaks and nails. Feather picking occurs (Figure 2.5) when a bird plucks their own feathers and is commonly secondary to poor husbandry, improper diet, or underlying medical and/or behavioral conditions.

2.5.7 Poultry

Poultry refers to species of birds primarily raised for meat or egg laying. These include chickens, geese, turkeys, ducks, and quail. Poultry are typically fed commercial pelleted feed or grains, which are often supplemented with fresh vegetables or table scraps. Poultry require access to fresh water. They are often housed in groups but should not be so overcrowded that they cannot move about easily, as overcrowding contributes to disease, cannibalism, and injury. Enclosures should be free of hazards that could cause injury and should protect the birds from overheating or freezing.

Poultry can suffer from viral and infectious diseases and parasites. They may also experience medical emergencies related to retained eggs, viral or infectious diseases, and parasites. All avian species may carry reportable diseases that require coordination with government agencies.

2.5.8 Reptiles

This is a large group of cold-blooded animals and includes snakes, lizards, turtles, and tortoises. Most snakes and some lizards and turtles are carnivores or insectivores, while iguanas and land tortoises are vegetarian. Every species of reptile eats a slightly different diet. For reptiles who eat prey, the size of the reptile determines the size of the prey they should be fed. Most snakes kept as pets are fed mice or rats of varying sizes, while smaller snakes and lizards are fed a variety of insects. These "feeder animals" are available at most pet shops and by mail order and may be fed live or frozen. Many types of lizards require fresh greens in addition to their insect diet. Because of their slow metabolism, adult snakes may only eat once every two or three weeks. Smaller or younger snakes need to eat more often, usually twice a week. Most lizards and herbivorous reptiles need to eat every day. Reptiles require constant access to fresh, potable water. Reptiles must have a habitat that provides the heat and light that mimics their native ecosystem. To a reptile, proper heat and light is as essential as food and water. Reptile enclosures need to offer a temperature gradient, with a warm area for the animal to bask and increase its body temperature and a cooler area to mimic the shade. As cold-blooded animals, they rely on external sources for body heat and will die without the proper enclosure temperature. Additionally, without adequate heat support, many species of reptiles (Figure 2.6) cannot properly digest their food. Heating options for enclosures include under-tank warming mats, electrical heated basking stones, basking lights, and ceramic heating element bulbs. Aside from heat, some reptiles need ultraviolet (UV) light. This wavelength of light is necessary for calcium metabolism. In enclosures without UV light, reptiles often develop debilitating bone diseases, loss of muscle function, and altered metabolism. The reptile habitat should be free from hazards, excess waste, and spoiled food. It should provide a hiding and sleeping area and appropriate climbing accessories for the species. Many reptiles are susceptible to bacterial and fungal infections, which can cause painful ulcers. It can be very difficult to recognize serious illnesses and disease conditions in reptiles, and whenever possible investigations involving

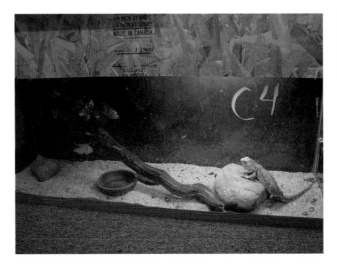

Figure 2.6 Inadequate lighting and heat in reptile enclosures can lead to skeletal diseases and nutritional deficiencies. *Source:* Oregon Humane Society.

reptiles should include a veterinarian familiar with treating them. Poor husbandry and diet commonly lead to a variety of medical conditions, including dysecdysis (improper shedding) and metabolic bone disease, which can lead to brittle bones that break easily.

2.5.9 Unusual Exotics

Monkeys, large cats, wildlife, and animals typically seen in zoos are also discovered as "pets" when investigating animal cruelty. Laws at both the state and federal level may apply to these animals, in addition to laws applicable to the care and husbandry of all animals. Unusual exotic animals are rarely domesticated and can be difficult and dangerous to assess and handle. The owner is responsible for providing a diet appropriate for the species in type, quality, and quantity. They should have access to clean, potable water. They should not be subjected to extreme temperatures or temperatures the species is not adapted to. Enclosures should be secure, free of hazards and waste, provide shelter and shade, and room and accessories designed for the animal to exercise and express its natural behaviors. Wild exotic animals are especially prone to stress-induced behaviors in captivity such as self-injury, fighting, and cannibalizing cage mates and offspring. When approaching cases involving exotic wild animals, include other agencies with oversight such as the United States Department of Agriculture (USDA) and state fish and wildlife agencies. Arrange for experts such as zoologists or zoo veterinarians to assist with all handling, capture, and assessment of these animals.

2.6 Basics That Apply to All Animals

Another basic requirement that applies to all animals, regardless of the species, is the understanding that veterinary care is required to relieve an animal's suffering. Any sick or injured horse, ferret, turtle, or animal of any species that is injured, sick, and suffering must be offered relief through medical care, treatment, or euthanasia.

Any animal that is old, disabled, pregnant, nursing, or juvenile may require special care due to their weakened or debilitated state (Figure 2.7). Owners are required to provide that care so that animals with these types of special needs do not suffer. In simple terms, the minimum care required

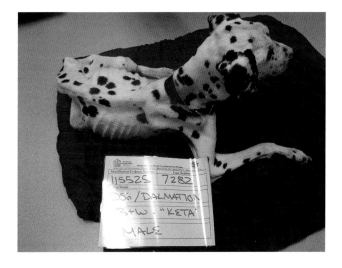

Figure 2.7 Animals in a weakened or debilitated state require veterinary care to address pain and suffering. *Source:* Oregon Humane Society.

for animals at a specific life stage or condition is often over and above what would be considered adequate or minimum care for an average healthy adult animal of the same species. Examples of provisions that must be made for these animals might include extra calories and supplements, reinforced shelter or additional heat support, and padded stalls or bedding to prevent pressure sores or provide for parturition and raising young.

Some cases, like cockfighting and farmed animal investigations, require coordination with the State Veterinarian whose role is to consider public health risks from zoonotic diseases (transferable from animals to humans). Diseases such as avian influenza, brucellosis, and rabies carry a risk to humans and testing or reporting may be warranted.

2.7   Putting Your Basic Knowledge to Work

Rely on your knowledge of animal basics to inform you when you approach an animal cruelty investigation. If an animal looks ill or injured, call on what you know about the required minimum care of animals and start to identify what is missing. At the beginning stages of an investigation, it is not required that you know what exact disease, injury, or illness an animal is suffering from, only that the animal is suffering or not being provided shelter, nutrition, or veterinary care as required by law. Once you have established that fact, then applying the Five Freedoms can guide you as you evaluate the animal's environment and look for adequate food, water, shelter, and sanitation. Does the animal's enclosure provide for its needs for exercise and freedom from urine and feces? Are there hazards in the environment that have resulted in injury to the animal? Is it able to maintain an appropriate body temperature? Who are the local animal experts that can assist you in further evaluation of the circumstances if necessary? The more you learn about the basic needs of animal, the more confident you will become as you respond to animal cruelty cases, and the more thorough your part in an investigation will become.

References

1 Animal Legal Defense Fund (2020). 2020 U.S. state animal protection laws rankings. https://aldf.org/project/us-state-rankings (accessed 30 May 2021).

2 Elischer, M. (2019). The Five Freedoms: a history lesson in animal care and welfare. MSU Extension 4-H Animal Science, Michigan State University https://www.canr.msu.edu/news/an_animal_welfare_history_lesson_on_the_five_freedoms (accessed 30 May 2021).

3 ASPCA (n.d.). Five Freedoms. https://www.aspca.org/sites/default/files/upload/images/aspca_asv_five_freedoms_final1.ashx_.pdf (accessed 30 May 2021).

4 Animal Welfare Act, 1966 (USA).

5 Polak, K.C., Levy, J.K., Crawford, P.C. et al. (2014). Infectious diseases in large-scale cat hoarding investigations. *Vet. J.* 201 (2): 189–195. https://doi.org/10.1016/j.tvjl.2014.05.020.

3

Fundamentals of All Cases
Linda Fielder

It should come as no surprise that the basic needs of animals described in the previous chapter play a critical role in every animal cruelty investigation.

Without food and water in sufficient amounts, a horse cannot sustain its body weight and will become emaciated over time. A cat's wound or illness left untreated will cause pain and may result in death. Without a shelter that allows for maintenance of body temperature, a dog may freeze to death outdoors. Once we understand the basic needs of animals, we can begin to understand how the absence of those necessities becomes the indication of neglect or abuse to vigilant observers and initiates an investigation.

In the example of the dog with no shelter, the investigative team of police officers, veterinarian, and animal control officers will piece together the evidence of neglect, which led to the dog perishing in the cold. How was the shelter inadequate? How long had the dog been outdoors? How low was the temperature the night the dog died? Did the dog's body condition, breed, or hair coat provide protection or make it more vulnerable? A successful investigation begins with a keen understanding of the animal's needs and fills in the blanks regarding how those needs were or were not being met in the days, weeks, or months prior to the case coming to rest on the desk of the investigator or veterinarian (Figure 3.1).

A thorough investigation is an attempt to leave no stone unturned when searching for the evidence of a crime. It includes physical examination, interviews, scene searches, photographs, diagnostic imaging, pathology, and much more. The investigation sets out to assure the prosecutor there is no other excuse for or reason that the animal became ill/injured/deceased but by the commission of the crime of animal neglect or abuse and provides a narrative that leads to the identification of the individual(s) responsible for said crime.

3.1 Interdisciplinary Roles

Every investigation is more comprehensive and able to withstand examination by the defense when it employs the skills and expertise of all the practitioners for whom this book is written. The law enforcement professional utilizes their skills of interviewing suspects and witnesses, identifying evidence, and noticing and documenting conditions relevant to the investigation. Veterinarians

Animal Cruelty Investigations: A Collaborative Approach from Victim to Verdict^{TM}, First Edition.
Edited by Kris Otteman, Linda Fielder, and Emily Lewis.
© 2022 John Wiley & Sons, Inc. Published 2022 by John Wiley & Sons, Inc.
Companion website: www.wiley.com/go/otteman/victimtoverdict

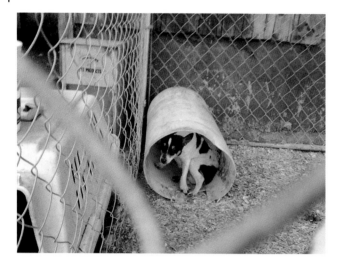

Figure 3.1 The shelter pictured here does little to provide protection from the elements. *Source:* Oregon Humane Society.

are valuable when assessing the crime scene. They also provide clinical expertise in diagnosing and treating victim animals and are qualified to explain how the animal experienced pain, what intervention or actions may have changed its condition, and how the investigator's findings were relevant. Animal welfare and shelter professionals may offer resources to owners that prevent an animal from suffering and eliminate the need for a criminal citation. They can also provide excellent environments for victim animals to heal and rehabilitate and keep accurate records around all aspects of those animals' care and movement. The prosecutor applies the laws of the state to the facts of the crime report and the supporting evidence and documentation that comprises the case file and makes the best possible use of witnesses when the case proceeds to the courtroom. When all the professionals involved are using their skills and training together, they support each other in the process of moving a case along from the scene of the crime to the trial.

3.2 Environment

Many investigations begin with the report of an animal living in an inadequate environment. Animals confined to a pen, a crate, a stall, or tethered by a chain may suffer illness and injury as a result of their inability to get away from their feces, or standing water, or other unsafe or unsanitary conditions present in their environment.

An environment marked by excess feces and urine, standing water, or thick mud can cause painful issues, including ulcerated sores on the feet and hocks, infection, which may progress through the skin and into the bone, hoof and skeletal abnormalities, a high incidence of miscarriage and death of neonates, injuries caused by an animal's repeated attempts to escape the environment, gastrointestinal disease, and parasite burden. These are only some of the conditions animals may develop as a result of living in a squalid environment and which contribute to a conclusion that the animals are suffering from criminal animal neglect.

So many aspects of an animal's environment are relevant to a criminal investigation. The environment includes the high and low temperatures an animal is exposed to, access to shelter or shade from the elements, the provision of reasonably clean and dry bedding, and the physical space to shift positions, stand, sit, and lie comfortably, with flooring that does not injure or entrap an animal's feet or limbs.

In the case of a physical abuse or animal fighting investigation an animal's environment will also contain evidence vital to the investigation. Implements used to strike a victim animal, blood spatter, or indicators of a physical altercation or struggle may all be visible in the environment and subject to the keen eye of the investigator. Equipment used to condition animals for fighting or supplies to treat wounds are often discovered hidden or in plain view within the environment of a dog- or cockfighter.

The opportunity for evaluating an animal's environment is often time sensitive. You may not be granted access to view the area where an animal is kept or may only see it for a brief time during an initial site visit. Knowing how the environment impacts the health and well-being of an animal is crucial to ensuring you notice important aspects of the environment in the time you are given. In the case of a search warrant execution, more time may be available for the assessment of the environment. Photo and video recordings preserve the conditions for later review by investigators, veterinarians, prosecutors, defense attorneys, and judge and jury.

When examining an animal's environment be sure to look for and record what is present as well as what is missing. For example, if the enclosure is wet with standing mud and rainwater, but there is no drinking bowl or trough with potable water the animal can access, this must be noted in the record. By specifically indicating that you did not see any water trough or container available to the animal, this overcomes the notion that you may have neglected to notice a water container that was clearly present in the pen or stall.

Generally, when responding to reports of an unacceptable environment, the investigator should assess the following components:

- Shelter: Is it safe and appropriate for the species and number of animals? Can they maintain a normal body temperature, and does it provide protection from wind, rain, cold, heat, and standing water?
- Confinement (fences, cages, stalls, chains): Does the method of confinement contain hazards or harmful components such as broken wires, rust, damaged floors, or doors? Is the chain so tight as to cause wounds on the animal's neck? Does the size and design of the enclosure allow for the animal to stand, move, rest, and sleep comfortably? Does it restrict their movement and expression of natural behaviors such as cleaning themselves, stretching, eating, and drinking?
- Surrounding areas (yard, room, pasture, barn): Are there dry areas where the animal can walk, sit, lie, and eat away from standing water, feces and urine, contaminants and other hazards. Is there mud, downed trees, machinery, vehicles, or other dangers within reach of the animal and on which it could injure itself or become trapped or entangled?

3.3 Sanitation

Sanitation is a component of an animal's environment that often comes up as a significant factor in animal cruelty cases. Animals, like humans, prefer to live, sleep, raise their young, and eat in environments that are free from urine, feces, and other contaminants. When animals are confined in cages, pens, stalls, or even houses without attention to sanitation in the form of human intervention, their enclosures quickly become saturated with waste. This creates an unsanitary environment that is not only extremely unpleasant for the animal, but also subjects them to injury and illness. In practical terms, we do not mean that *sanitary* environments are sterilized and germ free, but we are expecting domestic animals to be kept in such a way that they can get free from their own waste. Constant exposure to feces and urine causes scalding wounds and accompanying infections, fumes from ammonia in urine-soaked enclosures (Figure 3.2) lead to respiratory and eye irritation, and all manner of parasites proliferate in areas where feces build up over time.

(a)

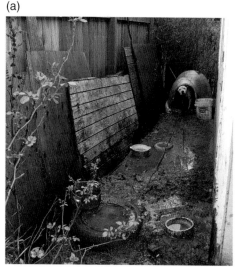

(b)

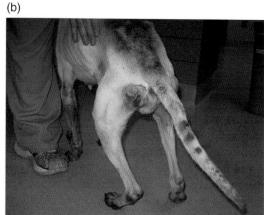

Figure 3.2   The multiple wounds and abscesses on the dog in this photo can be attributed to the conditions within her run and shelter. *Source:* Oregon Humane Society.

3.3.1   Some Considerations Regarding Sanitation

3.3.1.1   Stalls, Kennel Runs, Litterboxes

Areas where animals defecate and urinate need to be maintained. They should not be overflowing with waste so that animals must stand in or on their waste when confined within or accessing these areas. A buildup of waste attracts insects and harbors parasites. Animals within these environments are often heavily parasitized and may suffer from wounds or ulcers with maggots present in the surrounding fur or wool.

3.3.1.2   Ammonia/Urine

If the smell of ammonia is overwhelming in the home or area where the animals are housed, this is a hazard for both humans and animals and can damage respiratory function, sinuses, and eyes. Contact with urine on the skin causes chemical burns and ulcers, and can lead to infections over time.

3.3.1.3   Contaminated/Spoiled Food, Dirty Food, and Water Receptacles

The area and containers where animals eat and drink need to be safe and reasonably clean (Figure 3.3). Contamination from feces and urine, rotten food, chemicals, or other environmental contaminants poses an immediate risk to an animal's health. Parasitic infections, bacterial, and protozoal diseases are spread by animals ingesting the infectious agent while eating or drinking.

3.4   Food and Water

A good investigator always checks for food and water. However, as is the case with so many aspects of animal cruelty investigations, there are many factors at play to consider when assessing these two critical requirements.

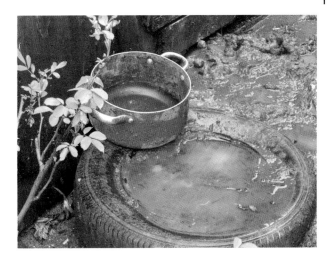

Figure 3.3 Contaminated food and water pose health risks to animals. *Source:* Oregon Humane Society.

Food and water must be of a quantity and quality that is beneficial to the animals. A canary who is fed only parrot food will not be able to break open the large seeds and gain adequate nutrition from his diet even though his bowl is always full. Likewise, if a horse has overgrown teeth that have not been maintained in some time, the horse will roll its hay or grass into a ball in its mouth repeatedly and eventually drop it. The horse's teeth lack the flat surface that allows it to grind the hay or grass into pieces it can swallow. A horse with this problem can starve to death in a pasture full of grass. A dozen cats may have access to a large hopper of dry food, but the group has established a hierarchy in which a percentage of older, weaker cats are denied access to the food by younger, more dominant ones. Water bowls and troughs may be full, but on closer inspection, there is no water service to the property, which could mean the animals are at the mercy of the rain to provide the water they need to sustain life.

Food and nutrition are areas where human ignorance often precedes animal suffering. The role of the veterinarian, animal control officers, and law enforcement in educating owners about proper nutrition should always come first when responding and identifying a problem. Many times, individuals take on pets or livestock without properly researching their care and feeding requirements.

3.4.1 Assessment of Food and Water

3.4.1.1 Accessibility

Are there enough food and water receptacles for the number of animals? Can all the animals reach the containers? Is there a hierarchy within the population leading to resource guarding and lack of access? Is there running water on the property or are the animals dependent on rainwater? Are receptacles and water sources frozen over?

3.4.1.2 Type and Amount

Is the food appropriate for the species? Are the animals actually eating it? Is there a store of food on hand that gives you confidence that the owner can provide the amount of food the animals require daily? Is the food expired or stored where it has become contaminated by insects or rodents?

Note: It is common to investigate starvation cases where the owner assures you the animal has access to food but is not interested in eating. In these cases, you can offer the animal a treat or some food or ask the owner to feed the animal, in order to confirm the owner's statement. A thorough examination and diagnostics by a veterinarian will aid in confirming if starvation was due to an underlying medical condition or inadequate amount of food. More information about investigating starvation cases is included in Appendix A.

3.5   Nutrition

As pets grow or age, recover from illness, or nurse litters of offspring, their nutritional needs change with their conditions. The first response to these cases should include educating the owner about the nutritional requirements of animals and enacting a plan for bringing the conditions up to muster, if the owner's resources and the animal's conditions allow.

While we know food is important, even vital to sustaining life, nutrition is the combination of carbohydrates, fats, fiber, minerals, proteins, and vitamins that support growth, reproduction, maintenance, and performance. The vast science of animal nutrition revolves around the livestock industry and food production where exact standards are set that will provide optimal and predictable weight gain and finishing. Although food animal nutrition is based on food production science, much information is available about the nutritional needs of all species of animals kept as pets and in zoos as well [1].

Diet and nutrition support every basic function of the body. Today there are commercially prepared diets available for most of the animals we keep as pets, from fish and rabbits to dogs and cats. Manufactured pet and livestock food is regulated by the US Food and Drug Administration (FDA) and the Association of American Feed Control Officials (AAFCO) [2].

Especially within the pet fancier's community, there is much debate about what makes an "adequate" or "high-quality" diet, and opinions differ wildly about the best options available to owners. For the purpose of evaluating nutrition in the field, the following observations can be helpful when assessing nutritional status:

- Is the type and quantity appropriate for the species and size/age of the animal?
- Is food being offered at the appropriate frequency?
- Is it fresh and stored properly?
- Are there factors related to nutrition that need special attention (allergies, illness, age, etc.?)
- Is the animal interested in eating the food and is their body condition appropriate?

Just like human infants, juvenile animals require more frequent feedings and a more nutrient-dense diet. Their mothers also need additional calories to support nursing and recovery (Figure 3.4). Geriatric animals or those recovering from injury or illness may need a special diet they can both tolerate and that will support their healing. They may benefit from accommodations as to how they are fed, or may need to be separated from other animals while feeding. Again, by educating the owner and monitoring compliance and progress, many of these cases can be resolved satisfactorily without the need to issue criminal citations.

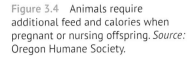

Figure 3.4 Animals require additional feed and calories when pregnant or nursing offspring. *Source:* Oregon Humane Society.

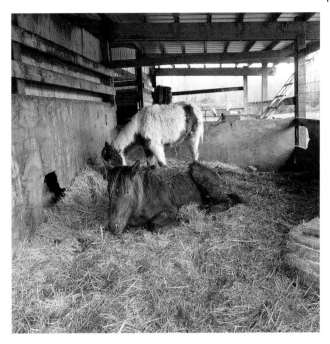

3.6 Documentation

Documentation is critical to the success of every investigation. Approach every interaction with the mindset that "if it isn't documented, it didn't happen." This is especially important in animal cases because the victims cannot speak; therefore, they cannot testify to the level of care and treatment they received. The investigator must be able to fill in the blanks.

Make detailed notes immediately after site inspections and interviews. When possible, record interviews so you have an exact account of what was said. Months and sometimes years will pass between the time an investigator submits a report to the courts and the day that case is heard at trial. Your notes, reports, photos, and recordings will serve you well, as you recall the facts on the witness stand.

Documentation is critical (Figure 3.5) when establishing facts about an animal's environment and access to resources like food and water. Always utilize photos and video whenever possible both to illustrate the conditions and to remind you of your findings. Make note of food in storage, the expiration dates of feed, the number of food and water bowls or troughs compared with the number of animals, the animals' demeanor when presented with food or a treat, and the body condition of the animals at issue.

Sometimes we feel compelled to collect food and water samples for testing, especially in cases where the food and water are fouled or expired. Lab testing can determine the nutritional characteristics of a bale of hay or identify chemicals or toxins in the water supply that might render it nonpotable. Keep in mind that sample collection, storage, and submission processes can be very specific and so investigators must be trained in those procedures and have the proper equipment on hand when utilizing these diagnostics, in order for them to be of value at trial.

(a)

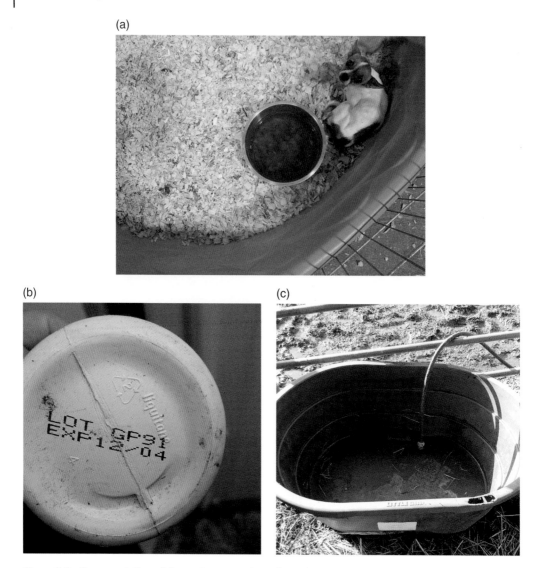

(b)

(c)

Figure 3.5 Documentation of the environment through accurate notes, photography, and video is a critical component of every animal cruelty investigation. *Source:* Oregon Humane Society.

3.7 Body Condition

We have already used the term "body condition" several times in this chapter. Body condition refers to the amount of fat stores and the presence of muscling in an animal. Body condition scoring is a hands-on procedure originally developed as a method for assessing cattle used in food production. According to the species of animal being assessed, specific points on the animal's body are felt and observed for the presence of fat. The findings are then used to assign a score to each animal, which serves as its "body condition score" (BCS). Since its development, body scoring has been applied to almost every type of livestock and pet animal, as a way to assess the body that is much more accurate than simply looking.

As you know, many animals have thick, curly, or matted hair coats, dense feather coverings or even dark colorations, which can prevent an accurate assessment of body condition by sight alone. While no one will testify that body condition scoring is a foolproof method for analyzing animal fat stores, BCS charts serve the important role of setting a standard for the ideal body condition for the species, as well as the degrees on either side of that standard ending in emaciation or obesity.

3.8 Documenting Body Condition

It is helpful for staff conducting investigations to be trained in several species' body condition scoring methods. Knowing the bony points of an animal where fat stores are first depleted, such as the tail pins, the hip joints, and the ribs; these also serve as the key areas to observe when noticing the condition of an animal you cannot touch. It is important to make note in your reports of whether you assessed the animal using your hands or if you were unable to touch it. Here is an example of a statement regarding observations from a distance, "I was unable to enter the paddock where the horses were kept. Their coats were wet and from a 20-foot distance I could easily count each horse's ribs and the tail pins were prominent on all four horses."

Be sure you are documenting body condition according to the standard and not compared with other animals on the property. Universities around the country have published body condition scales, which are available online.[1] Include a copy of the chart you utilized on site and refer to it as the standard you used when you write your reports. Share it with any veterinarians or other experts who will be examining the animals, so everyone is referencing the same body condition assessment scale in their examinations.

Photo and video documentation of body condition is very important and must not be overlooked. Familiarize yourself with the points on the body used to assess body condition and include those points in your videos and photographs. Make sure the light is adequate to display an accurate representation of what you see with your eyes, taking care not to exaggerate or underrepresent the body condition. Include five views of each animal (front, back, each side, and from above).

If an animal has a thick hair or feather coat, it can be helpful to use your hands when photographing, both to move the hair aside and as a caliper around the spinal column (Figure 3.6) (on a dog, for example) or to demarcate the prominent chest or keel bone of a bird.

3.9 Dental, Foot, and Hoof Care

In the wild, animals exist in their native terrain for which their bodies, including their feet and hooves, have specifically evolved over time. The same is true for animals' teeth. In their natural environment, an animal's teeth would become worn from foraging through grasslands or hunting and eating their prey. In captivity, where the conditions for which these animals were evolutionarily designed are not present, owners must intervene to provide maintenance services on their animals' hooves (Figure 3.7), nails, teeth, hair coats, etc. It is the responsibility of an owner to know what is considered routine maintenance or wellness care for the species of animals they own, and to

---

1 For example, see Body Condition System. https://www.library.tufts.edu/vet/images/bcs_dog.pdf, accessed 30 May 2021.

(a)

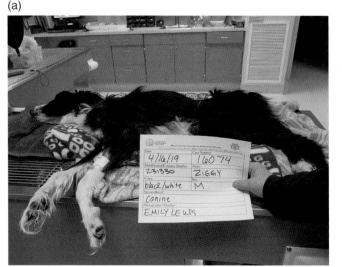

(b)

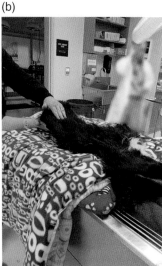

Figure 3.6   Photos should accurately represent the animal's body condition. *Source:* Oregon Humane Society.

provide that care often enough that conditions do not become painful or dangerous for their pets or livestock.

When responding to animal cases, it is important for the investigator to make themselves familiar with the type of routine care the animals in question should be receiving. Some issues, particularly dental problems, may not be immediately noticeable at first glance and will require a closer look at the animal, if it is willing, or by a veterinarian using sedation. Because conditions arising from lack of dental, hoof, and coat care are so common and can become so painful, even debilitating, this is an area worth the investment in time and research so that you are able to identify the issues, educate the owner, and, when necessary, articulate the evidence of criminal neglect.

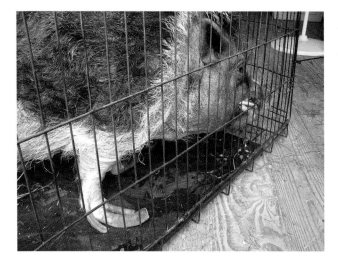

Figure 3.7   Many animals, such as the pot-bellied pig in this photo, require regular hoof and dental care to prevent painful overgrowth. *Source:* Oregon Humane Society.

3.10 Veterinary Care, Medications, and Treatment

There are several reasons an individual might fail to provide veterinary treatment for an ill or injured animal. More "passive" reasons include a lack of education about or understanding of the seriousness of an animal's condition. Financial insecurity (limitations or constraints or choices) may play a part, as can a lack of transportation, language barriers, geography, and many other contributing factors that create obstacles for the animal owner. A failure to provide veterinary care can also be deliberate and with knowing disregard for an animal's suffering. It is important that the investigation sheds light on the details surrounding the owner's action or inaction in providing medication and treatment to their animal. Animal cruelty citations can result from an owner's failure to provide medical treatment to relieve pain and suffering.

When investigating cases involving the care and treatment of a sick or injured animal, the investigator will attempt to learn what, if any, treatments have been given, as well as what medications have been utilized by or prescribed to the owner to administer to the animal. By interviewing the owner and examining the medications, you can draw your own conclusions about whether the treatment, or lack of treatment, is evidence of animal cruelty.

When examining medication presented by the owner as evidence they are addressing (Figure 3.8) the animal's condition, look closely for the following:

- If prescribed, is the medication specified for the animal in question?
- Is the medication expired?
- Is there evidence the animal has been receiving the medication (number of pills missing, liquids or ointments are open and obviously have been used)?
- Are there accompanying vet records or other instructions to the owner regarding the condition and medication?

It is always a good idea to photograph the medication with the amount used and expiration date visible.

In many cases, the initial interaction with the owner will lead you to mandate that they seek veterinary care for an animal within a certain amount of time, after which you will return to confirm that the owner has followed your instructions, the animal is receiving adequate treatment, and is on the mend. Outcomes like this are ideal and demonstrate the important role of animal

Figure 3.8 Examine medication closely for prescription information, expiration date, and evidence of use. *Source:* Oregon Humane Society.

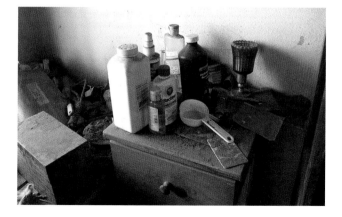

control and law enforcement officers as educators and community caretakers. This approach is successful in nonemergent cases, in which the officer is truly able to conduct rechecks, and the owner can provide the care and treatment recommended by the veterinarian to address the injury or condition. Some communities offer programs that provide qualifying pet owners with accessible and affordable veterinary care. In many investigations you will find that the owner wants to do the right thing for the animal but does not have the means to do so. Subsidized programs often provide the help pet owners need to care for their animals adequately, and ultimately preserve the bond between animals and owners by keeping the pet out of the shelter.

3.11 Nonaccidental Injury and Trauma

Investigations of traumatic injury and physical abuse of an animal require a swift response and keen interview skills. Because evidence of abuse such as bruising, limping, and wounds can heal quickly, it is important to facilitate veterinary examination of the animal and interview witnesses and suspects as soon as possible after receiving the report. A veterinarian will be able to uncover injuries through examination, X-ray, and other diagnostics. Their medical record and reports along with photos, videos, and test results can guide the investigator to ask questions that will shed light on the facts that led to the animal's injury or death. Likewise, information the officer gleans from interviewing witnesses and suspects can guide the veterinarian in his or her examination and diagnostic plan.

Nonaccidental injury cases can include drowning, burning, asphyxiation, beating (Figure 3.9), sexual abuse, shooting, and torture. The list is as long as the list of injurious and assault crimes humans commit toward one another. People who commit these crimes toward animals may also be abusing family members or committing other crimes in the community. Many are in need of professional mental health assessment and services. Animal abuse cases should never be set aside because the victim was "just a cat" or the owner "lost their temper," when disciplining their puppy.

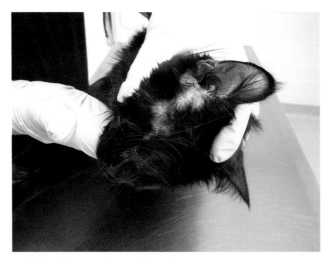

Figure 3.9 There is a well-established link between animal abuse and other violent crimes. *Source:* Oregon Humane Society.

3.12   The Link Between Animal Cruelty and Crimes Against Humans

You have learned about the Five Freedoms and know that animals suffer and feel pain, and you understand these crimes must be investigated on their own merit, but we must also remember that people who willfully harm animals rarely stop there. Results of many studies have established the link between animal cruelty and human crimes. Linked closely to domestic violence, cruelty to animals is now recognized as a valid "predictor crime" of spousal and child abuse [3]. According to a 1983 study, 88% of homes in which child abuse was investigated also had identified instances of abuse of animals within the home [4].

Always be alert to the possibility of other victims in any animal investigation. Abusers frequently harm the family pet as a method of controlling their human victim [5]. These are not uncommon scenarios; they are at play within every community across the nation. By enforcing animal protection laws, in addition to saving the lives of animals, the investigator is disarming the cycle of physical violence within families and communities.

3.13   Emergency Issues

Unfortunately, many animal welfare calls initiate with an animal in crisis. In these cases, it is important the investigator respond with the humane care of the animal foremost in their mind but remembering that their investigation will require them to pay attention to all the elements discussed in this chapter. A livestock animal that is down and unable to stand on its own, or a dog with a gunshot wound, is an example of a case that must be addressed in the moment to provide care to the animal, whether through an emergency aid warrant exception, exigent seizure, or the owner's swift and immediate action. Some counties may allow animal control officers to utilize impoundment in these situations. Regardless of the means, the investigator must ensure that the animal receives care.

It is always more difficult to find resources and create plans in the middle of an emergency. Establish partnerships in animal control, law enforcement, animal rescue and sheltering, and the veterinary community, so when help is needed you will have these contacts available to you.

References

1 NRCS (n.d.). Livestock nutrition, husbandry, and behavior. https://www.nrcs.usda.gov/Internet/FSE_DOCUMENTS/stelprdb1043065.pdf (accessed 24 May 2021).

2 US FDA (n.d.). Center for veterinary medicine. Product regulation. https://www.fda.gov/animal-veterinary/animal-food-feeds/product-regulation (accessed 25 May 2021).

3 Arluke, A., Levin, J., Luke, C., and Ascione, F. (1999). The relationship of animal abuse to violence and other forms of antisocial behavior. *J Interpers. Violence* 14 (9): 963–975.

4 DeViney, E., Dickert, J., and Lockwood, R.(1983). The care of pets within child abusing families. https://www.wellbeingintlstudiesrepository.org/acwp_awap/15 (accessed 26 May 2021).

5 Ascione, F.R., Weber, C.V., Thompson, T.M. et al. (2007). Battered pets and domestic violence: animal abuse reported by women experiencing intimate violence and by nonabused women. *Violence Against Women* 13 (4): 354–373.

4

Initial Investigation and Assessment
Linda Fielder

Cases of animal neglect and abuse may originate with the anonymous report of an owner kicking their dog at the park, or a call of concern for an emaciated cat the next-door neighbor sees from their window. A veterinarian may report an owner's failure to provide essential medical care for a horse with severe dental issues, or an appliance repair technician may call upon finding birds in horrendous conditions during a service call to the home of an animal hoarder.

Regardless of where a report originates, the resulting investigation is guided by the knowledge of the basic needs of animals, and the application of that knowledge to the animal and its surroundings.

Animal cruelty investigations are often compared to homicide cases because of one important shared element: the victim cannot speak as a witness to the crime. Because of this, the investigator shoulders the responsibility of assembling the evidence thoroughly and precisely, through use of all his senses, through photographs and documentation, research, and interviews to piece together the elements of the crime and work the case through from report to resolution.

4.1 Types of Reports

Reports of concern for an animal's welfare generally fall into one or more of the following categories:

- Emaciated animal(s)
- Inhumane/inadequate living conditions
- Injured or ill, lacking veterinary care
- Physical abuse or killing of animal(s)
- Animal fighting
- Sexual abuse of animal(s)
- Overworking or inhumane training methods, exhibition, or exploitation of animals
- Hoarding or overcrowding (Figure 4.1).

A working knowledge of your state's statutes, as well as county or jurisdictional ordinances that apply to animals, is vital when receiving and investigating reports of animal cruelty.

Animal Cruelty Investigations: A Collaborative Approach from Victim to Verdict™, First Edition.
Edited by Kris Otteman, Linda Fielder, and Emily Lewis.
© 2022 John Wiley & Sons, Inc. Published 2022 by John Wiley & Sons, Inc.
Companion website: www.wiley.com/go/otteman/victimtoverdict

Figure 4.1 Many reports concern animals living in inadequate conditions that can be observed from the public's view. *Source:* Oregon Humane Society.

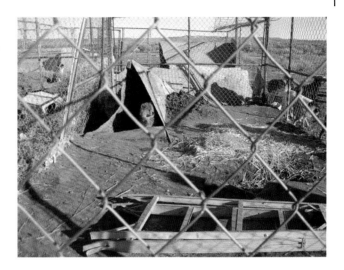

4.2 Anonymous Reports

While it is always preferable that the reporting party identifies themselves, anonymous complaints should not be disregarded as they are usually legitimate. The reporting party often wishes to remain anonymous because they fear retribution by the suspect, who may be a neighbor, family member, or associate. If an anonymous complaint is detailed and reasonable, it is in the agency's and the animal's best interest to initiate a site visit or investigation.

4.3 Required Information

In order to provide a response, the following information, at a minimum, is necessary:

- Date and time the witness observed the incident/conditions.
- Explicit address/location/directions where the incident occurred, including a description of the property, building, vehicles, and any other information the reporting party can provide that will guide the investigator in finding the animals and/or the suspect.
- Number and type of animals involved, including descriptions such as breed and color.
- Why the reporting party believes the animals are being neglected or abused.
- Any information the witness can provide about the owner/suspect, such as name, physical description, place of work, vehicle description, and license plate number.
- Can the animals or their conditions be viewed from the road or public property?
- Are there any other witnesses to contact?
- Has this incident been reported to any other agency? If so, what agency and when?

After your agency receives the report, it is prudent, if staffing and resources allow, to confirm the address, review online maps of the property, search relevant websites or social media posts that might be related to the incident or suspect, and generally verify any information provided that might inform you about the incident prior to contacting the suspect or performing a site visit.

4.4   Response Triage

It is all too common that animal control, law enforcement, and animal welfare organizations are working with limited resources, personnel, and equipment. Due to these circumstances and others – including vast geographic response areas, weather, holidays, etc. – an immediate or same-day response to a report may be impractical or impossible. A system for triaging reports can help ensure that investigators attend to the most critical cases as soon as possible. When developing a triage matrix for your organization, it is important to set realistic response goals based on your agency's staffing and resources. A sample triage matrix might look like this:

Red (immediate response): Deceased or dying animal, or emergency such as a dog confined in a hot car, a horse stuck in flooded pasture, organized animal fight in progress, animal crime with human crime investigation in progress (such as domestic violence).

Orange (response within 24 hours): Abandoned animals without food or water, emaciated, ill, or injured animals, physical abuse with injury.

Yellow (response within 48 hours): Inadequate shelter (not life-threatening), poor sanitation, hoarding/overcrowding, physical abuse (no injury observed), overgrown hooves, or lack of grooming.

4.5   Legitimate or Not? How to Decide

Unfortunately, as is the case with any agency that accepts reports from the public, some accounts that are filed with your office will be false or exaggerated, which is both a frustration and a time waster for responders. These calls can be the product of a family feud or dispute among neighbors and may be completely unfounded. Most states have laws in place that prohibit false reporting.

In other cases, the witness may disagree with the way an animal is being housed or trained, but the reality is that the owner is providing minimum care for the animal, as required by the laws in your state. As an example, the reporting party believes that a dog should not be secured by a chain to an outdoor doghouse. While most of us would agree that dogs are companion animals that should not live on a chain, in most states this is within the law, if all the components outlined for the provision of minimum care and shelter are being met.

Though sometimes while obtaining information needed to generate a case it will become clear the call is false or unfounded, most of the time a site visit is required to make that determination.

4.6   Responding to Calls: Initial Site Visit

4.6.1   Using All Your Senses

The moment the property or location of the report comes into view, you will begin using your senses of sight, hearing, smell, and touch to gather information for your case.

As you approach the location, be aware of any animals you see outdoors. Livestock animals may be easily visible, and you can assess the condition of their available pasture, make note of their behavior, and start to count the number of animals visible. A hoarding case may offer clues to what lies inside a home or outbuilding by the smells and sounds emanating from within (Figure 4.2).

Figure 4.2 The number of cats in this window offers a glimpse into conditions inside the home of an animal hoarder. *Source:* Oregon Humane Society.

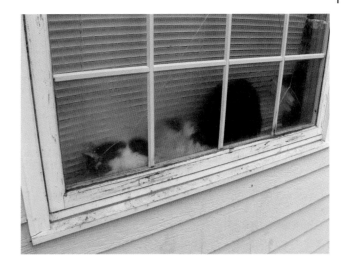

4.6.2 Attempting Contact: No One Home/No Answer

All attempts by an investigator to contact an owner and gain access to the animal(s) must be done through avenues within the laws of your state regarding a citizen's expectation of privacy and private property. Consult with your agency and your prosecutors to determine how your state's laws will guide your decisions in this regard.

If you knock on the door of a residence and no one is home or no one will answer the door, your investigation does not end there. You have already taken notice of what you could see, hear, and smell from your location in the driveway and on your walk to the door. Side yards, back yards, and any areas behind a door or a fence, such as barns and sheds, are generally considered off limits without consent or a search warrant; therefore, do not be tempted to have a look around in these areas. Such a decision is not only dangerous but is most likely unlawful.

To further your investigation, leave a card and instructions for the owner to contact you immediately regarding a concern for their animal(s). Agencies often find it useful to have printed notices that allow space to communicate with the animal owner, and which also clearly identify your agency and provide (Figure 4.3) contact numbers and email addresses.

Figure 4.3 Notices should be easy to read and posted in a conspicuous place. *Source:* Oregon Humane Society.

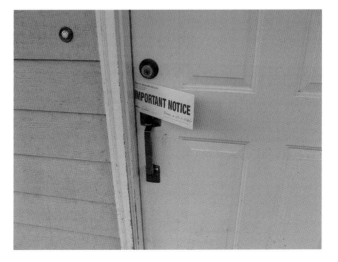

Make sure to record in the case file the date and time you attempted contact, as well as your notes regarding observations. This may be a good time to attempt contact with neighbors who may be a witness to the animal(s), and you can leave a card with your contact information on those attempts at contact as well.

It is vital that you are responsive when a witness or a subject calls or emails regarding a case. Make sure your voicemail message includes your name and title, as well as the days you are on shift, and an alternative contact within the department for urgent matters. Utilize auto reply email features that will notify subjects if you are off shift and when they can expect to hear from you. Check your voice mailbox and email at least twice a day and follow up with contacts in a timely manner during your work week.

4.6.3 Attempting Contact: Responsible Party Is Not Home/Is Unavailable

It is not uncommon that the person who answers the door is not the person who owns or is responsible for the animal(s) at issue. If this is the case, collect the name and contact information for this person, who may be a spouse, a roommate, or a family member. Write down your contact information and ask them to give it to the subject. If they refuse, you can post the notice and contact information on the front door, much as you would if no one answered. These individuals usually do not have authority to show you around a property when the animal owner may have an expectation of privacy. If they do feel compelled to offer information about the animal(s) or your investigation, be sure to record those details in the case file, along with the individual's full name, and the date and time of your exchange.

4.6.4 Attempting Contact: Owner Is Home/Contact Successful

If the animal owner is home and willing to speak with you, it is time to employ your interview skills (see Chapter 5) along with your knowledge about the fundamentals of animal care (see Chapters 2 and 3) to determine the following:

- Who is responsible for the care of the animal?
- How long have they had the animal?
- How long has the animal been in that condition (thin, injured, improperly housed, etc.)?
- Ask the owner to describe their procedure for feeding, cleaning, and medicating the animal.
- What other animals does this person own or care for? Do others co-own or assist with care?
- What, if anything, has the owner attempted to remedy the situation?
- Who is their veterinarian? When did this animal last see a veterinarian and what was the reason for the visit?
- Is the animal in immediate danger or at risk of death?

Ideally the responsible party will prove cooperative, in which case you should attempt to view the following:

- The animal(s)
- The animal's living environment
- Available food and water
- Any medication or vet records associated with the animal.

In nonexigent cases, in which you have a degree of confidence the owner can and will work to remedy the situation for the animal(s), you may choose to educate the owner and make recommendations for correction. We will discuss this process in Chapter 8.

4.6.5 Attempting Contact: Owner Is Uncooperative

In some instances, despite your best effort and utilization of the techniques for rapport-building, a subject may be uncooperative. The subject may initially agree to show you the animal or its environment but become agitated or uncomfortable as you pose questions to him or her. They may appear defensive or belligerent or deny the animals are in any way neglected, ill, or injured. This response can be especially true in cases involving suspected intentional abuse. Always make note of a subject's statements, including those in which they deny neglecting or abusing an animal. You should also include facts about the subject's demeanor and body language. For example, if the subject begins pacing and yelling when questioned about a particular animal, make sure to include those behaviors in your case notes.

Cases in which the owner is uncooperative may escalate to a search warrant and seizure. If you have reason to believe the animals are suffering, at risk of death, or that the subject may remove or alter the evidence including the animals, a search warrant can be a viable option for a rapid response. These types of cases will be discussed in more detail in Chapter 9.

4.6.6 Unable to Make Contact

If your attempts to make contact prove unsuccessful, you may have to explore other methods for conducting your investigation. Repeated visits to a property offer opportunities to notice if there is actually anyone living at the reported location. You may see your written notices stacking up on the door, with no indications anyone has been home since your investigation began. This could mean that the resident uses a side door or garage entrance and has not seen the notices, no one is living at the residence, or the subject is simply coming and going and has chosen not to retrieve or respond to your notices. Other indicators such as the location of vehicles, foot tracks in the snow, or accumulating mail or garbage can all lend clues about whether someone is ignoring your attempts to make contact. Oftentimes persistence pays off – if a subject begins to realize that you will continue to visit them until the matter is resolved, they may eventually decide to answer the door. If not, there are other investigation methods you can employ that may inform your next steps up to and including application for a search warrant. Consider talking with the complainant again, interview neighbors, other witnesses, or follow up on other information you have learned that could prove helpful. In most cases it is not appropriate simply to close a case because you cannot make contact, so be persistent and think outside the box about ways to compel the subject to talk with you or other ways to verify the legitimacy of the report and complete your investigation.

4.6.7 Exigent Circumstances

First responders to reports of animal cruelty, or criminal activity in general, may find themselves faced with an animal in need of emergency veterinary care without which death is imminent. You *must* invest the time to understand from the prosecutors in your jurisdiction what actions you can take to aid the animal in that moment, as well as preserve evidence of the crime of animal cruelty (see Chapter 9 for additional nuances of the emergency aid and exigency exceptions [Figure 4.4] to the warrant requirement). Again, if you are acting as a representative of any state agency, it is your duty to understand what your state law permits in these emergency situations.

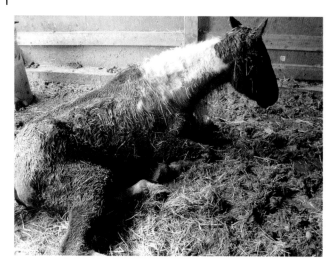

Figure 4.4 Understand what the laws in your state specify about providing emergency aid to an animal in critical condition, such as this downed horse. *Source:* Oregon Humane Society.

4.6.8 Cross-Reporting and Other Vulnerable Individuals

Animal cruelty investigations frequently uncover evidence of other crimes or human health and welfare concerns. Children, family members, partners, and the elderly can be victims of abuse in much the same way animals are. Children, disabled individuals, and the elderly are all particularly vulnerable to neglect, if they depend on others for their daily care and support.

You may be mandated by law to report concerns for human welfare to the appropriate agencies, and even if you are not a mandatory reporter, it is prudent to contact human welfare agencies anytime you are aware of the potential for human neglect or abuse, during the course of your animal investigation. Make a list of all appropriate health and human welfare agencies in your response area, as well as code enforcement, fire marshals, and any other agencies that can respond to these types of concerns so you will be able to contact them without delay.

5

Witness and Subject Interviewing

Linda Fielder

A thoughtful and thorough interview provides valuable information to support an animal cruelty investigation. The subject of the interview may be a witness or a suspect. Law enforcement and animal control officers are the most common interviewers; however, veterinarians, veterinary staff, and animal shelter employees may find themselves conducting interviews when animal cruelty cases present themselves in their clinic or shelter. An investigator or veterinarian who asks thoughtful and open-ended questions, understands the importance of building rapport with the subject, and conducts the interview in a respectful and ethical manner will gain useful insight into the facts of the case.

The interviewer bears the responsibility of asking questions that are direct, specific, and easily understood. They must listen to, understand, and ask for clarity when the need arises. A great interviewer is adept at formulating follow-up questions that encourage the subject to elaborate and offer additional details. A useful subject interview serves as a roadmap for an investigation. By following up on information provided by the subject, the investigator gathers the building blocks of the case which will support or refute the evidence of the crime.

5.1 Preparation for the Interview

The more prepared and organized you are going into an interview, the better the case will be served by the information you gain. Start by taking the time to review the information you have available to you prior to meeting with the subject. This may be the initial report, veterinary records, social media posts, other interview notes, or transcripts. Reviewing everything available will give you the opportunity to formulate questions that will allow the subject to fill in the blanks and provide direction for further investigation or next steps. Look for elements of the crime that will need to be proven, statements that demonstrate motive, and references to evidence that is missing or does not add up.

Animal Cruelty Investigations: A Collaborative Approach from Victim to Verdict™, First Edition.
Edited by Kris Otteman, Linda Fielder, and Emily Lewis.
© 2022 John Wiley & Sons, Inc. Published 2022 by John Wiley & Sons, Inc.
Companion website: www.wiley.com/go/otteman/victimtoverdict

5.2   Interview Location and Setting

Be thoughtful when selecting an interview time and location. Is this interview best conducted in person or by phone? In-person interviews are usually preferred, but if timelines and schedules preclude such a meeting then a phone interview is better than none. When conducting a phone interview, always make sure to ask questions that will verify the identity of the person you are speaking to – note accents, word choices, and other distinguishing verbal characteristics to help you recognize that you are actually speaking to the subject and not someone else. Note the ways you verified the subject's identity in your report so the interview is accepted as valid.

Make sure the subject is able to speak to you without distractions. Interviewing a subject at their workplace may make them self-conscious or may not allow them to fully focus on your interaction, due to noise and interruptions. The same may be true in a household where there are many family members present. Depending on their involvement in the case, a subject may feel nervous about meeting at a law enforcement agency and might be less likely to cooperate fully with the interview in this setting. The location of the interview should never create an environment where the subject might feel trapped or detained.[1] With all these factors in mind, determine a meeting place where the subject can speak freely, without fear of being overheard, and without distractions.

You should also be certain that you, the interviewer, will not be interrupted by phone calls, coworkers, radio transmissions, or other distractions during the interview. Take steps to eliminate these possibilities to the extent possible in advance of the interview.

Many interviews are conducted in the moment during a site visit, when responding to a report of potential abuse or neglect. In these settings you may be able to inspect the animal(s), their surroundings, and other elements that will provide evidence in your case. Specific questions and recommendations for these types of interviews are contained in Chapter 4 as well as in Appendix A.

5.3   Miranda and Consent

When a suspect is interviewed by law enforcement or other agent of the state in a custodial setting, the Fifth and Fourteenth Amendments of the Constitution afford them due process rights (privilege against self-incrimination, right to counsel) [1]. The Supreme Court of the United States has found that, prior to questioning a suspect in that setting, you must provide them with warnings of their constitutional rights [2]. If you are a law enforcement officer, you have been trained on Miranda warnings and the circumstances in which they should be given, but a court could decide to hold any individual acting as an agent of the state to the same standard. Miranda warnings must be given in order to question a suspect in a custodial setting [2]. Whether a setting is considered "custodial" is determined by an assessment of all the circumstances, such as the location, the duration, the statements made, or physical restraint [3–5]. A court will evaluate whether a reasonable person in those circumstances would have felt free to leave [6].

Similarly, if the suspect makes a confession, a judge will evaluate the circumstances of that confession to determine if it was voluntary and admissible. A confession is defined as "any confession of guilt of any criminal offense or any self-incriminating statement made or given orally or in writing" [7]. The court can look at factors, such as the timing of the confession in the context of the

---

1 Note that this section discusses interviews in which the individual is free to leave. There are strict laws that govern parameters of custodial interviews, see Section 5.3.

arrest or arraignment, or whether the suspect knew the nature of the offense, or whether the suspect had been advised of their right to an attorney and did they have an attorney present [8].

If a suspect chooses to waive their rights and decides to respond to your questions without an attorney present, they can also choose to reassert them at any time during the interview. A suspect has the right to remain silent and not answer any questions. A suspect is also constitutionally protected when they decide to answer some questions but invoke their right to remain silent on other questions [9].

A suspect has a right to an attorney and the minute they request an attorney all questioning must cease. Although the suspect "must unambiguously request counsel," [10] such "that a reasonable police officer in the circumstances would understand the statement to be a request for an attorney" [10], there is no set terminology for this request. Statements such as "I think I should get a lawyer" and "[m]aybe I should talk to a lawyer" have been upheld as invocations of a suspect's right to counsel [11, 12]. If you improperly continue to question a suspect after they have requested an attorney, that part of your interview will be inadmissible as evidence. Be aware of your surroundings and the statements made by the person you are questioning at all times as they will be scrutinized later in court.

5.4 Building Rapport

There is a wealth of training materials and research available around the importance of building rapport with an interview subject. Studies have determined that particular verbal techniques as well as reading body language and "mimicry" are helpful in establishing trust, which in turn invites the subject to speak more openly, producing an interview product that is more accurate, detailed, and helpful to the investigation [13, 14].

Many individuals will be nervous and anxious at the prospect of being interviewed, regardless of whether they are a suspect or a witness. You can mitigate this through your demeanor and by beginning the interview with some deliberate conversation, aimed at putting the subject at ease.

The interviewer should invest time into building a rapport that may alleviate some of the subject's anxiety. It may be tempting to start with "small talk" about the weather or the local sports team, and while this may do some good, really trying to relate to the subject through a sincere mutual connection will produce more meaningful results [15].

Interviews are heavy with questions. Establishing a connection is a time for you, the interviewer, to humanize yourself to the subject by telling them something about yourself, ideally something they can relate to. For example, if you approach a subject who is working on their car's engine, you might offer up a story about a car repair that vexed you in order to illuminate a common experience. It has nothing to do with the details you will be questioning the subject about shortly, but it goes far to build trust and foster open communication. It is also a time for you to show empathy, an important trait to display to interview subjects [16].

Your body language also influences the subject's willingness to open up to you. Some subjects will not immediately respond to your efforts to build rapport and you will need to continue to make intentional efforts to connect throughout the interview. Adopt a casual posture, with hands and arms relaxed and visible. Indicate that you are listening by showing interest, making eye contact, nodding, and so forth. *Mirroring* is a behavioral technique in which the interviewer subtly copies a subject's mannerisms and tone, as a way of building trust and showing understanding. This is especially helpful when supporting a positive interaction. In situations where a subject becomes angry or volatile, you can often subdue them simply by adopting a demeanor that is the opposite of theirs. If they begin to yell, you might lower your voice and slow your speech in response, which will then encourage the subject to mirror you [17].

Time invested in learning and practicing rapport-building strategies is worthwhile. As you learn new techniques, practice them in casual settings with friends and family, and gauge their responses as a way of knowing what to expect in the field.

5.5 Ask Clear and Direct Open-Ended Questions

After you have reviewed all materials available and determined the goals of the interview and the information you are seeking to gain from the subject, you may prepare your questions. When possible, questions should follow the timeline of the case, though in some cases questions may address details that happened even before the timeline of events relevant to the crime. For example, you might begin by asking about how a witness first met the suspect and the nature of their relationship prior to any of the events you are investigating. You want your subject to feel as comfortable speaking with you as possible by the time your most important questions are posed to them. Facilitate this by allowing the subject to give you some background in their own words and without interruption.

Interview questions should be open-ended. Open-ended questions are ones that cannot be answered with "yes" or "no." They require an answer, as well as an explanation, and will supply you with important details to consider in your investigation. Open-ended questions draw out information. They also do not feed information to the subject by telling them in advance the information you are seeking.

Consider the following examples of an interview following a report of a man kicking a dog:

Example A
INTERVIEWER: "Did you witness the suspect in an angry and intoxicated state yelling at and abusing the dog in the parking lot?"
WITNESS: "Yes."
INTERVIEWER: "Did you see the suspect kick the dog in the parking lot last Wednesday?"
SUBJECT: "No."

Example B
INTERVIEWER: "What happened in the parking lot between the suspect and the dog last Wednesday?"
WITNESS: "I was leaving my shift at the bank, and I saw a man and a woman across the parking lot. The woman was crying, and the man was grabbing at her little brown dog's leash. The man fell down twice and was unsteady on his feet, but he managed to get the dog away from her, falling to the ground a third time in the process. The man was yelling at the dog. The woman was crying. She got into a black car and got on her cell phone."
INTERVIEWER: "What happened next?"
WITNESS: "The man stood up and picked up the dog by the leash. It was hanging a couple of feet off the ground and making an awful sound. He tried to kick it but missed and then he slammed the dog down against the pavement at least three times. The dog got away from the man and kind of crawled back to the woman in the car and she picked it up and drove away."

Example B began with open-ended questions and led to the witness supplying the investigator with some valuable details they can follow up on:

- While the man attempted to kick the dog, he failed in this and actually committed other cruel acts toward the dog (hanging, slamming).
- Who was the woman with the dog?
- Who did she call on her cell phone?
- Because the witness disclosed that they work at a bank, the investigator can follow up with the business to review security footage of the parking lot on the date and time of the incident.

It is important to note that this witness is not going to know *why* the suspect was harming the dog, so it is not necessary for them to speculate on this. The value of this witness is their detailed account of *what* happened and not *why*. The statement above should serve as a foundation for the interviewer to pose additional, more detailed questions about the length and type of leash the witness saw, any particular words they could hear the suspect yell, and who else might have been present in the parking lot or seen this incident through the bank window.

You should not expect that any one interview will provide all the information you need to finalize an investigation. On the contrary, the most valuable interviews provide information that guides you to more sources of information and additional witnesses. In the case above, knowing the witness worked at a bank that most likely collects round-the-clock surveillance video footage pointed the investigator to a recorded account of the incident for analysis.

5.6 Suspect Interviews

The importance of setting the subject at ease, establishing rapport, and building trust is no less important when the subject is the investigation's suspect than when they are a witness. While the ultimate goal of the suspect interview might be to obtain a confession, this should not be the driving motivation when structuring the interview. There may also be times when an investigator is faced with interviewing a suspect in a case in which it is seemingly obvious, due to the other evidence at hand, that the individual most certainly committed the crime, but this decision may only be made by the courts and the duty of the investigator to interview the suspect with integrity and impartiality remains unchanged.

After you have introduced yourself, established rapport, informed the suspect of their rights, and explained why they are being interviewed and what to expect, it is time to allow the suspect to provide you with their account of the incident at question. Begin by posing an invitation to tell their story and allow them time to collect their thoughts. Try not to interrupt or ask clarifying questions during the suspect's narrative, allow them to pause to gather their thoughts as needed, and resist the urge to fill their silence with questions. As the suspect offers you their story, you will most likely identify pieces you will want to examine more closely. Once the suspect has said their piece with minimal interruptions, it is time for you to pose clarifying questions, introduce evidence or elements of the investigation that the suspect may have left out of their account, and address any blatant misinformation. Even when digging deeper and posing questions that may cause discomfort for the suspect, remember to ask questions in an open-ended way and treat the suspect with respect. Your job is to probe and challenge the suspect's account, as needed, while striving for accuracy and truthfulness.

In cases with multiple suspects, interview each suspect separately, if possible, and clarify any "we" statements made during the interview. It is important to document each suspect's individual culpability for the violation you are investigating. Ask direct questions about their participation in the incident or role in the care of the animal. If a suspect continues to use "we" statements in discussing the circumstances leading to the alleged violation, try to narrow your questions in order to get a statement that does not involve other suspects. For example, if an emaciated dog is discovered in the care of three brothers who live together and one of the brothers responds to your questioning, "We all were in charge of buying the dog food." You should then ask clarifying questions like, "When was the last time *you* bought the food?" or "When was the last time *you* fed the dog?" Ensuring that you have statements specific to each suspect's involvement in the situation is crucial for prosecutors in a case with co-defendants.

5.7 Reading Body Language and Detecting Deception

You have likely watched television shows in which highly trained detectives identify a murderer based on the way the suspect glances to the left or purses his lips during a critical point in the interrogation. The science around micro expressions as an indicator of deception has connected minute changes in eye movement, respiration, or mouth movement to lying and deception. A less scientific understanding of body language can be beneficial to investigators, without extensive specialized training, if you think about it as the physical cues a person's body transmits in response to stimuli. An individual displays body language when the stimuli they are interpreting is pleasant or unpleasant. When assessing body language, pay attention to not just the way the person carries themselves, but also look for changes in pitch and speech patterns, eye contact, and the words they use. In response to a pleasant conversation a person will lean forward, nod in agreement, stay on the subject, and usually speak in complete sentences. If a conversation is unpleasant, the subject may display a more closed-off stance, shift their weight, and even turn away partially or fully from the speaker. They may gesture in a more exaggerated fashion than the situation calls for, their voice assuming a higher pitch. They tend to stutter, give incomplete answers, change the subject, or draw others into the conversation. A subject's body language may be relaxed and open at the beginning of an interview, and then begin to display signs of discomfort as the questioning continues. Do not assume this is always a sign of guilt, but be alert to changes in body language that can inform your strategy and result in a more productive interview.

It is helpful to make note of significant body language cues when writing your report after the interview. If the subject suddenly clenches their fists and turns away from you during questioning, this is a significant change in behavior that should be recorded [18].

5.8 Confessions

When a suspect confesses to neglecting, killing, or otherwise harming an animal, they are taking responsibility for their actions. When possible, an investigator should request the suspect to submit a signed statement, which, along with their confession, outlines the suspect's actions, and identifies their motive. Confessions are useful, but only if the confession is the truth. There are multiple reasons a suspect may choose to confess to committing a crime before, during, or after an interview. In some cases, the suspect may be overwhelmed with remorse and guilt for their actions. They may know the evidence you possess against them is insurmountable. There are also reasons a suspect may offer up a false confession. They may be protecting someone else or trying to create a diversion from additional crimes.

5.9   Ending the Interview

If at any time during an interview the subject voices a desire to seek counsel, have their attorney present, or otherwise engage legal advisement, a law enforcement officer must stop the interview immediately and cannot arrange for further questioning until the subject has had an opportunity to obtain counsel. Make sure you have a clear understanding from the prosecutors you work with what actions or words suffice as a request for counsel. This is a constitutional right and courts construe what constitutes a request for counsel very broadly.

5.10   Documenting the Interview

All interview notes must include the subject's name, address, and contact information. Record the date, time, and location of the interview as well as the names and addresses of any other individuals present during the interview. While audio or video recording is the most accurate and desirable method for collecting and preserving the information gained during an interview, it may not always be practical or possible. When relying on your notes and recollection of the interview, it becomes even more important that your interpretation of the information provided by the subject is accurate. Ask clarifying questions and repeat the subject's statements back to them to check for accuracy as you make a written record of the interview.

5.11   Additional Resources and Training

Strong interview skills are developed through training, practice, and by observing seasoned professionals. There are excellent trainings available through law enforcement agencies and organizations, and numerous techniques have been developed around interviewing, reading body language, detecting deception, and many other aspects of the subject interview. Because the interview is so vital to the development and prosecution of criminal cases, time and resources spent developing your interviewing skills and increasing your knowledge will be rewarded in the field.

References

1 Constitution of the United States, Amendment 5 1791 (USA); Constitution of the United States, Amendment 14 1868 (USA).
2 *Miranda vs. Arizona*, 86 St. Ct. 1602, (1966).
3 Then, L. (2015). Applying the 'cuffs: consistency and clarity in a bright-line rule for arrest-like restraints under Miranda custody. *Fla. St. U. L. Rev.* 42: 843.
4 *Thompson vs. Keohane*, 116 S. Ct. 457, (1995).
5 *Howes vs. Fields*, 132 S. Ct. 1181, (2012).
6 *United States vs. Kim*, 292 F.3d 969, (2002).
7 *Corley vs. United States* 556 U.S. 303, (2009).
8 United States Code Annotated, title 18, Pt II, chapter 223, s 3501(b) 1968 (USA).
9 *United States vs. Jumper*, 497 F.3d 699, (2007).
10 *Davis vs. United States*, 512 U.S. 452, at 459, (1994).

11 *Wood vs. Ercole*, 644 F.3d 83, (2011).

12 *Abela vs. Martin*, 380 F.3d 915, (2004).

13 Bailenson, J.N. and Yee, N. (2005). Digital chameleons: automatic assimilation of nonverbal gestures in immersive virtual environments. *Psychol. Sci.* 16 (10): 814–819.

14 FBI (2016). Interrogation: a view of the science HIG report. https://www.fbi.gov/file-repository/hig-report-interrogation-a-review-of-the-science-september-2016.pdf/view (accessed 26 May 2021).

15 Collins, R., Lincoln, R., and Frank, M. (2005). The need for rapport in police interviews. https://www.researchgate.net/publication/27826896_The_Need_for_Rapport_in_Police_Interviews (accessed 6 August 2021).

16 Biss, M. (2014). Philosophy Documentation Center. Empathy and interrogation. *Int. J. Appl. Philos.* 28 (2): 277–288.

17 Frank, M.G., Menasco, M.A., and O'Sullivan, M. (2008). Human behavior and deception detection. In: *Wiley Handbook of Science and Technology for Homeland Security* (ed. J.G. Voeller). Hoboken, NJ: Wiley http://dx.doi.org/10.1002/9780470087923.hhs299.

18 Matsumoto, D., Skinner, L., and Hwang, H. (2014). Reading people: behavioral anomalies and investigative interviewing. https://leb.fbi.gov/articles/featured-articles/reading-people-behavioral-anomalies-and-investigative-interviewing (accessed 6 August 2021).

6

The Veterinarian's Role in Animal Cruelty Investigations

Kris Otteman

6.1 The Veterinarian is an Important Partner in Animal Cruelty Investigations

A veterinarian's participation in an animal cruelty investigation is important. The veterinarian is positioned to report on and testify to the overall health and welfare of the animal(s) and has the training, experience, and credibility required to speak to the pain and suffering an animal experienced, and uncover evidence to help determine how an animal died or was injured, or whether sufficient care was given to protect the health of an individual or group of animals.

Veterinary expertise is often required to help answer legal questions as to whether an animal victim's injuries were reckless, intentional, or knowingly committed. Investigations benefit from the participation of a veterinarian who can and will provide information that others involved cannot be expected to contribute.

Veterinary forensics is the use of veterinary medical and animal knowledge to identify, collect, and assess information vital in determining whether a crime involving an animal was committed; in some cases, how, when, and by whom. Veterinarians evaluate evidence in all aspects of animal health and husbandry. Questions about appropriate housing, sanitation, life stage care, and access to veterinary care provide the base of information necessary for law enforcement to investigate a potential crime. Veterinarians crack the code on many complex issues such as time, manner, and cause of death or injury, and can provide information that will be used to rule in or out a criminal act.

Entities that call on the veterinary profession to provide assistance may include law enforcement, prosecutors, agricultural experts, animal care experts, animal control agencies, humane societies, and so on. Services that veterinarians provide in animal cruelty investigations include: assisting in the investigation itself by aiding in identifying important questions and observations for the investigator to consider; assistance at an animal crime scene or in processing evidence including live or deceased animals from a crime scene; communicating results of findings, which may include email and reports; witness or expert testimony; and planning and oversight of medical and behavioral care for animals involved in an investigation or otherwise in care in poor condition or injured as a result of animal cruelty (Figure 6.1).

Animal Cruelty Investigations: A Collaborative Approach from Victim to Verdict^{TM}, First Edition.
Edited by Kris Otteman, Linda Fielder, and Emily Lewis.
© 2022 John Wiley & Sons, Inc. Published 2022 by John Wiley & Sons, Inc.
Companion website: www.wiley.com/go/otteman/victimtoverdict

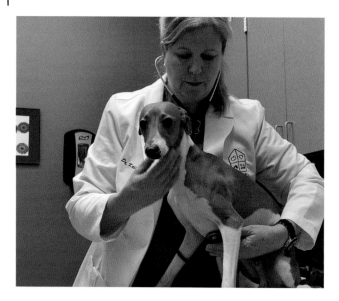

Figure 6.1 The veterinarian's role includes evaluation of the behavioral and medical status of each animal. *Source:* Oregon Humane Society.

Veterinary forensics digs deep into potential mysteries around animal injury or death and draws conclusions about potential criminal acts, while mirroring the normal process veterinarians use in clinical practice. The veterinarian gathers subjective and objective information, makes an assessment, and delivers a plan for next steps (subjective, objective, assessment, and plan [SOAP]). This information ultimately results in a final opinion and report that is provided to the agency leading the investigation or in some cases directly to a prosecutor or defense attorney.

The need for veterinary forensics is substantial and the lack of access by law enforcement to draw on this expertise is often a limiting step in addressing animal cruelty investigations. When veterinary resources are not available, communities suffer significant risk of negative consequences to people and animals. Veterinarians in every type of practice have relevant knowledge and talent needed in this field. By engaging in forensics and developing an understanding of how to contribute they become an asset to the process.

Remember, while the veterinarian is vital to the fight against animal cruelty, they are not alone in protecting the welfare of animals. Every state has criminal laws that require a minimum standard of care and law enforcement, and prosecutors are charged with upholding and enforcing these laws. Therefore, interdisciplinary cooperation between the veterinarian, law enforcement, and prosecutor is crucial.

Combining veterinary expertise with a review of the applicable laws in cruelty case investigations often reveals the cause and effect of human actions or lack of actions toward animals. When an animal is found to be unhealthy or to have died of a disease or injury, the veterinarian's findings and the legal requirements for care provide guidance as to whether the circumstances that contributed to the animal's illness, injury, or demise meet the standard for criminal prosecution. For example, in the case of an emaciated dog suffering from cancer and receiving appropriate medical care, there is no maltreatment under the law, while in the case of an emaciated dog chained to a tree in the backyard, forgotten and without provision for adequate nutrition, there is maltreatment, and the action is criminal by violation of the law's requirement to provide minimum care. The veterinarian's role in solving the case is to examine the evidence and determine the cause of the animal's condition.

In addition to providing services as part of an investigation the veterinarian or veterinary staff may be the first to receive a report of or to recognize animal cruelty. Many states have laws that require veterinarians to report suspected animal cruelty and, in some states, veterinarians are immune from criminal and civil action for reporting a concern, if acting in good faith. When confronted with potential animal abuse or neglect a veterinarian must consider the ethical, legal, and obligatory aspects of reporting suspected cruelty and take appropriate action.

6.2 The Veterinarian's Oath

Upon graduation with a doctorate in veterinary medicine the new graduate swears an oath of dedication to the profession. This oath was first authored in 1965 and was modified in 2010 to include the words "welfare" and "prevention . . . of suffering" [1]. This small change has far-reaching meaning for the profession. Not only are veterinarians responsible for expertise in animal and public health, but they are also obligated to protect the welfare and prevent the suffering of animals (Box 6.1).

Box 6.1   Veterinarian's Oath

Being admitted to the profession of veterinary medicine, I solemnly swear to use my scientific knowledge and skills for the benefit of society through the protection of animal health and *welfare*, the *prevention* and relief of animal *suffering*, the conservation of animal resources, the promotion of public health, and the advancement of medical knowledge.

I will practice my profession conscientiously, with dignity, and in keeping with the principles of veterinary medical ethics.

I accept as a lifelong obligation the continual improvement of my professional knowledge and competence.

The oath underscores the duty of the profession to aid in responding to animal cruelty. It is the veterinarian's responsibility to report cruelty when suspected, and to intervene before the potential for neglect in a client's animals becomes criminal. Animal welfare is the proper treatment of animals. According to the American Veterinary Medicine Association: "Ensuring animal welfare is a human responsibility that includes consideration for all aspects of animal well-being, including proper housing, management, nutrition, disease prevention and treatment, responsible care, humane handling and when necessary, humane euthanasia" [2]. In each instance of examining an animal, a crime scene, or other evidence, the guidance provided to the veterinarian by the veterinarian's oath and the relevant law provide clarity to direct the actions of the veterinarian.

6.3 How Veterinary Forensics Differs from Traditional Veterinary Medicine

Owing to the advancement and increasing specialization of veterinary medicine and the recent expansion of the crucial role veterinarians play in the fight against animal cruelty, the field of veterinary forensics has emerged. This specialized area within the profession is gaining

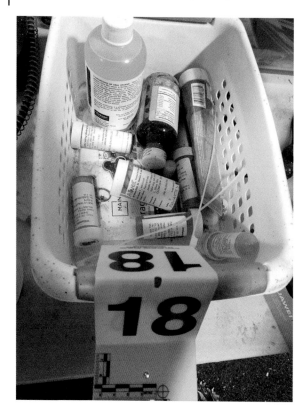

Figure 6.2 The forensic veterinarian's role includes examining physical evidence and reporting on its significance. *Source:* Oregon Humane Society.

tremendous recognition, while establishing knowledge and practices that benefit humans and animals in communities around the world.

Forensics is defined as gathering evidence to evaluate whether a crime has occurred [3]. The veterinary exam, which is well defined by academic training and practice, becomes a forensic exam when the information gathered is used in this manner. Thus, any veterinary exam could be used as evidence in a legal matter. Medical records and opinions of veterinarians are scrutinized by colleagues, clients, and others as a matter of normal business. The significant difference in a forensic exam is that the information included may involve additional detail and organization of information such as housing, behavioral observations, extensive medical history, and husbandry. Ancillary reports, photos, physical evidence, witness statements, investigators notes, and other items not traditionally reviewed in clinical practice may also become part of the forensic examination report (Figure 6.2). The field of veterinary forensics also varies from other specialties in that it is not commonly a full-time focus in everyday veterinary practice, but rather a skill that all practitioners may need to draw on as part of their clinical and community duties when the need arises or when they are called upon.

6.4 Veterinary Confidentiality and Medical Records Requests

Maintaining confidentiality protects privacy of individuals and respects legal boundaries. Details about individuals or ongoing investigations are not to be shared by professionals unless permission is given, or it is necessary to further the investigation. Failure to understand and respect these boundaries may have an adverse effect on the outcome of an investigation and the legal process involving a case. During animal cruelty investigations, questions about the boundaries of confidentiality and what information may be shared, with whom, must be answered correctly.

In the practice of veterinary forensics, there are several aspects of confidentiality to consider. During an ongoing investigation, the information gathered inclusive of all statements, reports, photos, videos, or other evidence is to be protected and only shared with individuals who are working directly with you on a case. This includes scribes, technicians, laboratory staff, photographers, and even shelter or rescue operations staff. When authoring reports and engaging with others who assist you, make note of these individuals' contributions and involvement by documenting this in the report.

When caring for live evidence in Protective Custody or stored evidence, maintain strict chain of custody practices with the appropriate record of individual involvement. Be proactive and inform others who are assisting you that investigations are confidential. Be clear about the boundaries of discussing the findings, posting on social media, or talking with uninvolved staff or other parties.

Clear direction regarding communication helps to maintain confidentiality and reduce the potential for dissemination of inaccurate information. Record th details of who was involved in communications and what directions they were given in your notes for the case.

In the event medical records from another agency or veterinary practice are needed, use a standard format for requesting records, and include these records in their original format with the final report, preferably as an attachment. Individual states have laws pertaining to veterinary record confidentiality. Record requests may be made without client permission, depending upon the state [4]. The licensing board in each state or country is a good resource for current laws or rules regarding records requests.

6.5 Public Information Considerations

Animal cruelty investigations are of high interest to the public and the media. Veterinarians serving on a case must avoid talking with the media, until the case is adjudicated. If sharing information with the public is necessary, use a secondary resource, such as someone from the public relations department or from practice management to talk with the media. These individuals must have basic media communications skills and understand the boundaries regarding what can be discussed when an investigation and case is ongoing. Law enforcement and prosecutors are an excellent resource if you are not sure what the boundaries are in terms of discussing a case and need help determining who should talk to the media and what, if any, information may be released. In some cases, talking with the media about the status of a case or alerting the public about needing leads and a reward may be helpful. Know how and when to provide this information to the media ahead of time so a mistake is not made under pressure and in the middle of an active news story. See Chapter 14 for additional information about media relations.

The veterinarian may provide information for release that is approved by the law enforcement representative for the case such as breed, age, medical findings, or details about how the animal was found. This information may be used for the reward via a public information officer or other party (Box 6.2). By checking with law enforcement before providing information, the risk of jeopardizing the case by releasing confidential or investigatory information is eliminated.

In most cases, it is impossible for a veterinarian to remain completely anonymous when reporting or assisting with an investigation. While these situations may be emotionally charged and challenging, advocacy for the animal(s) involved, consideration of other aspects of human involvement such as child welfare or elder abuse, and the veterinarian's obligation to confront the findings fairly and accurately based on their knowledge are required.

Box 6.2   Case Example

Case example:

News release to media:

$2000.00 reward offered for information leading to arrest of persons responsible for an animal abandoned in Washington Park Forest. A two-year-old terrier cross was found abandoned in a crate in a public area on Saturday. If you have information about this case, please contact Sheriff Jones at 503-555-1122.

The forensic examination of evidence provides the essential insight with which law enforcement and the criminal justice system will act but is not the decider of the suspect's guilt or innocence. Inform colleagues and clients about the veterinarian's obligation to recognize, report, and assist with the fight against animal cruelty, and that the veterinarian is not judge and jury in these cases, but rather called upon for expertise. Generally, the public expects veterinarians to be animal advocates and sees veterinarians as reputable and trustworthy. Failure to act casts a shadow on the reputation of a clinician, while acting on behalf of an animal is the expectation of the public. Do not allow fears about client confidentiality or retaliation prevent you as a veterinarian from acting, when necessary, in an animal cruelty case. Consult with law enforcement or the prosecutor if you have specific concerns regarding anonymity, safety, or public information.

6.6   Conflicts of Interest

A conflict of interest may occur when there is a competing professional or personal interest making it difficult for an individual to follow through with their duties in an impartial manner. A conflict of interest becomes an issue if the appearance or evidence of bias arises and can be used to discredit a veterinarian in court. The most common scenario in which concern about a potential conflict of interest may surface is with the veterinarian–client or veterinarian–employee relationship.

In community practice, veterinarians are paid by clients to diagnose and treat their animals. In the event a veterinarian suspects a client of potential animal neglect or abuse, the doctor may question themselves as to whether objective and impartial opinions regarding the situation are possible. An individual's loyalty is to the truth and the law first. The oath sworn upon graduation to protect animal health and welfare also lights the path forward in circumstances that may seem unclear. Remember that in many states and countries reporting animal cruelty is required and affords financial and legal protection for the doctor involved. Many times, the veterinarian is the sole advocate for the animal that has suffered maltreatment and, much like the teacher or the doctor, in the case of children, is the professional with the knowledge and obligation to detect and report abuse. Act on your concerns and move forward with reporting and investigating appropriate suspicions whenever necessary. When the investigation is completed, if bias is a concern other veterinarians may be asked to review evidence in the case to ensure elimination of this concern. Avoid being offended by this situation, but rather view this as the appropriate safety net and second opinion that will lead to a fair and legal outcome in each case. This obligation goes both ways: you could be called upon to be the reviewer in some cases as well.

Situations in which a veterinarian must consider recusing themselves from involvement may include those in which the doctor has an ownership interest in the animal(s) being investigated or is the subject of the investigation. Employee–employer relationships may also have an impact on an investigation. If the employment relationship makes it difficult to ensure impartiality and thorough analysis of the situation, the veterinarian should not be involved in this type of case. This may occur when an employee of a veterinarian is a suspect or somehow involved in a cruelty investigation. Details with consideration for privacy requirements about these relationships, such as the employee's status (hired, fired, in good standing, and so on), must be provided to the investigator, who is often a good resource in identifying potential conflicts of interest.

A suspect in an animal cruelty case may very well be a current or past client of the veterinarian assisting in an investigation or reporting potential cruelty. Again, provide details about these relationships to the investigator. Client information about services provided and financial transactions are all relevant. This includes work previously completed and paid for or failure to pay for services. Any other issues that have arisen with the professional relationship must be fully disclosed. Previous records of providing services or a client's failure to pay do not necessarily conclude that a veterinarian cannot provide an expert opinion without bias. Exchange of money for veterinary services and failure to pay are all considered to be part of the routine business of veterinary medicine, and a credible veterinarian would be expected to hold financial dealings separate from their opinions on the animal's health and welfare. Always disclose this information to investigators to ensure full transparency.

The possibility of a conflict of interest is considered on a case-by-case basis and may occur even when nothing improper, illegal, or unethical has occurred. Assuming the veterinarian can maintain objectivity and fairness, the next question is will others believe the veterinarian's opinions to be true? Unless a clear conflict is uncovered by an investigator, the answer to this question is yes. Transparency to the investigating agency is crucial in all cases. Be certain to explain relationships, prior or current business dealings, or any other information that may be relevant to the investigation.

6.7 Be Familiar with the Laws

Law enforcement and prosecutors depend on veterinary expertise when determining if there has been a violation of law. Familiarize yourself with the laws in your state so you are aware which are relevant, and what specific requirements reside within each law. An officer may be investigating a "skinny horse" due to neighborhood complaints that she appears to be malnourished, only to find out from an involved veterinarian that the horse is geriatric and under care for a chronic condition resulting in adequate care but diminished condition. A police officer may not know the appropriate body appearance of dairy versus beef breeds of cattle and so on. A veterinarian answers these questions based on an understanding of the laws' requirements for care.

State statutes differ in the language used to describe animals, standards of care, abuse and neglect, and how specific categories, such as livestock or exotic animals, are defined. The knowledge and experience of the veterinarian guides law enforcement in determining whether a violation of a statute has occurred.

6.8 How to Find and Build Knowledge in the Area of Animal Law

Technology provides easy access to relevant governmental laws and regulations that every veterinarian must know. Staying current only requires time and access to technology or a printout of the latest information. The laws of your state or country that are relevant to animals are published on a regular basis and are worthy of a detailed study. Consider reviewing these annually and keeping a tabbed paper copy handy as a reference when you are working on a case and writing reports. Reach out to other experts in your area to learn more about the laws and how they are applied to animal cases. These experts include prosecutors, defense attorneys, animal control officers, veterinarians, and law enforcement professionals. Sources for finding the latest accurate information include state practice acts and veterinary medical associations. Federal laws can be found on American Veterinary Medical Association or government websites. The Animal Legal Defense Fund (ALDF) maintains an organized database of current animal protection laws [5].

6.9 Understand What the Prosecutor and Law Enforcement Need to Know

6.9.1 Animal Neglect

Neglect laws specifically call out the basics of animal care, including food, shelter, water, and access to veterinary care, and are species specific in some areas (Figure 6.3). The veterinarian evaluates the evidence, including animals in some cases, and assists in determining whether or not failure to meet the legal standards for care has resulted in neglect. For example, 40 cats living in a hoarding situation may have access to plentiful food and water but are so severely flea-infested they are dying of anemia (blood loss). In this case the animal owner met the standard of care for food and water, however, did not meet the standard for sanitation or veterinary care, and as an outcome of this failure the cats suffered or died.

6.9.2 Animal Abuse

Laws may include language that describes an individual's mental state, such as "intentionally," "recklessly," or "knowingly" with regard to causing harm to an animal (Figure 6.4). The veterinarian's examination of evidence and knowledge can help the investigator determine whether the injury to the animal was intentional or accidental. Veterinarians understand the force required to break a dog's femur, for example, and can provide an opinion as to how the injury occurred. Degree

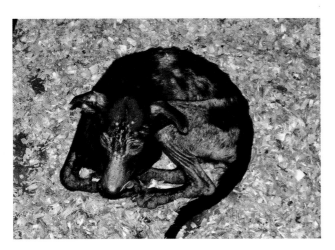

Figure 6.3 Evaluating overall animal husbandry and access to veterinary care is a key responsibility of the veterinarian in matters of potential animal neglect. *Source:* Oregon Humane Society.

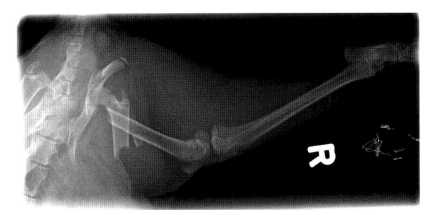

Figure 6.4 Veterinarians assist in ruling in or out the reported causes of injury or illness by answering the question as to whether or not the "story" aligns with the findings. *Source:* Oregon Humane Society.

of injury and the animal's ability to recover are also part of the veterinarian's assessment. In a case of aggravated animal abuse, the charge may stand if the animal is killed or permanently injured but be a lesser charge if the animal can fully recover from the incident.

6.10 How Animal Cruelty Investigations Surface and Become Active Cases

Investigation of animal cruelty or neglect cases begins with a report from one or several sources. Private citizens are the eyes and ears of our communities and the most common reporters of suspected animal crimes. Local agencies responsible for investigating or referring these cases compile the information and determine what complaints to act upon. Most complaints are collected via phone or website reporting mechanisms. Private community practice and specialty practice veterinarians are also on the front line in recognizing and reporting animal neglect or abuse. Veterinary professionals, including doctors and staff, are more fluent in recognition and reporting of animal cruelty in recent years and may initiate a report that leads to an investigation. Other sources include humane agencies, animal control organizations, agriculture affiliates, social workers, and other in-home vendors such as meter readers and repair personnel who may notice and report an animal at risk or suspicious activities.

Some agencies are dedicated to the investigation of animal crimes and others are a specialized department within an organization. All government law enforcement agencies, whether local, state, or federal, are sworn to uphold all laws including those relating to animal theft, abuse, and other protections. Animal control agencies are on the front line in cities and counties to enforce animal cruelty laws in some jurisdictions and to educate on animal ordinances such as barking or managing stray dogs, cats, or other animals. Animal control agencies may be called upon to evaluate and lead or partner on investigating and responding to potential criminal animal crimes.

A wide range of concerns are reported for investigations, some of which fall into the category of an enforceable law, while others do not. For example, keeping a dog on a tether in a yard without shelter may not be against a code or law in some areas and is a violation of the law in other geographic areas. Common concerns include sanitation, husbandry, shelter, starvation, hoarding, abuse, lack of socialization, and organized fighting. These reports are typically evaluated and triaged by the organization to which they are reported. Agencies prioritize response based on legal requirements and resources available. Being accessible and willing to help is one of the most important attributes the veterinarian brings to the fight against animal cruelty.

References

1 American Veterinary Medical Association (n.d.). Veterinarian's oath. https://www.avma.org/resources-tools/avma-policies/veterinarians-oath (accessed 6 August 2021).

2 American Veterinary Medical Association. (n.d.). Animal welfare: a humane responsibility. https://www.avma.org/resources/pet-owners/animalwelfare (accessed 30 May 2021).

3 Merriam-Webster (n.d.). Medical definition of Forensics. https://www.merriam-webster.com/medical/forensics (accessed 27 May 2021).

4 AVMA (n.d.). Confidentiality of veterinary patient records. https://www.avma.org/advocacy/state-local-issues/confidentiality-veterinary-patient-records (accessed 27 May 2021).

5 Animal Legal Defense Fund (2020). 2020 U.S. state animal protection laws rankings. https://aldf.org/project/us-state-rankings (accessed 30 May 2021).

7

The Veterinary Exam and Treatment Plan

Kris Otteman and Zarah Hedge

The practice of veterinary medicine in the United States and around the world is evolving quickly, as technology and specialization influence the way services to animals and their owners are delivered. The spectrum of veterinary medicine is tremendous, and the variety of disciplines that have emerged has transformed the knowledge and types of intervention made on behalf of most living species on the planet. From beekeeping and the health of honeybees and pollinators to marine mammal rehabilitation, animal production, preservation of endangered species, surgery, chemotherapy, and wellness care, the skills, knowledge, and wisdom expected of and delivered by the veterinary profession has never been so broad or so impactful. With this diversity in specialization, and realization of the advantage of the expertise provided by veterinary medicine in the fight against animal cruelty, veterinary forensics has emerged as a new field and is gaining tremendous ground, while establishing knowledge and practices that benefit humans and animals locally, nationally, and globally. The utilization of veterinary expertise to evaluate evidence to rule in or rule out a crime is now considered a vital part of any animal cruelty investigation.

The veterinarian's traditional training and experience provide the foundation of knowledge and expertise necessary to evaluate circumstances regarding the physical health, emotional well-being, husbandry, and other aspects related to animals and their condition. Specialized training and resources are becoming available in the field of veterinary forensics and should be used to build upon the foundation all veterinarians possess as an outcome of their academic training and practical experience. Textbooks, published articles, lectures, and online training on topics related to the veterinarian's role in animal cruelty investigations are available to bolster any veterinarian's knowledge.

Examination and analysis of animals, both live and deceased, as well as material related to their care, health, and environmental circumstances are essential parts of almost every animal cruelty investigation. When approaching the exam and analysis of animals and related materials – feed, housing, medical records – the veterinarian must prepare by studying the laws and codes pertaining to the care of animals in the area in which they are working and utilize a standard and systematic approach to the evaluation and documentation of findings. Having been trained to examine and assess findings in a standard subjective, objective, assessment, and plan (SOAP) format prepares the veterinarian to transfer clinical training and skills directly to the assessment of animals for forensic evidence. It is not the veterinarian's duty to be judge and jury, but rather to provide accurate, high-quality, and comprehensive information that becomes part of the overall investigative process and adjudication of a criminal case.

Animal Cruelty Investigations: A Collaborative Approach from Victim to Verdict[TM], First Edition.
Edited by Kris Otteman, Linda Fielder, and Emily Lewis.
© 2022 John Wiley & Sons, Inc. Published 2022 by John Wiley & Sons, Inc.
Companion website: www.wiley.com/go/otteman/victimtoverdict

The veterinarian's role in evaluation of animals and related evidence in a cruelty case is an essential piece of the puzzle in the fight against animal cruelty. The impact and far-reaching consequences to society as a result of cruelty to animals are well known. In their oath of service, veterinarians swear that they will strive to meet the obligation to participate in this important work by contributing to the health and welfare of animals.

7.1 Request and Review Evidentiary Material

Live animals or remains of animals may be presented for forensic evaluation, and veterinarians may be asked to review all types of evidentiary material including medical records, photographs, videotape, email, food, medications, habitat, and so on. A request to review and comment on photos, reports, or medical records without an animal is sometimes requested as a part of an investigation and aids those assigned in determining next steps or evaluating whether a crime may have occurred.

When a law enforcement agency or other industry partner requests an exam and assessment of any type of evidence, it is prudent to ask for any related documentation such as: police records, photos, witness statements, and other materials related to the case. This information becomes part of the data the veterinarian works with to form an opinion or conclusion. Ask the person requesting the evaluation what the expectation is for format, for providing your opinion, and the timeline within which you are working. In many cases a summary email of your findings is adequate when evaluating photos (Figure 7.1) or other physical evidence; in other cases a more formal report may be required. It is appropriate for the veterinarian to request all available previous medical information and review it prior to the exam. Include previous veterinary records, laboratory results, and radiographs in your overall evaluation of each situation when possible.

Create a timeline that summarizes key events prior to starting an exam, participating in processing a crime scene, or evaluating any type of evidence. This foundational information serves as documentation and a reference to create reports. In some cases, law enforcement or prosecutors have collected information that is relevant, such as other medical records. In other cases, the veterinarian will need their assistance and instruction as to what information is helpful. It is the investigator's responsibility to request and gather the information for the veterinarian to review.

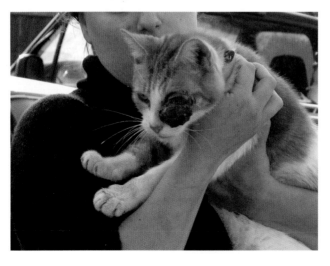

Figure 7.1 Evaluating photos of animals and their environment is an essential part of the veterinarian's role in animal cruelty investigations. *Source:* Oregon Humane Society.

Gathering medical history is important in all cases, but the police officer or investigator may not know this. Inform this individual of the importance of medical history, if available, and how to get this information so that they can proceed with this task.

7.2 Initial Steps

The veterinarian is the expert in evaluating physical health, medical history, husbandry, and behavioral characteristics of the animal. It is the veterinarian's responsibility to provide expertise in evaluating the environment in which the animal has been living, and in assessing the injuries to an animal, including how and when they occurred. Combining all this information into a meaningful and accurate conclusion establishes the veterinary forensic exam, which may then be a part of the evidence presented to the court in a criminal case of abuse or neglect (Figure 7.2).

If the veterinarian's findings and opinions are used at trial, they may be provided in written form or in live testimony depending upon the circumstances and the request of the investigator or prosecutor. This may occur months to years after the time of the initial evaluation. An excellent process for documenting and collecting details provides assurance that, when called upon, the veterinarian will have the information available and accurately recorded, in such a manner that the report is essentially timeless.

7.2.1 Relevant History

7.2.1.1 History of Ownership of the Animal and Animal Identification

It is important to establish who has owned the animal(s) involved, for how long, any ownership transitions that have occurred, and to document carefully any identifying features of the animal. If possible, identify and consider anyone else who is responsible for the daily care and husbandry of the animal, as it may become relevant in ruling in or out nonaccidental injury and neglect, and identifying the party responsible. Questions about ownership origin and history may include how many people own

Figure 7.2 Thorough and well-documented examination of all evidence is the foundation for establishing an opinion regarding potential abuse or neglect. *Source:* Oregon Humane Society.

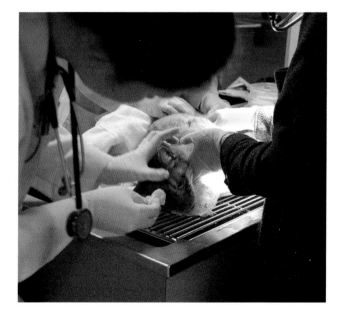

the animal, is the animal under the care of an agent or other responsible party, is there a boarding agreement involved, how was the animal obtained and when and by whom, and so on.

Document in writing and with photography any collars, harnesses, halters, or other items found on the animal or with the animal, including fit (loose, tight), type and material, tags, microchip, and tattoos. Include kennels, containers, and other related items. Then crosscheck findings with available ownership records. Photograph and measure identification and all items found with the animal (Figures 7.3 and 7.4).

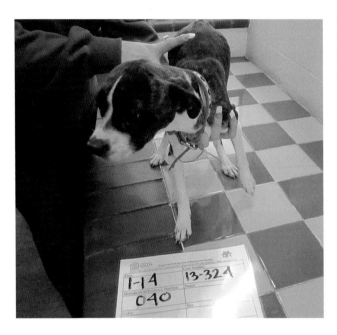

Figure 7.3 Take multiple views of significant findings. In this case the dog's body condition and loose collar is seen in this photo. *Source:* Oregon Humane Society.

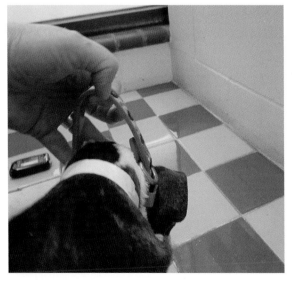

Figure 7.4 This photo clearly depicts how loose the dog's collar has become with weight loss. *Source:* Oregon Humane Society.

7.2.1.2 Medical History and Care Provided

Gather and review all available medical history and include a short summary of this information in your report. Create a timeline of medical history and events that illustrate the key findings. Attach or retain previous medical records that are referenced in your report. Document your medical and behavioral findings in the usual SOAP or other electronic medical records format that you are accustomed to and include a standard animal cruelty investigations form used for note taking during initial live or deceased animal exams. Once the exam is complete, use all this information to generate your final report that you will submit to authorities. This report must include exam findings, husbandry evaluation, timeline, conclusions, and relevant information you have gathered in these initial steps. This same document will be your reference for supplemental reports and in testimony at grand jury, trial, or before a judge. Further discussion of the recommended sections of a final report are covered in Chapter 12. Additional details about documentation of specific areas of the exam and other evidence are to follow.

7.2.2 Overview of the Physical Exam Process for Live Animals

Throughout the process of examination and evaluation of evidence keep in mind that the final goal is to conclude, if possible, how the findings relate to the laws in your state. As in all clinical duties carried out by a veterinarian, objectivity and integrity form the basis for the final assessment and documentation of findings and conclusions.

By creating a standard and systematic approach to the evaluation and documentation of findings in each animal cruelty case presented, the veterinarian provides a report that is objective, consistent, thorough, and high quality. Veterinarians are trained to examine and assess findings in a standard and consistent format. This methodology prepares the veterinarian to transfer clinical skills directly to the analysis of animals for forensic evidence.

A final opinion, even if inconclusive, is an essential part of a veterinary forensic report. It may be possible to rule in or out a gunshot for example, but in the same instance it may be impossible to determine the exact time or cause of death. Summarize and conclude what you know and explain what you cannot conclude and why.

7.2.2.1 Preparing for the Exam

Animal cruelty investigations are rarely scheduled events, but in most cases a few hours or minutes of preparation time are available. Checklists, forms, and necessary basic equipment kept in a specific area or in a kit that is mobile and easily accessible will eliminate last-minute prep that can be fraught with forgotten essential items.

Most everything needed to create a comprehensive exam kit is standard equipment in a veterinary hospital or inexpensive to acquire. Exam tools include a stethoscope, otoscope-ophthalmoscope, and thermometer. Supplies to have at the ready include sample collection supplies for blood, feces, and urine, and labels and packaging materials. Evidence collection supplies to have organized include paper envelopes, polyester swabs, permanent marker, and sample containers and tubs. Beyond the basic exam equipment, the essentials required are photographic equipment, an evidence placard, examination record or form, evidence log, and an appropriate scale. Verify the scale for accuracy and record the time and date of this inspection. If you are processing multiple animals, stop and check the scale on a regular basis to ensure accurate readings. Additional details about the use of photography and evidence collection are included in Chapter 10.

A checklist of basic equipment, forms, and items to include to prepare for live animal exams are included in Appendix B.

7.2.2.2 Important Guidance for Photographing Examination Findings

Include photographs of all significant findings as part of the documentation during the physical examination. Supplement still photos with video when appropriate. Each photo no matter how blurry, bad, or irrelevant must be submitted with the discovery to a prosecutor. Do not delete photos or alter original photos. Take as many as you need to illustrate thoroughly your findings without wasting time on unnecessary video or photos. Include the following views in photographs during the physical exam, as available and relevant. Always use an evidence placard to identify the animal and the case. Include the following photos for all cases:

- Far, mid-range, and close-up photos that demonstrate the overall appearance of an animal including identifying features (Figures 7.5–7.7).
- Capture five views (Figures 7.8 and 7.9) (front, back, each side, and from above) that clearly show the overall condition of the animal and demonstrate important aspects of the animal's presentation such as coat markings, sores, or other visible abnormalities.
- Photographs and video that demonstrate behavior, appetite, ability to eat, and other relevant findings.

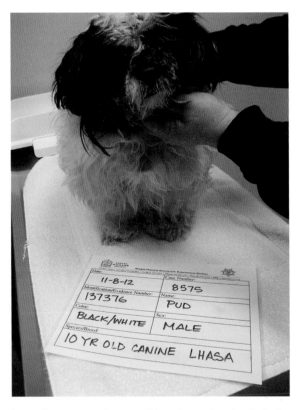

Figure 7.5 Far-range photos demonstrate the overall location and scale of a lesion on an animal body. *Source:* Oregon Humane Society.

Figure 7.6 Mid-range photos provide context and detail. *Source:* Oregon Humane Society.

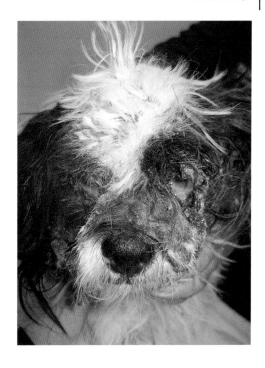

Figure 7.7 Close-up photos reveal details that are not visible in other views, such as margins of a wound, or presence of hair and debris. *Source:* Oregon Humane Society.

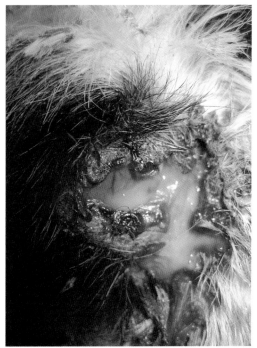

- Mid-range and close-up photos of lesions, injuries, or any abnormality with measurements when appropriate.
- Photographs that demonstrate relevant immediate changes such as grooming and matt removal, or wounds that are sutured or bandaged.

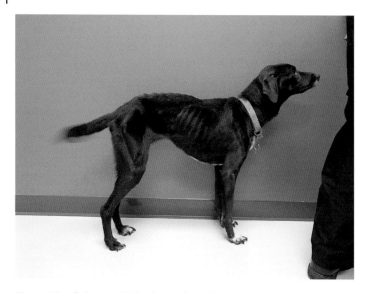

Figure 7.8 Collect multiple views when photographing animals. This photograph captures the dog's identifying features as well as her poor body condition score. *Source:* Oregon Humane Society.

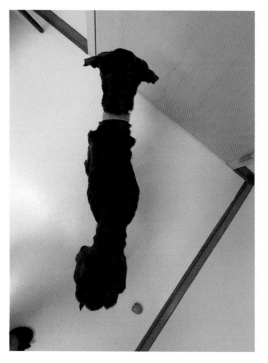

Figure 7.9 The aerial view of this dog clear demonstrates her emaciated condition. *Source:* Oregon Humane Society.

- Ancillary and related materials such as embedded or loose collar or halter, teeth that have been removed, or claws that were damaged or not trimmed.
- Medical supplies, medications, and food and supplements related to the animal being examined.

- Include normal and abnormal. If one eye is normal and the other damaged, document both with photography and explain the difference you are seeing.

In short, be thoughtful and concise with photography but do not spare photos at the expense of failing to illustrate a relevant finding.

7.2.2.3 The Physical Exam: Quality, Consistency, and Efficiency

The forensic exam of a live animal includes the systematic aspects of a traditional physical exam of an animal with several critical, noteworthy differences. In documenting the exam use available charts and diagrams to assist you in capturing the details you are finding. Include observations, conclusions, and make detailed notes of relevant findings. Document what is *found* and what is *not found*. For example, a penetrating wound is discovered with an entry and exit wound, but no evidence of the projectile is found during necropsy or on full body radiographs.

Use a standard exam process and form to input your findings (written or electronic), to ensure that details and steps of your exam will be thorough, and the probability of forgetting a simple step such as recording a temperature, or a microchip scan are less likely to occur. A checkbox system for input of findings that denotes normal or abnormal findings adds efficiency and provides a guide that will help the clinician complete accurate exams, even when many animals are involved (see Appendix B for an exam form).

Include exam assistance and a scribe when necessary and possible, especially in cases with multiple animals. Take into consideration the order and importance of a thorough examination. If anesthesia or sedation is required to complete portions of the exam, plan your approach such that all the aspects of the exam that will benefit from being done during this time are completed efficiently. Oral, ophthalmic (eye), otic (ear), and dental exam, for example, are easily completed during sedation or anesthesia for radiographs, as are blood and fecal sample collection.

7.3 Examination Key Elements

The information in the next few sections was drawn from [1].

7.3.1 Section A: Documentation, Identification, Examination

7.3.1.1 Animal Identification

Clearly identify the animal using a written description that is thorough, including age, sex, breed, weight, and color. Document any identifying details such as tattoos, ear tips, tags, or microchip numbers. Unique identifiers assigned to each animal should include a patient number generated by software or manually assigned, and a case number provided by the agency in charge of the case, and a unique evidence identifier. See Chapter 9 and 10 for further information about unique evidence identifiers.

Example:

- Adult canine, intact female, light brown, smooth coated, terrier mix with no other markings.
- Scanned with microchip scanner and AVID chip 1234567890 found on dorsum of neck between shoulder blades. Photograph taken of number displayed on the scanner.
- Patient ID: 12345678 Case Number: 2244. Animal known as Sparkie and listed on the animal inventory as "S.".

7.3.1.2 Begin Photographic Documentation and Continue Throughout Process

Document and photograph the animal prior to starting your exam and continue this documentation as necessary throughout the examination. Include video documentation when needed to illustrate key aspects of the animal's condition.

Examples:

- An emaciated animal's willingness to eat and drink when the opportunity is provided.
- Abnormal gait or inability to stand on overgrown feet.
- Lack of grooming and sanitation with mats that impede ability to walk, see, eat, or hear.

7.3.1.3 Physical Exam Findings

Document the following details on individual records and in the final record for each animal's initial exam:

- Weight in kilograms or pounds or estimated weight (i.e. livestock)
- Temperature
- Pulse
- Respiration (rate, quality, effort, sounds)
- Capillary refill time and mucous membrane color
- Hydration level based on clinical assessment
- Otic and ophthalmic exam notes
- Findings by system including:
  - Integumentary
  - Cardiovascular
  - Respiratory
  - Musculoskeletal
  - Gastrointestinal
  - Urogenital
  - Neurological

Document each system as normal or abnormal and, if abnormal, include an explanation for this finding. When writing the initial report and including physical exam findings, explain the normal range and species differences. For example, if this is an equine and canine mixed case and the normal heart rate range for horses is 36–40, and for dogs is 80–140, include this information and an explanation as to the species and size difference, so that these basic data are not left open to interpretation.

In cases with multiple animals, consider summarizing the animal identification and key elements of the physical exam findings. This provides an efficient way to communicate overall findings and create a snapshot of specific relevant case findings.

For example, entering body condition score (BCS) for all animals involved in a large case into a summary or a spreadsheet and then calculating an average illustrates the overall condition or demonstrates how some animals' body condition was adequate while others' were not.

7.3.1.4 Radiographic Examination

Radiographs provide useful baseline information in most cases, and it is surprising what may be unexpectedly discovered as a result of a good series of radiographs. In some cases, such as gunshot wounds or fractures, additional specific radiographic studies may be helpful.

Take whole-body diagnostic images whenever possible for any case of suspected nonaccidental injury or repeated trauma cases in small animals. These cases benefit from whole-body views, which may reveal unsuspected findings that are relevant. Multiple broken ribs or healed fractures of ribs (Figure 7.10) or long bones that cannot be detected on a physical exam will surface on radiographs and allow for an estimation of age of injury.

Accurate and complete labeling of each radiograph is essential and includes the animal's unique identifier and clinic name. In some situations, imaging is not available and, if this is the case, make notes regarding the circumstances.

7.3.1.5 Body Condition Score

When completing the physical exam it is essential to assign a BCS using a published system (Purina or Tufts) and include this in the documentation for each animal [2–6]. Include the definition of the score established and, if possible, include pictures that demonstrate the score you have assigned. Whenever possible, the BCS determination should include a "hands-on" assessment (Figure 7.11) of each animal. Explain the relevance of this finding as it relates to the overall condition of the animal.

7.3.1.6 Injuries

Evaluate the entire animal for acute or chronic injuries and scars, and document these using standard language, descriptions, and templates that show the outline of ventral, dorsal, and side-view aspects of the animal when needed. Measure injuries, including size, circumference, and depth, and describe color and appearance. Estimate time of injury and document any drainage or bleeding. Use drawings and photos to further illustrate your findings. In documenting scars, use the same principles of templates, drawings, and photos. Scars that indicate previous injury may be cause for follow-up radiographs of the area in which the scar is found. As an example, in the

Figure 7.10 Radiographs reveal unsuspected findings that are relevant, such as evidence of both fresh and healed rib fractures in this cat who presented with a rear leg fracture. *Source:* Oregon Humane Society.

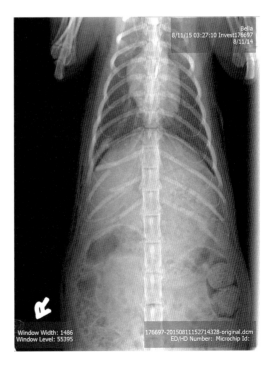

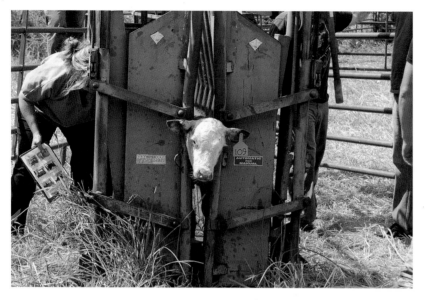

Figure 7.11 Hands-on body condition scoring is a valuable tool for most species. *Source:* Oregon Humane Society.

instance of dogfighting injuries with scarring to head and forelimbs, damage to facial bones and the long bones of the forelimbs may be visible radiographically.

7.3.1.7 Use Sight and Smell

Use sight and smell to further describe exam findings. Urine-saturated matted fur and scalding of skin, staining of hair, pressure marks or sores from confinement, chronic infection from embedded collars, and other findings all require description that includes the smell and sight and how these are linked to the animal's suffering and harm. Document and collect samples if foreign substances are detected by odor, sight, or otherwise. This may include accelerants, pollutants, or other debris, such as plant material, or projectiles, such as an arrow or pellets. To collect and preserve samples, cut hair with scissors and store in a labeled paper envelope. Any samples that are damp or organic must be stored in paper or cardboard containers that are not airtight so they do not become moldy thereby changing the viability of the sample as evidence (see Chapter 10 for further information about evidence packaging).

7.3.1.8 Coat Condition and External Parasites

Breed- and life stage-specific information about the appearance, odor, and care of the animal's fur or feathers, and relevance of these findings is important. Otherwise healthy kittens that are flea infested may be suffering from life-threatening anemia. Lack of grooming by owners and the dogs themselves may result in loss of vision, chronic skin and ear infections, and even severe injury caused by entanglement of extremities in matts that leads to strangulation, vascular necrosis, or loss of toes or limbs. Poor husbandry, including inappropriate temperature and humidity can lead to dysecdysis (improper shedding) in reptile species, which can also cause strangulation, vascular necrosis and loss of digits or limbs. Describe and photograph coat condition and the type and quantity of parasites seen including location, ratio of live or dead, and the significance of these findings. Consider scanning the entire body with an alternative light source in cases in which you may find bodily fluids or disease that will be highlighted with this technique.

7.3.1.9 Feet, Claws, Paws, Hooves

Examine, document, and swab the extremities of the animal as needed, making note of normal and abnormal findings. Include photos of overgrown claws or hooves, and infections or other findings. Poor hoof care of an equine becomes a life-threatening emergency when it causes the cannon bone to rotate and sometimes protrude through the bottom of the foot. Overgrown claws in dogs and cats may be evidence of overall neglect, or in some cases simply a missed trimming that can be easily taken care of and is not a criminal violation. Torn and shredded toenails in dogs or cats (Figure 7.12) may result from vehicular trauma and being dragged. Cat nails may shred because of the animal hanging on while being pulled along the carpet or other fabric or from being thrown and using claws to "hang on." Typically, shredded nails because of vehicular trauma will be broken and contain dirt or other road-related materials. Nails that are shredded because of the animal hanging on most commonly retain shreds of whatever material the claw contacted to stop the force or pull away. Consider looking for skin, blood, fabric, and fibers. Take photos of this damage and collect and clip toenails for analysis of DNA or fiber if relevant. Label and store in paper envelopes. Take care in documenting the appearance, deviation from appropriate or normal, and the consequence for the animal of these findings.

7.3.1.10 Oral Exam

Document a thorough oral exam whenever possible. Include a description of the teeth, gingiva, and oral mucosa, and use a dentition chart and a species-specific numbering system when documenting. Describe tooth loss, damage, calculus, odor, and relevance to the health of the animal. Estimate the time that is required to accumulate tartar, or for teeth to abscess and fall out. Explain the relevance of findings, such as chronic stomatitis or chronic upper respiratory tract infection with pharyngeal drainage that may impede the animal's ability to smell or eat for example. Describe dental fractures and damage in detail and with photos.

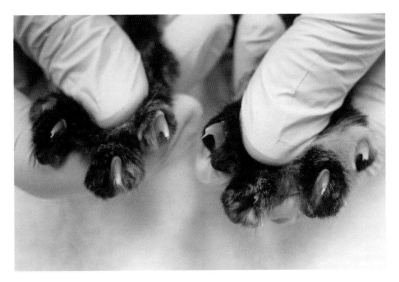

Figure 7.12   Evidence gathered from feet or claws can contain important details. Shredded nails indicate an attempt to escape and can contain valuable information about the environment and event. *Source:* Oregon Humane Society.

7.3.1.11 Sample Collection

Collect relevant samples during the physical exam including screening for infectious disease, baseline laboratory tests, fecal, urinalysis, or other specialized tests as deemed necessary. Review results of fecals prior to administration of anthelmintics to ensure proper documentation of types of parasites and incidence.

7.3.2 Section B: Behavior Observations

The physical exam process is an excellent time to document each animal's overall attitude, comfort, pain score, and demeanor. Reporting observations about behavior and the relevance to the animal's condition is an essential part of a thorough exam. Include observations and assessments of the animals as a group or herd if relevant, and individually whenever possible. Document behavior using written observations, photography, or video. Make certain when possible that no external noise, including people talking, is included during video used in a forensics examination.

Information about proper socialization or the lack of socialization, abnormal behavior as a result of confinement or boredom that causes stereotypic behavior, fear, or pain responses all give insight into the overall health and care of the animal. Use current knowledge about how to evaluate an animal's temperament and behavior in the exam room, home, or shelter environment, or even at a crime scene, and document this in addition to the medical findings.

Behavioral assessment contributes to determining a prognosis for future behavioral care, rehabilitation, and placement of the animal if this becomes necessary.

Include details and descriptions and explain how you evaluated the animal using a standard format for this process each time an exam is done to maintain quality and consistency in the process.

Examples of behavioral observations relevant to establishing standard of care and overall conditions the animal has lived in:

- Dogs found kenneled, cowering, and hiding in small kennels at a crime scene that are unsocial, unable to walk without fear outside of their enclosure, and do not have any experience in responding to a collar or leash have all the hallmarks of being unsocial, unhandled, and undomesticated. These observations may be relevant in describing a hoarding or breeding operation.
- A dog that cowers when a hand is raised to pet her may be exhibiting a behavioral indication that she has been abused by striking or has had negative experiences that condition this response.
- Circling within a kennel by dogs or stall "weaving" by a horse may indicate the animal has been held in this confined housing for an excessive amount of time resulting in abnormal behaviors.

Examples of how behavioral knowledge assists in analysis of cause of injury:

- A veterinarian's knowledge about normal behavior can also help to affirm or deny a rendition of events as to how an animal was injured. Do the reported series of events align with known animal behavior that is relevant? A cat thrown by an individual out of anger would not typically flee from that person by running past them unless there was no other route. A cat found strangled by a leash off a balcony may require further investigations to determine nonaccidental injury versus a cat who allegedly jumped off the second story and caught her leash, resulting in strangulation. A cocker spaniel with a fractured femur presented as a result of "playing ball in a small apartment" is not consistent with normal canine behavior or the force required to fracture a healthy femur; thus further investigation reveals the dog having been thrown down the stairwell.

These are examples of how behavioral observations and assessment can relate directly to cruelty investigations. Knowledge about animal behavior is an essential part of solving the forensic puzzle.

Behavioral observations from a crime scene report provide valuable insight into overall assessment of the case, including the cause and effect of findings that otherwise would be challenging to determine (Box 7.1).

Box 7.1   Example

Example: In a herd of 30 horses known to be housed together long term and receiving approximately a quarter of the calculated food required daily, you find 24 have a BCS of 1–2 and 6 have a BCS of 6. Your behavioral observations include herd attributes such as stallions competing for food, and foals and mares being pushed and fought away from the manger, thus unable to access daily nutrition.

Dogs held in groups may exhibit resource guarding and food aggression, leaving the smallest or least aggressive with wounds and starving.

The history of the animal's behavioral characteristics, observations made while in care, and those collected during examinations and treatments are all relevant aspects of a cruelty case.

7.3.3   Section C: Evaluating Pain

Pain is defined by the International Association for the Study of Pain [7] as "an unpleasant sensory and emotional experience, associated with actual or potential tissue damage, or described in terms of such damage." Pain is a complex experience that involves both sensory and emotional components. Because our patients cannot express pain verbally, we must rely on our understanding of their behavioral cues to alert us to their pain. Pain is an important piece to document in every case and aids in demonstrating the severity of the cruelty. An owner's failure to provide veterinary care to their animal(s) may lead to prolonged pain and suffering. While an individual's response to pain may differ based on myriad factors (age, health status, species, etc.), it is reasonable to assume that if a condition is painful to humans, it will also be painful to animals. There are charts for dogs and cats that can be used as a guide for perceived pain with various conditions.

Behavioral signs of pain can include changes in body language (including squinted eyes, head down, crouched, or hunched position), absence of normal behaviors (like grooming, playing, mobility), or presence of abnormal behaviors (like aggression, vocalization, reduced activity, loss of appetite, and hiding). These behaviors can be species specific, and it is important to understand normal behaviors and those associated with pain in the particular species being examined and worked with.

Pain, whether acute or chronic, should be evaluated, treated, and documented. Pain scores are evaluated and assigned based on physical exam and behavioral observations and applied consistently, using a known pain score technique when possible.

7.3.4   Section D: Additional Diagnostics

In today's clinical world there are many diagnostic tests and services available to veterinarians. When approaching a forensic exam remember that a physical exam and behavioral assessment coupled with what you know about the history and presentation of the animal are the foundational data points required. Next, decide how to approach additional diagnostic tests most efficiently, thoroughly, and realistically (Figure 7.13).

Choose diagnostics that are relevant in an individual case or in a multi-animal case based on your knowledge and assessment of all the data you have collected thus far. Perform appropriate

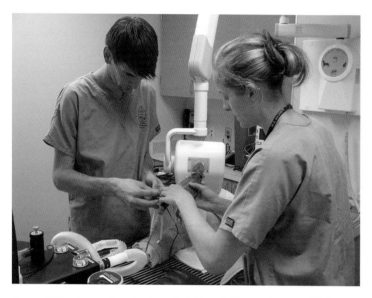

Figure 7.13   Approach selection of additional diagnostic tests efficiently. *Source:* Oregon Humane Society.

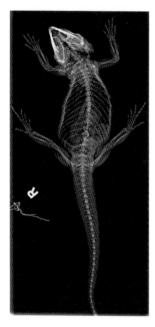

Figure 7.14   Radiographic density as demonstrated via imaging may illustrate metabolic bone disease. *Source:* Oregon Humane Society.

screenings that are relevant to the region, species, or breed-specific conditions or diseases (Figure 7.14).

Opt for tests that will provide the most information with a realistic eye on expense. To say that cost is not relevant in assisting with cruelty cases is naive, and in many cases initial findings, physical exam, and history guide the veterinarian to accurate conclusions. Do not leave out necessary tests and jeopardize your reputation or report but be prudent and explain your decisions in your reporting. If resources for baseline diagnostic testing are not available, clearly document this and describe what the plan and implications of not having these data may be (Box 7.2).

Customize the diagnostic plan with the goal of determining the cause of the animal's condition and circumstances in mind. Focus on tests that will best assist in developing a treatment plan and opinion about prognosis. When examining an individual animal presented with suspected starvation, the clinician must rule out other causes of emaciation, thus a case such as this requires complete blood count, serum chemistry panel, fecal, urinalysis, and survey radiographs, as well as observations while in care to assess appetite, swallowing, and digestive capabilities. Whereas in assessing a large population of felines from a hoarding case, surveillance of the population with fecal analysis and respiratory

---

Box 7.2   Example

Example: In the 74 cats examined in the Smith hoarding case fecals were not completed due to lack of access to laboratory funds. A course of comprehensive flea and tapeworm treatment was prescribed based on the physical observation of fleas and the high probability of intestinal tapeworms. A course of dewormer for feline ascarids was administered to each cat based on the probability of the presence of these parasites. This treatment is safe and effective.

---

polymerase chain reaction (PCR) panel testing of 30% of those who are ill will guide clinical decisions and assist in determining if these tests are necessary in all patients.

Chain of custody in sample collection, handling, and evaluation is important in any forensic exam. When possible, collect and run laboratory samples in-house with documentation as to who assisted or provided the expertise to do the test and who documented the results. Doing diagnostic tests this way improves chain of custody compliance and eliminates the need to verify who, what, when, and where the sample was handled outside of your control and the need to call on outside laboratory employees to testify. When samples are sent out of house and the chain of custody cannot be verified, the results may be excluded from testimony and therefore may impact the outcome of a case.

7.3.4.1 Other Tests or Screenings

Consider screening for toxins, analysis of feed or supplements, or other environmental substances as appropriate. Resources for specific testing include conventional veterinary diagnostic laboratories, veterinary colleges with laboratory testing capabilities and specialty testing availability, and private agencies that specialize in testing, such as detection of chemicals or DNA analysis in animals. Confirm that the laboratories you choose to use are familiar with animal evidence samples and can adhere to chain of custody requirements and documentation.

7.3.4.2 DNA Analysis

For DNA analysis in an investigation use a commercial DNA sampling kit whenever possible. As an alternative a sexual assault kit used for humans contains the necessary items and is readily available. Always consult with the lab you intend to use for analysis ahead of time for specific guidance regarding how to collect and preserve the sample. Store this material in a secure area until sending it out for analysis. This is useful in analysis of familial genetic information and may also be used in comparisons done by criminalists.

7.3.5 Section E: Special Considerations

7.3.5.1 Evidence Packaging

Evidence collected during live animal exams or scene processing must be labeled, preserved, and protected in accordance with standards established by law enforcement professionals. This includes items collected during the exam such as toenails, teeth, matted fur, or nonbiological items such as collars or harnesses.

When collecting specimens such as blood or urine, use the proper chain of custody documentation and keep samples stored in a secure location until they are processed. Make a note of who did the processing or where the samples were sent by using a log or other document that serves as a reference.

(See Chapter 10 for additional detailed information on evidence collection and processing.)

7.3.5.2 Multi-Animal Cases

When processing cases with multiple live animals, consider appropriate population screening and data collection using ready-made forms and spreadsheets, and decide what diagnostic plan is necessary for each animal. The direction given by the veterinarian in charge or by the investigating agency based on resources, as well as the nature of the case, may all weigh into determining the need for overall screening tests and individual testing. Ultimately the veterinarian is the decision maker.

Once triage and initial examination of a population are complete, the veterinarian is responsible for formulating a plan that may include follow-up diagnostics on select animals or a representative number within the population to provide necessary data and evidence related to the care of the animals and the investigation of the case.

7.3.5.3 Animals That Cannot Be Handled Safely

Be prepared to document and care for animals that a veterinarian may not be able to initially complete a physical exam on or care for without sedation or anesthesia owing to safety concerns. This situation can occur with any species ranging from wild horses to unusual species in the reptile family, to aggressive dogs, and feral cats.

When dealing with animals that cannot be safely handled, provide safe housing and habitat that minimizes stress, delivers proper nutrition, can be cleaned properly, and allows for frequent and thorough observations of the animals so that notes can be made about conditions. Use video and photography as appropriate. If immediate treatment or diagnostics are needed and cannot be done with normal restraint, consider the use of sedation or anesthesia. In using these methods, create a safe plan for administration, delivery of services, documentation, and recovery. This may be the only way, for example, to attend to wounds or to overgrowth of hooves on an equine victim or attend to the immediate care requirements of seized feral dogs who are injured or must be safely vaccinated for rabies to be held in care. Consider the safety of the people and the animals involved in all cases and be creative about how to document the conditions found and deliver the necessary care.

7.3.5.4 Diagrams

Charts and documents that illustrate findings are immensely helpful in case documentation. Consider including standard dental documentation, skin findings such as stab wounds, abrasions, hair loss, or other visually definable findings. Creating a diagram that illustrates where and under what conditions animals were found helps deepen the reader's understanding of your findings. Include standard forms and grid paper in your investigations kit so that you are prepared with these tools as a supplement to your documentation.

7.3.6 Section F: Documentation

7.3.6.1 Tips for Summarizing Overall Findings

Upon completion of the live animal exam all findings are collected using individual exam forms, follow-up exam notes, laboratory or radiographic findings, and other important medical and behavioral information, and can then be used to create a meaningful summary. If more than one animal is involved in the case, an analysis of the findings is created by organizing this individual information in a manner that provides an overview of the characteristics and analysis of the population. All this information becomes part of the veterinarian's forensic report and conclusions.

For example, in a hoarding case of 120 cats, each cat will have an individual medical and behavioral examination report and all the relevant data for the population are collected in a spreadsheet that is then used to summarize the overall findings within the population. Data may include age, sex, breed, description, weight, feline leukemia virus (FeLV), feline immunodeficiency virus (FIV) testing results, BCS, illnesses found, and diagnostics used. Summary assessments are helpful and illustrate the overall impact to the population as well as the individual animals (Box 7.3).

Box 7.3   Example

Example of note in final report: The 120 cats in the Smith hoarding case were 85% adults (over six months of age), 75% female, all intact (not spayed or neutered), and 35% tested positive for FeLV on their initial snap ELISA (enzyme-linked immunosorbent assay) test. I diagnosed severe upper respiratory disease in 75% of the cats and kittens by physical exam. We completed respiratory disease panels on 30% of the population, with 100% of these samples showing positive results for herpes, calicivirus, and mycoplasma.

In the summary the author pulls all the data and opinions into a concise, clear, and reader-friendly dialogue that illustrates the overall themes and summarizes findings. This section also explains how the author is developing opinions or conclusions, and explains the impact and prognosis for the animals involved. The intent of the summary is to educate the reader about what the findings mean to the animal(s) by taking all the detailed clinical information that has been collected and explaining its relevance (Box 7.4).

Box 7.4   Example

Example: 118 large breed dogs and 33 horses were examined after a search warrant execution. All the dogs were weighed and assessed by a veterinarian trained in body condition scoring, using the Purina Body Condition System. The dogs' body body condition scores ranged from 1 to 3 with an average for the population of 2. Of the 33 horses all were examined and assigned a body condition score of 1–9 using the Heineke method. The average BCS in this group was 5 with 10 of the adults scoring at 5 or above.

Summarizing data, by calculating percentages of the population with specific findings, such as dental disease, retrovirus infection, upper respiratory illness, or emaciation, illustrates the overall health of the population as well as the individual animals.

7.3.6.2   The Veterinarian's Report and Conclusion

The conclusion of the written report includes the veterinarian's analysis of the situation from an animal health and welfare perspective and clearly describes the veterinarian's opinion as to how the evidence supports this opinion. Clearly state the final opinion regarding the impact to the animal(s), their prognosis for recovery, care required, and to state relevant knowledge of the laws governing animal health and welfare and how the findings relate to these laws.

All the work done to review, analyze, and evaluate evidence, including written communications, reports, and other documents, photography, videography, physical examination details, and information gathered onsite, is brought together in the form of a well-organized and logical report that includes the *heading, introduction, narrative, findings, summary*, and a *conclusion*. This report is then submitted to law enforcement, or in some cases directly to a district attorney.

When compiling your report, select a consistent format with which you become familiar and proficient. Always include layman's terms as a part of the written text. The use of technical and layman's terms together ensures that findings are clear, do not require significant translation, and helps avoid misinterpretations. Remember, your report will be read and utilized by law enforcement professionals, lawyers, possibly grand jurors, judges, or citizen jury members. Keep this in mind when you write, and include descriptions and language that translates for these individuals (Box 7.5).

Box 7.5   Examples

Example(s): The dog was severely emaciated (skin and bones, exhibiting severe loss of body fat and muscle) with a BCS of 1 (a normal/healthy BCS for a dog this age is 5–6).

The kitten presented with severe scleral hemorrhage of the right eye (rupture of blood vessels on the white surface of the eye) and a broken lower right mandible (jawbone).

The introductory and narrative portion of the written report includes information relating to how the case was presented, who is involved in requesting the veterinarian's services, time, date, and other information. The findings section of a report includes all the data and detail collected including physical exam findings and general laboratory findings. The summary brings the findings to conclusion. Once the body of the report is completed, wrap up with a final succinct statement of findings and conclusion. This is the area of a report in which to address the impact to the animal's physical health and welfare. Include physical findings and husbandry information that had a positive or negative impact on the animal, and address the behavioral and emotional needs of the animal. Explain whether or not pain and suffering occurred and whether it is ongoing or not. Address exam findings and communicate your opinion regarding the prognosis for a full, partial, or no recovery. Articulate whether the animal has suffered permanent injury or died as a result of a particular action or inaction. Succinct language in this area of the report gives the reader a clear understanding of the case and provides law enforcement, a prosecutor, or a defense attorney with information necessary to formulate the next steps.

Be specific and tell the truth. Include all medical and behavioral findings. If the femur was broken causing severe pain and lack of use of the leg, and the prognosis for healing is excellent, this is the place to say so. If the leg was damaged beyond repair and had to be amputated, causing chronic pain and changes in the animal's behavior or abilities, say so.

Bringing all the findings together to form your expert conclusion is essential. This is the bottom line. Do not create a cliffhanger. If you do not know what happened, or cannot conclude, say that, and say why. If you know what happened, but you are not sure how, say so. If you are certain about what happened, and what the outcome will be, say so. Review what you know about the entire situation and include your assessment of whether the care given met minimum standards, or whether temporary or permanent damage to the animal occurred. You can also describe in detail the severity of neglect, absence of veterinary care, or evidence of intentional abuse. Call attention to the specific statute that is relevant in the case if appropriate (Box 7.6).

(See Chapter 12 on report writing for additional information.)

Box 7.6   Example

Example: In the absence of external accidental damage such as trauma from a vehicle which would cause scraping, skin damage, or other abrasions, these injuries and the cause of death are consistent with blunt force and sharp force trauma to the dog that was delivered in an intentional manner by a person. The initial trauma that the dog suffered caused severe pain and damage to his body. The subsequent multiple stab wounds resulted in fatal damage to his body, and he died of pulmonary collapse and blood loss. These injuries are consistent with Aggravated Animal Abuse, ORS 167.322.

7.4   Ongoing Responsibilities of the Veterinarian

Consultation, development, and supervision of treatment plans also fall under the veterinarian's purview. Depending upon the circumstances of the case an animal may remain in care or hospitalized and require detailed plans for treatment or surgery, or may be rehabilitated and rehomed once released.

7.4.1   Treatment Plans

When animals come into the care of a shelter or veterinary hospital as an outcome of an animal cruelty investigation, the status of the animal must be clearly communicated to the veterinarian because ownership status or Protective Custody may impose boundaries regarding decisions regarding the care and availability for adoption of the animals. Regardless of the legal status of the animal, the veterinarian's treatment plan must include all reasonable measures to save the life of the animal and address and prevent suffering. This includes medical care, surgery, and even euthanasia when necessary. If ownership is in question, limbo, or still assigned to a private individual, the veterinarian must develop treatment and care plans that include relieving suffering and improving the medical and behavioral well-being, but do not perform elective and nonessential services such as sterilization or microchipping.

Caretakers rely on the veterinarian's plan to instruct them on individualized care. Make certain that treatment plans are developed and communicated in a timely and thorough manner. Never allow an animal involved in a neglect or abuse case to go without the proper access to veterinary care once in custody.

Treatment plans also include recommendations for rechecks as needed and timelines for continued veterinary services. The resources of the agency providing the care are an essential part of the response and must be used judiciously and with open and frequent communication regarding decisions and the associated cost.

With clear relinquishment of ownership and approval by the law enforcement or prosecutor partners on the case, the animals become free to move toward adoption if possible and restrictions for nonessential services are generally removed.

7.4.2   Recheck Exams

During an animal's continued care the veterinarian is responsible for establishing an appropriate plan for follow-up and recheck exams. Continued recording of the on-going care and status of the animal may become part of the case file and requires the same quality and thoroughness of process used during the initial exam (Box 7.7).

Box 7.7   Example

Example: A dog found emaciated and with a body condition score of 1 with no underlying causes of weight loss, such as neoplasia or renal failure, and a willingness to eat and drink normally and gain weight will be confirmed by the veterinarian as a starvation case. A dog found in the same condition but with documented palliative medical care provided by a veterinarian will likely not be deemed a cruelty case.

All recheck and follow-up treatment plans for Protective Custody animals are handled as any other medical care for animals would be, keeping in mind that record keeping and detailed medical notes are paramount. It is important that medical staff and veterinarians follow their prescribed treatment plan to the letter, including recheck exam dates. A missed or tardy medical recheck could be interpreted as a careless or negligent misstep. Often the initial veterinarian attending to the case and ordering the treatment plan is not available to provide the follow-up. This does not jeopardize the care or the case but emphasizes the importance of following the plan or documenting changes in the plan that are ordered in subsequent treatment and care.

Monitoring the rehabilitation and progress, as well as addressing any decline in condition, is the veterinarian's responsibility during the animal's entire stay in Protective Custody. Remember, these animals may be exposed to infectious disease and common shelter illnesses at any point during their evidentiary hold. Animal shelter staff and foster caregivers must be made aware of how and when to contact the veterinarian for emergency and follow-up care.

7.4.3   Supplemental Reports and Updates to Case Partners

If animals remain in care, set a regular interval to provide a summary update to the law enforcement professional involved, or to the prosecutor. These updates can be in the form of a written supplemental report, if there is significant information to relay, or concise emails reminding these individuals what is happening with the animals. Examples of the need for supplemental written reports include laboratory or necropsy results, euthanasia decisions, or movement of animals to foster care. These reports are always provided in writing as an email or a new document, depending on the content and the preference of the prosecutor. It is essential to maintain a regular flow of information to the regulating agency and the prosecutor. A veterinarian's initial and on-going findings may influence additional charges or guide a law enforcement partner's further actions on the case. The prosecutor is the individual with ultimate responsibility for the evidence once charges have been filed and, for that reason, needs to be fully aware of any changes/updates.

7.4.4   Emergency Treatment, Euthanasia, and Necropsy Decisions

When an animal involved in a cruelty investigation presents in severe, life-threatening distress, it is the veterinarian's responsibility to make an assessment and address the needs of the animal immediately. Delivery of urgent or emergency care is appropriate and necessary in some cases, and lack of clarity around the next steps that will be taken in the case should not stand in the way of the doctor advocating for treatment and relief of suffering immediately. The veterinarian must make the necessary moves to get the animal the medical care needed and direct a plan for diagnostics as needed. In most cases, pain relief and delivery of hydration or appropriate medications provide stability and relief to the animal while the next steps in the case are determined, and a long-term prognosis and plan can be created. The worst outcome in a situation such as this would be that first responders to a case stall in decision making and prolong the suffering of an already neglected or abused animal.

In the case that immediate euthanasia appears to be the only possible next step, the veterinarian should document with photos and written notes why this conclusion was drawn, and decision was made. In this instance euthanasia may be carried out in accordance with American Veterinary Medical Association (AVMA) euthanasia [8] guidelines. The veterinarian should then decide if a forensic necropsy is warranted. It is advised in most cases that this is in fact an important next step and will establish overall medical findings.

Whenever possible, significant medical developments and plans, euthanasia decisions, and necropsy plans shall be made in consultation with the lead animal cruelty investigator and/or a lead prosecutor if one is in place.

7.4.5 Documentation of Cost of Care

In any animal cruelty investigation thorough and accurate recording of the cost of the investigation of the case and the care of individual animals and groups or populations of animals is an important part of the medical record. Financial information may be requested as part of a court case for purposes of establishing whether care was sufficient, or for reimbursement or restitution purposes, or for the veterinary practice or agency involved to use for budgeting and planning. Regardless of the reason, this information may be requested, so it is prudent to proactively track this as a part of your involvement in the case from the initial exam, through on-going treatment, and until final disposition of the animals.

If a cruelty or neglect case is adjudicated, the court may have the authority to award restitution to the individuals or agencies who provided care to the animals involved. For this reason, and for budgetary analysis, careful tracking of expenses related to the animal's care is an important activity and another item that must be included in the regular updates to law enforcement or the court. Expense tracking may include boarding fees, treatments, medical care, necropsy, laboratory expense, supplies, and all other items and resources used to provide care to the animals. These expenses are tracked at cost to the agency providing the care, which includes inventory and staff expenses. The agency or individual veterinarian providing the services for law enforcement may invoice the agency as they would any other client and that agency may try to recover the expense in award of restitution or other means. Whenever possible, determine who is paying for services ahead of time.

Veterinarians and agencies providing the care must not count on this court awarded payment as it is up to the court to decide how much, if any, restitution is owed and/or ordered to be paid. Reimbursement for services in part or in full is not guaranteed. Reimbursement requested is calculated based upon the cost to the agency or individual who provided the services. The court will decide whether or not to order restitution in the form of money and the amount and payment schedule. When this occurs, it will be documented as part of the court order given to the individual convicted of the crime and when it is established that the services were provided and not paid for in any other manner.

7.4.6 Conclusion: Bringing it All Together

Draw on your training, knowledge, and clinical experience to approach a forensic exam of a live animal. Use a standard format, when possible, for collection of information and have the proper tools and equipment or check lists at the ready.

Remember to document using words that describe sights, sounds, smells, impressions, and conclusions that illustrate your findings to the layman and nonmedical reader. Keep in mind that documenting what you *do not find* may be as important as what you do find in some cases.

The veterinary opinion about what the animal experienced, felt, endured, or lost because of abuse or neglect gives voice to the situation. The impact of animal cruelty goes beyond the animal and may have devastating consequences for children, seniors, domestic partners, and others in our communities. The veterinarian and those confronting an animal cruelty case are the experts that can bring fairness to an accusation and advocacy to an otherwise silent victim.

References

1 International Veterinary Forensic Sciences Association (2020). Standards document for the forensic live animal examination. https://www.ivfsa.org/wp-content/uploads/2021/05/IVFSA_Veterinary-Forensic-Live-Animal-Exam-Standards_Approved-2020_With-authors.pdf (accessed 6 August 2021).

2 Purina Mills (n.d.). Body condition scoring. https://www.purinamills.com/2.purinamills.com/media/PDF/CampaignsAndEvents/Horse-Body-Condition-Scoring-Sheet.pdf (accessed 21 May 2021).

3 Merck, M.D. (2008). Appendix 21 Tufts animal care and condition scale. In: *Veterinary Forensics* (ed. M.D. Merck), 291–292. Oxford: Blackwell Publishing Ltd https://onlinelibrary.wiley.com/doi/pdf/10.1002/9780470344583.app21 (accessed 21 May 2021).

4 Tufts (n.d.). Body condition system. https://www.library.tufts.edu/vet/images/bcs_dog.pdf (accessed 30 May 2021).

5 Tufts (n.d.). Nutrition and body condition. https://www.library.tufts.edu/vet/images/bcs_horse.pdf (accessed 30 May 2021).

6 Teng, K.T., McGreevy, P.D., Toribio, J.-A.L. et al. (2018). Strong associations of nine-point body condition scoring with survival and lifespan in cats. *Journal of Feline Medicine and Surgery* 20 (12): 1110–1118. https://wsava.org/wp-content/uploads/2020/08/Body-Condition-Score-cat-updated-August-2020.pdf (accessed 6 August 2021).

7 IASP. (n.d.). IASP guidelines – IASP. https://www.iasp-pain.org/Guidelines?navItemNumber=648 (accessed 27 May 2021).

8 American Veterinary Medical Association. (2020). AVMA guidelines for the euthanasia of animals. https://www.avma.org/sites/default/files/2020-01/2020-Euthanasia-Final-1-17-20.pdf (accessed 27 May 2021).

8

Setting Expectations and Monitoring Compliance
Linda Fielder

Not all investigations result in a criminal citation. One of the most important roles of the investigative team is that of advocate and teacher. In many cases investigators, veterinarians, and animal welfare professionals use their expertise to guide and educate owners on proper nutrition, adequate shelter, necessary medical care, and humane training methods as a first line of response to reports of neglect and abuse.

To say all animal owners will do better if they know better is unrealistic, but when you begin by educating an owner on the steps they must take to provide proper care for an animal, you also set a foundation for a criminal citation should the owner fail to rectify the situation in a timely and appropriate manner.

In order to resolve a case through education, investigators must set clear and reasonable expectations for the owner and then be diligent in monitoring and confirming follow-through. Managing these cases can be time consuming. They require commitment and the same attention to detail in the recording of progress and compliance as cases where citations are issued right out of the gate. These cases can also be the most rewarding, and a positive resolution for both the animal and the owner reminds us of the reason animals and humans share such strong bonds.

8.1   Education and Guidance vs. Citation

Certain types of cases will always be dealt with as a crime when they are discovered. Animal fighting, animal sexual abuse, and willful physical abuse of an animal are examples of cases where education in lieu of citation is not appropriate. These cases require law enforcement's attention to and acknowledgment of not only the severity of the animal crime, but also the connection to other serious crimes that occur simultaneously.

These types of cases are best worked through the cooperation of multiple agencies. Animal fighting goes hand in hand with drug and firearm dealing, racketeering, and even human trafficking. Animal sexual abuse often occurs alongside sexual abuse of minors and child pornography. Physical violence toward animals has a well-documented link [1] to intimate partner violence and child abuse. Cases must be worked carefully, as the individuals known to participate in these

Animal Cruelty Investigations: A Collaborative Approach from Victim to Verdict^{TM}, First Edition.
Edited by Kris Otteman, Linda Fielder, and Emily Lewis.
© 2022 John Wiley & Sons, Inc. Published 2022 by John Wiley & Sons, Inc.
Companion website: www.wiley.com/go/otteman/victimtoverdict

crimes are dangerous and the stakes are high when their crimes are uncovered. We will cover each of these types of cases in more detail in Appendix A of this book and list the agencies that must work in partnership with you throughout the investigation.

8.2 Passive Neglect and Lack of Resources

On the other end of the spectrum, investigations often lead us to animals without adequate shelter, in need of veterinary care or grooming, or not receiving food of the proper quantity or quality. In many of these cases the animal's owner is unaware of the issue, or if they do recognize the problem, they lack the resources to make the necessary changes. Financial barriers are some of the most common reasons owners fail to provide minimum care to their animals. An individual may have a strong bond with their pet but have no extra income to pay for veterinary care to treat an illness or disease that left untreated will result in suffering and possibly even death. These types of cases can cause frustration and heartache for investigators.

Veterinary care for pets may be out of reach for individuals living in poverty. Poverty coupled with housing restrictions may mean dogs and other pets live outdoors, without adequate shelter from the elements. In homes where animals are not spayed and neutered, they reproduce until owners find themselves overwhelmed by litter after litter of offspring they now must provide for. Livestock owners may be faced with mobility or other issues as they age that prevent them from providing the same level of husbandry and upkeep for their stock that they were able to for years prior.

When evaluating these types of cases consider whether this situation is best addressed through criminal citation, education and monitoring, or some type of community resource to help the owner correct the issues affecting their animals (Figure 8.1). Consider a solution for the problem at hand as well as the likelihood that, once resolved, the individual will be able to provide proper care for their animals in the long term. A one-time donation of hay to a horse owner who has fallen behind due to loss of employment may be the assistance that individual needs to get back on their feet. Conversely, the same donation would do little to correct a situation where the owner has become disabled and can no longer care for their horses that have been underfed and chronically neglected for months to years. A thorough interview will aid you in determining which path to explore.

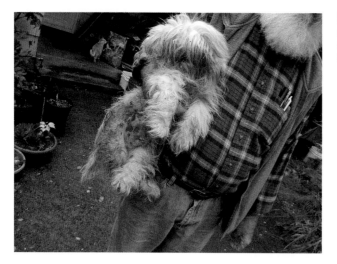

Figure 8.1 Many cases can be resolved through education and compliance monitoring. *Source:* Oregon Humane Society.

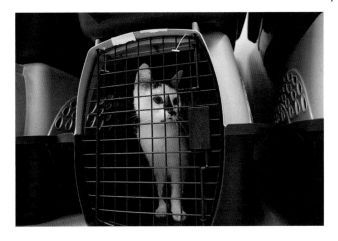

Figure 8.2 Subsidized programs that provide spay/neuter and veterinary care help owners overcome financial barriers. *Source:* Oregon Humane Society.

Some communities have programs in place that can give aid to animal owners experiencing financial hardship, homelessness, domestic violence, or illness. They may be connected to a non-profit organization, animal shelter, veterinary clinic, or neighborhood food bank (Figure 8.2).

Become familiar with these resources in your community and then be thoughtful about referring animal owners to them. These types of organizations operate with limited funds and are not the cure-all for every neglect case, but in those cases where there is a likelihood that the owner will be able to continue to provide care for their animal after receiving assistance to spay and neuter their pets, accessing veterinary care, or constructing an appropriate shelter, they can be a solution that improves the situation at hand, maintains the human–animal bond, and keeps the pet out of the shelter.

In the case of a 13-year-old poodle living with a senior owner on a fixed income, the best outcome for the animal, when discovered in a matted condition but otherwise healthy, may be to connect the owner to resources that offer assistance with grooming services, rather than issue the owner a criminal citation on the spot. In this case, the investigator acts as a community steward and even though the case may require some monitoring and follow-up before it is closed, odds are the outcome will be favorable for the animal, the owner, and the investigating agency.

Sometimes owners find themselves overwhelmed by the cost of caring for too many animals. In these cases, you can help with rehoming by engaging the services of animal shelters and encouraging the owner to rehome some or all of their animals. This helps reduce the financial burden on the owner and removes the animals from an environment in which their needs were not being met.

8.3 Education

In this age of technology, when seemingly everything you need to know is just a click of the mouse away, you might believe there is no reason a pet owner should be ignorant to the type of care an animal requires. While it is true an abundance of information is readily available through the internet, keep in mind it is also full of contradictory information, that utilizing technology is still beyond many people's reach, and that while the internet is a source of information about animal care and husbandry for many, it has also become a robust marketplace for buying, selling, and giving away animals.

Thorough interview techniques can shed light on whether a failure to provide proper care is most likely due to the owner's lack of knowledge about the animal's needs, or willful or reckless negligence. If you feel the owner may truly lack adequate knowledge, you might take the opportunity to offer guidance and education.

Law enforcement and animal control officers, veterinarians, and animal welfare professionals can educate owners on the aspects of minimum care for animals they are familiar with. It may be well within your area of expertise to educate an owner about providing a rabbit with an enclosure that is safe, clean, allows for exercise, and provides adequate shelter from the weather. If the animal in question happens to be an exotic reptile you have never seen before, rather than guess or misinform the owner, refer them to a veterinarian who treats reptiles or another reputable expert.

Animal care and control professionals are constantly working to increase their knowledge about care and husbandry, which helps them educate owners in the field. Veterinarians are animal experts trained to diagnose and treat illness, injury, and disease, and provide animals with preventative care such as worming and vaccinations to keep them healthy. If the case involves an animal that is sick or injured, make sure the animal is seen by a veterinarian for treatment. Resist the temptation to offer medical advice or endorse home remedies for ill or injured animals in lieu of veterinary care. Always ensure that sick or injured animals are seen by a veterinarian familiar with the species in question.

8.4   Setting Expectations

When is it appropriate to set expectations and allow subjects time to correct situations before elevating the case to the level of criminal citation or seizure? Most importantly, the animals involved must not be in immediate risk of serious injury or death. In areas of the country where winter temperatures fall below zero, an investigator would address a dog without adequate shelter very differently in January than they might if they investigated the same case in May.

When you have determined the animal is not in immediate danger and you feel it is appropriate to allow the owner time to rectify the problems you have identified, make your expectations clear to the owner and confirm they understand what is expected of them as well as the timeline by which the corrections must be made. A standardized form, which allows you to record the issues in need of correction, is useful in making your expectations clear and providing a written record of your instructions to the owner (Figure 8.3). An example notice to comply form is included in Appendix C.

Using a horse with overgrown hooves as an example, you would take the following steps to set expectations:

- Determine the horse can stand, walk, and access food and water easily.
- Determine there is no immediate concern for serious injury or death.
- Ask the owner if they have a resource for farrier work and if they can commit to arranging hoof trimming for the horse within a set time (two to three weeks may be reasonable).
- Ask the owner if there are any barriers (finances, temperament of the horse, access to services) to providing the service within the time frame you have set.
- Relay your expectations to the owner verbally and in writing. Include contact information for any resources you have suggested and the approximate date you will return for a recheck. Take a photo of the notice to comply for your records.
- Ask the owner again if they are confident they can correct the identified issues within the time you have set, and let them know you will be checking on the horse to make certain care was provided.
- Make detailed case notes that include the information outlined above and set a calendar request or other reminder for follow-up.

Figure 8.3 Compliance notices are a useful way to communicate instructions for correcting issues.

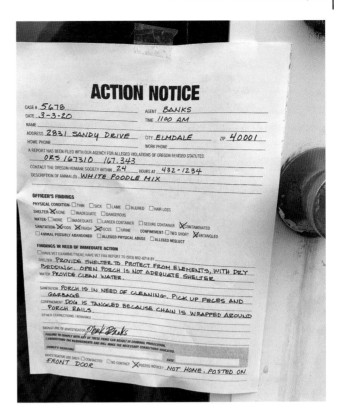

This procedure can be modified for most cases in which the investigator believes the owner can provide adequate care to the animal(s) within a certain period of time. This type of approach can prove valuable because it places the responsibility for coordinating or providing care on the owner and establishes that they are aware of the changes they are required to make to bring the level of care to an acceptable level. These approaches require follow-up and rechecks as well as a plan for next steps or citation if the owner does not follow through as suggested.

In most cases you can and should require the owner fix any violations that are causing immediate risk to the animal before you leave the premises. Empty water bowls and troughs should be filled with fresh potable water, hazards should be removed, and the area and the animal should be deemed safe before your departure. Most investigators carry fresh water and a small supply of at least cat and dog food in their rig in the event an owner is not able to fulfill those requirements in the moment.

8.5 What You Can and Cannot Require

If you are a code or animal control officer, you may be enforcing ordinances that place a limit on the number or type of animals a person living within your jurisdiction may possess. You may also enforce licensing or facilities permit ordinances, which can be effective tools in working cases involving more animals than an owner can adequately care for. If this is the case, it is usually within your authority to require an owner to reduce their number of animals if they are in violation of an ordinance. If there are no ordinances like this in your area, or your job does not include enforcement of such ordinances, you may be limited in your lawful ability to require that an owner dispossess themselves of their animals as a condition you would include in a compliance plan.

If you are not able to utilize a statute or ordinance to reduce animal numbers in a case, you can still encourage the owner to make that decision by offering resources such as relinquishment to a shelter or rescue. In some cases, it may seem like there are no options for rehoming or reducing numbers. Shelters may be full, or there may not be rehoming options for the type of animal you are dealing with, such as exotic birds or reptiles. These types of cases can be frustrating and require a greater investment of time and resources to bring them to an acceptable level of compliance, and in some cases seizure and citation will be the end result despite your best efforts. While you may not be able to require an owner to surrender or rehome their animals, you can make it clear to them that if they are unable to provide adequate care and shelter to the number of animals they possess, they are eligible for criminal citation.

8.6 Conducting Rechecks

In order for compliance monitoring efforts to be effective, the investigator must be able to conduct rechecks and determine if the care of the animals in question has risen to an acceptable level. Frequently violations can be rectified with one recheck. For example, a cat with severe dental disease will be made comfortable after a complete dentistry service from a veterinarian and it will only require proof of the procedure for you to close the case. It is the responsibility of the investigator to confirm the animal received the required care, which will allow for the case to be closed. If the situation involves multiple animals or issues that require ongoing care, follow-up and monitoring may be protracted. Before engaging in a compliance plan, be certain that your agency has the resources to follow up on the case within the timeline you have communicated to the owner.

A call to the treating veterinarian to confirm adequate care and treatment has been provided may be a simple way to conduct a recheck. In other cases, you will want to return to the owner's property to confirm visually that an animal has recovered, their shelter or environmental shortfalls have been corrected, or the owner has been able to reduce the number of animals in their care to a manageable number.

When conducting rechecks, utilize your interview skills to determine the proper steps have been taken as directed, and the owner fully understands what care must be maintained in the future. A one-time grooming appointment to relieve a dog of severe matting will need to be repeated going forward, to avoid the animal suffering from the same condition in six- or nine-months' time. Make sure the owner can verbalize your expectations for future care and understands the animal's long-term needs.

8.7 What If Nothing Improves or Conditions Worsen?

It is unrealistic to think that all cases can be resolved through education and compliance monitoring. Sometimes, despite your best efforts, owners are unwilling or unable to make the changes necessary to relieve an animal's suffering and avoid a criminal citation.

If you have set forth a compliance plan and at any point during your monitoring and follow-up feel the condition of an animal has worsened, or the time period for compliance has run out and nothing has improved, you may make the choice to issue a criminal citation or apply for a warrant to seize the animal(s).

All the notes, photographs, and documents related to your previous interviews, site visits, and phone calls will serve to make the case for the owner's negligence in providing adequate care for their animal(s). It can be helpful to create a timeline for the case that begins at the time of your first contact with the subject, includes all the resources and recommendations you provided, and what, if any, steps the subject took to correct the situation. Cases like these will be strong if you have created detailed notes, reports, and photographs that illustrate the history of noncompliance.

8.8 What About Animal Hoarders?

Animal hoarding is a complex manifestation of mental health disorders including but not limited to depression, obsessive compulsive disorder, post-traumatic stress disorder, and anxiety disorders to name a few. Hoarders keep a larger number of animals than they can adequately care for and fail to see or understand the suffering of the animals in their care. Hoarders may keep one species of animals or many. People often envision a house full of cats when they think of animal hoarders, but dogs, birds, livestock animals, rodents, and reptiles are also common victims in these cases.

Because the hoarder is disconnected from the severity of their animals' conditions, enacting a plan for education and compliance may seem futile and has a high chance of failure in the end. That is not to say that offering such a plan is always a bad idea. Because hoarders can be reclusive and suspicious of strangers, a monitoring plan can be useful in building rapport and determining the scope of the problems at hand. Through a period of regular site visits, offering of resources, and rehoming options, you may gain some compliance and even effectively help the subject to reduce their numbers or at the least be able to garner more information to inform a search warrant application should the case require it (Figures 8.4 and 8.5).

Figure 8.4 Animal hoarding cases are complex, resource intensive, and best approached through a multidisciplinary effort. *Source:* Oregon Humane Society.

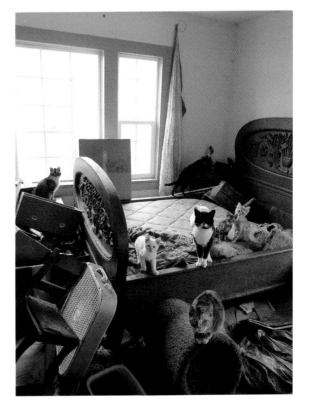

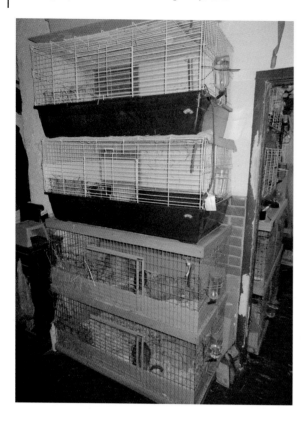

Figure 8.5 Animal hoarding cases may involve any species or variety of species. *Source:* Oregon Humane Society.

Hoarding cases are best approached as a multidisciplinary effort. The number or species of animals involved can easily overwhelm a single animal shelter or rescue. Care and planning are required to ensure the animal shelter or agency assisting with the seizure is capable of providing for the number of animals involved. Mental health and crisis intervention agencies and organizations often retain experts who can offer services and aid to the subject, which may enable the investigation to be more successful, and may also help prevent the hoarder from reoffending in the future. Hoarding cases are known to have a high rate of recidivism. They can be frustrating and sometimes overwhelming to address, however, they are often the culmination of years of chronic and extreme illness, starvation, injury, and neglect of many animals as well as humans living with the person suffering from hoarding disorder. You will find more information about responding to hoarding cases in Appendix A of this textbook [2].

References

1 Jegatheesan, B., Enders-Slegers, M.-J., Ormerod, E., and Boyden, P. (2020). Understanding the link between animal cruelty and family violence: the bioecological systems model. *Int. J. Environ. Res. Public Health* 17 (9): 3116.
2 Frost, R.O., Patronek, G., Arluke, A., and Steketee, G. (2015). The hoarding of animals: an update. *Psychiatric Times* 34 (4) https://www.psychiatrictimes.com/view/hoarding-animals-update (accessed 9 August 2021).

9

Search Warrants and Seizures

Emily Lewis

When criminal animal cruelty is discovered and persists, law enforcement is best advised to seek a search warrant as a means of pursuing the most thorough investigation into the victims and evidence of the violations. This chapter will discuss all aspects of requesting and executing a search warrant in an animal cruelty case. It will touch on the differences between a single animal case, a large-scale case, and cases involving livestock or exotic animals. Search warrants for animal cruelty cases require specialized considerations at every phase, from authoring of the affidavit through clearing the scene at the conclusion of the search warrant execution. It is important to take a deep dive into each of these phases to address the objectives and vulnerabilities present at each step across all disciplines. The search warrant and its execution are likely the first occasions for simultaneous collaboration by the three disciplines that are key to successful animal cruelty investigations – veterinarians, law enforcement, and prosecutors.

Both federal and state laws influence the parameters of search warrants and the circumstances that permit search and seizure without a warrant. Given the broad spectrum of nuanced interpretations across the country, this book will generally address exceptions to the search warrant requirement and how those exceptions pertain to animal cruelty cases but will focus primarily on the process of attaining and executing a search warrant as is generally best practice in these cases.

9.1 Exceptions to the Warrant Requirement in Animal Cruelty Cases

Americans enjoy a Fourth Amendment right "against unreasonable searches and seizures" in areas where they have a reasonable expectation of privacy, such as their home, their body, or their vehicles [1]. This right is preserved unless a law enforcement officer, or otherwise authorized agent, attains a search warrant, signed by a judge, to conduct a search and/or seizure. The reality of criminal investigations is that there will not always be the opportunity for officers to go through the necessary steps to procure a search warrant, and the law acknowledges this by carving out very specific circumstances in which search and seizure is legal in the absence of a warrant. It is important to note that these specific exceptions to the warrant requirement are reserved for those particular circumstances where there is not time to get a warrant and which, in the future, will be evaluated with that mindset in court. If there is time to get a search warrant, this is the course of

Animal Cruelty Investigations: A Collaborative Approach from Victim to Verdict™, First Edition.
Edited by Kris Otteman, Linda Fielder, and Emily Lewis.
© 2022 John Wiley & Sons, Inc. Published 2022 by John Wiley & Sons, Inc.
Companion website: www.wiley.com/go/otteman/victimtoverdict

action you need to take. Of the number of exceptions that have developed over the years, there are four most utilized in animal cruelty cases: consent, exigent circumstances, emergency aid, and plain view.

9.1.1 Consent

Consent is the most reliable of the exceptions that an officer can employ if certain measures are taken to document the consent. The exception is exactly as it sounds, an individual can allow, i.e. consent, to the search and/or seizure. There are factors that are important to keep in mind with this exception. First, the moment the person revokes their consent, or takes any action that indicates they are revoking their consent, the search/seizure must cease. Second, states may differ in their requirements of who can grant the officer consent. The federal standard, which is followed by many states, permits what is known as "apparent authority," meaning it appears to the officer who is getting the permission that the person has authority to grant consent for the area to be searched and items to be seized [2]. Some states do not adopt the federal standard and require that the person have "actual authority" to consent, which means it does not matter how it appears to the officer: if the person does not actually have the authority to consent to search or seizure of those areas, then the exception will be invalid and any evidence collected cannot be relied on in the case.[1] Third, consent cannot be coerced. Generally, coerce means "[t]o compel by force or threat" [3]. It would be prudent to check with your local prosecutor to understand how your state has construed what coerced consent looks like in order to avoid issues in your cases. Written or videotaped consent increases the likelihood that your reliance on this exception will withstand scrutiny by attorneys and judges who are evaluating the case.

In Appendix C there are "Consent to Search" templates specific to animal cruelty investigations. Most frequently you would utilize these when a suspect is consenting to a veterinary exam, or necropsy of their animal, or allowing you to come into their residence and search for evidence of the animal crime at issue. On occasion, you may encounter a suspect with whom you have built a strong rapport and who has a significant number of animals needing to be seized. Although this person may be willing to sign a consent form for you to search their home and take their animals, and even when that might seem like the most expedient way to further the investigation, be cautioned that often the capture of the person's animals may be more traumatic for them than they anticipated, thus causing them to immediately revoke their consent. This leaves you with the prospect of having to request a warrant at that time, and the resources prepared to process the scene and care for the animals will have been wasted. It is best, especially in those circumstances, to request and obtain a warrant ahead of time so that you can process the scene in a way that allows you to carefully search and seize the relevant evidence, without the risk of squandering resources.

9.1.2 Exigent Circumstances

Law enforcement officers may be in a position to rely on the exigent circumstances exception to the warrant requirement in their animal cruelty cases. This exception allows for a warrantless entry onto a property to search if probable cause for a crime exists in addition to exigent circumstances.

---

1 Oregon (*State vs. Will*, 885 P.2d 715, 719, [1994]; Constitution of Oregon, Bill of Rights, Unreasonable Searches or Seizures 1859 [OR]); Hawaii (*State vs. Lopez*, 896 P.2d 889, 901, [1995]; The Constitution of the State of Hawaii, Bill of Rights, Searches, Seizures and Invasion of Privacy 1968 [HI]); New Mexico (*State vs. Wright*, 893, P.2d 453, [1995], 460–461; Constitution of the State of New Mexico, Bill of Rights, Searches and Seizures 1911 [NM]).

Exigent circumstances have been defined to include among other things, harm to persons or property and destruction of evidence [1]. There is case law to support the assertion that the federal constitutional parameters support the seizure of animals who are suffering and facing imminent harm.[2] Check in regularly with your prosecutor to understand how exceptions such as these have been viewed by your local courts.

9.1.3 Emergency Aid

Whether the emergency aid exception to the warrant requirement applies to animals is very state dependent. Generally speaking, if an officer believes that someone is in immediate need of assistance, or if life or property needs preserving or protecting, the officer can make a warrantless entry to preserve or protect that life or property. If the officer encounters evidence of a crime while responding, the officer may seize that evidence [1]. This has been applied in animal cruelty cases where the officer reasonably believed that warrantless entry and seizure of the animal was necessary to protect the animal's life [4]. It is important to clarify that, while the exigent circumstances exception does require that the officer have probable cause of a crime to make a warrantless entry and seizure, this exception does not.

9.1.4 Plain View

Plain view is another exception to the warrant requirement that officers might rely on in an animal cruelty investigation. As with every exception there are very specific parameters around how it can be used, and each parameter will be scrutinized by the attorneys and judges reviewing the case. Generally speaking, if an officer, standing in a lawful location, identifies evidence of a crime, can determine that it is evidence of a crime without having to manipulate or explore the evidence, and if that officer can take the evidence into possession while still in a lawful location, that evidence is considered to be in plain view and the officer can seize it without a warrant.

The plain view exception, as is true with many other aspects of typical criminal investigations, is complicated by the unique fact that the evidence is a living being. This complication gives rise to questions such as can an officer standing on a public sidewalk call a neglected dog over to them from the suspect's garage or yard and still seize that dog under the plain view exception?[3] In the alternative, could the officer wait on the public way for the neglected dog to wander over and then

---

2 *State vs. Fessenden/Dicke*, 355 Or. 759, (2014); *Tuck vs. United States*, 477 A2d 1115, 1119, (2001); *Siebert vs. Severino*, 256 F3d 648, 657, (2001).

3 *State vs. Newcomb*, 359 Or. 756, 768–69, 375 P.3d 434, 441–442, (2016): "As an abstract proposition, we accept that a person who owns or lawfully possesses an animal, and who thus has full rights of dominion and control over it, has a protected privacy interest that precludes others from interfering with the animal in ways and under circumstances that exceed legal and social norms. Thus, for example, if a dog owner walks his dog off-leash down the street, and the friendly dog runs over to greet a passerby who pets it, that act of petting the dog would invade no possessory or privacy interest; a contact of that kind would fall well within social norms and conventions, even if by petting the dog the passerby discovers something concealed from plain view (e.g., that under the dog's thick fur coat, the dog is skin and bones to the point of serious malnourishment). On the other hand, if the passerby produces a syringe and expertly withdraws a sample of the dog's blood in the time that it would take to greet and pet the dog, that contact would violate the owner's possessory and privacy interests, even if the passerby did so for a valuable scientific study (e.g., whether local animals were infected with an easily transmitted virus); such a contact would fall well outside social norms and conventions. As those examples suggest, determining the existence of a constitutionally protected privacy right in property depends not only on the nature of the property itself, but also on the nature of the governmental intrusion and the circumstances in which it occurred."

seize it using plain view? Each state will interpret these circumstances differently and it is important to check with your prosecutor about how to navigate these circumstances successfully. Animals also complicate this exception because their poor body condition does not always equate to neglectful circumstances. If you are an officer intending to seize an animal in plain view because it has a poor body condition, you need also to be able to articulate why you have probable cause to believe that the animal's poor body condition is a result of criminal neglect.[4] As discussed earlier in this book, there are numerous reasons why an animal may be thin that are not due to criminal conduct on the part of the owner.

9.2 Prewarrant Considerations

There are considerations that need to be addressed prior to any warrant execution but dealing with the unique circumstance of living evidence results in several atypical factors that also need to be assessed prior to even the application for a search warrant.

9.2.1 Standard Considerations

9.2.1.1 Guard Dogs

From the first moment you think an investigation might need to be advanced using a search warrant, there are factors you need to start documenting in order to make that a successful venture, the first of which is guard dogs. If possible, make certain to note whether there are or likely to be guard dogs on the property. Even if an officer has not previously gained access to a location, there are indicators to look for that would help inform you of this likelihood. You may know the answer to this as part of your investigation but, if not, it may be worthwhile to ask neighbors, check with county dog licensing records, or simply observe the property in advance. If there are guard dogs or a likelihood of guard dogs at the location where you will be serving the warrant, a plan for handling that situation needs to be a part of your warrant execution strategy.

Serving a warrant on a property you know to have dogs, guard dogs or otherwise, without a nonlethal plan in place to address that issue is strongly discouraged and could be grounds for a lawsuit.[5] This is not to say that officer safety is not of paramount concern, but the optics of using lethal force against resident dogs in order to execute a search warrant in an animal cruelty case are not good. It is also worth noting that investment in training about dog behavior and body language has the potential to avoid precarious situations involving resident dogs

---

4 An example of this can be found in *State vs. Newcomb*, 359 Or. 756, (2016), where an officer seized a "near emaciated" dog under the plain view exception after seeing the poor body condition, learning from the suspect that she had no food on hand for the dog, and witnessing the dog eating nonnutritive items in the yard and dry heaving. Based on his training and experience he believed the dog was suffering from neglect.

5 *San Jose Charter of Hells Angels Motorcycle Club vs. City of San Jose*, 402 F.3d 962, (2005) – the court held that the shooting of dogs at two residences was an unreasonable seizure and an unreasonable execution of the warrants because exigent circumstances did not exist and because the officers failed to develop a realistic plan for incapacitating the dogs despite a week of planning. *Brown vs. Muhlenberg Twp.*, 269 F.3d 205, (2001) – the court found that the shooting of a pet is clearly unlawful when the animal "pose[s] no imminent danger and whose owners were known, available, and desirous of assuming custody." *Viilo vs. Eyre*, 547 F.3d 707, (2008) – the court held that it is a violation of the Fourth Amendment for a police officer to shoot and kill a companion dog that poses no imminent danger while the dog's owner is present and trying to assert custody over her pet.

without creating grounds for tragedy and litigation (see Appendix D for a list of courses and resources for training of this nature).

There are a few ways to approach the issue of guard dogs. First, if you have a good existing rapport with the suspect and feel safe doing so, make contact from the driveway or nearby the property (via phone or loudspeaker) and request that the dogs be contained. Another option would be to include professional animal handlers in your warrant service team to capture the dogs safely immediately upon your entry onto the property.

Finally, if an officer fears for their safety, there are other means of defending oneself before resorting to a firearm. Use of oleoresin capsicum (OC) spray or other aerosolized deterrents is one nonlethal way to respond to an aggressive dog [5]. Another option would be to use an electronic control device (ECD), like a TASER®, to subdue an aggressive dog. It is important to note that use of an ECD on an animal is not recommended and has the potential to seriously injure or kill a dog [5, 6]. ECDs should never be used on cats or other small animals [5].

Do not misconstrue this to say that using physical force, be it with a TASER® or pepper spray, can be the extent of your warrant service plan for guard dogs; in fact, it should be a last resort. The National Animal Care and Control Association (NACA) does not recommend ECDs as a method of capture and control, only as a means of self-defense when absolutely necessary [5]. The most prudent course of action is to try to contain the dogs in a way that does not injure them or any people in the process.

9.2.1.2 Cohabitators

Known cohabitators create another prewarrant consideration. Not only do suspects often have their family and/or roommates living with them in the house, but they can also have friends or acquaintances living in various accommodations around the property. This is of particular concern in livestock cases or locations with a lot of acreage, buildings, or other living quarters. These individuals are relevant aside from their place on the risk assessment checklist. It is important to know whether these third parties are connected in any way to the case, i.e. they are onsite animal caregivers. It is also important to note if any of the animals residing on the property could belong to them and not to the suspect(s) in the case. Finding this information out as part of the investigation that takes place prior to the search warrant service, rather than discovering cohabitators during warrant service, can improve scene safety and streamline the warrant service. Always be clear in your warrant drafting and in your preservice briefing whether or not the structures housing these third parties are subject to search and seizure or if they are not covered by the warrant that was issued.

On occasion while executing a search warrant you may discover a separate, additional animal crime at a cohabitator's residence on the property. If this situation occurs, the best course of action is to contact your prosecutor and inquire how they would like you to proceed. The warrant you are executing does not authorize seizure of any evidence from a different animal crime but there may be an exception to the warrant requirement that you could articulate or, more than likely, you could amend your warrant to include this new evidence.

9.2.1.3 Picture of the Property

Though it is not particular to animal cases, it cannot be said often enough – be sure to include a picture of the front of the property described in the search warrant in the search warrant itself. To avoid the potentially catastrophic mistake of serving a warrant on the wrong property, all safeguards must be utilized.[6] In more rural areas it can be difficult to capture a residence or a barn that is located farther back on the property. In these cases, you can include a photo from the public roadway and another from in front of the residence if you have been on the property through the course of your investigation and have a photo as a result.

9.2.2 Considerations Unique to Animal Cruelty Cases

Animal cruelty is a crime and the preparation for a search warrant execution in an animal cruelty case should follow the same protocol that search warrants follow in all other cases. Animal cruelty cases do have one glaringly obvious difference from traditional cases, though, the likelihood of living evidence. Owing to that factor, there are several additional considerations that law enforcement and prosecutors must evaluate prior to going forward with a search warrant.

9.2.2.1 Timing

With animal victims at risk there is always an underlying urgency in the process of attaining and serving a search warrant. If the facts of the case allow, include coordination and planning for the warrant in your timeline of when you seek to get the warrant signed and served. If your animal care partners need to find room for a potentially large number of animals, or if you need to locate a credible veterinary expert for an exotic species of animal, those tasks become much more difficult if you are operating within a five-day deadline to serve the warrant.

9.2.2.2 Species Variety

It is common for investigations into animal cruelty to begin with a report related to one, maybe two, species of animals. It is also common for investigators to discover additional species in the custody of the suspect, over the course of the investigation. Depending on what phase of the investigation a search warrant is being contemplated, you may have a clear idea of how many species will be at issue on the day of warrant service or may only have an estimate. In either circumstance, additional species might be found during the warrant service.

Do your best to get the most accurate estimate of how many and what species you will be dealing with on scene. If you are able, get this information from the suspect(s) during initial interviews, or make observations about the property, or items you can see in or around the home that might indicate other types of animals that could be present. Spend time reviewing the social media accounts of the suspects or other residents in the home and garner any information you can from those platforms about what animals are there. This is important because you want to be prepared with animal handlers and veterinary experts who can evaluate and address any type of animal you are likely to encounter during warrant service. Of course, there will be cases where you are unable to ascertain the number and species of animals on the property, but every possible method to do so should be pursued in order to avoid surprises and delay on the day of warrant service.

---

6 *Green vs. City of Phoenix*, WL 4016484, (2019), at 6–7 – the location listed in the warrant was incorrect and the warrant was served on the wrong location and the homeowner's dog was killed. *U.S. vs. Wagoner*, WL 6940506, (2020), at 3–11 – description in the warrant did not match the suspect's residence, warrant specified a different residence than the one actually searched. *Cohn vs. DeWeese*, WL 3906227, (2010) – the wrong address was on the search warrant and the descriptors in the warrant did not match the description of the wrongly searched residence.

9.2.2.3 Number of Crime Scenes

Each location where an animal is found on scene should be treated as a separate crime scene. The conditions between one stall and the next, one kennel or another, even one room to the next can differ drastically and in ways that are relevant to the crimes you are investigating. It helps to know, if you can, ahead of time approximately how many crime scenes you will be labeling and processing when you serve a warrant. As an investigator, if a suspect has agreed to walk you around their property during the initial phases of your investigation, be sure to note or make a map of how the property is arranged and where the animals are being kept.

If you do not have the benefit of drawing on past visits to the property, there are other ways to prepare yourself for the number of crime scenes you may encounter. Viewing an aerial map of the property can be extremely helpful in cases involving livestock, commercial breeding operations, and animal fighting cases. From an aerial map you can identify structures and get a rough estimate of how many animals or pens could be contained in that structure. If there are outdoor dog runs or pastures, you will be able to see those as well. Aerial maps can reveal potential water sources to animals with access to the entire property. In animal fighting cases, you will see circles where dogs or birds are tethered, and this can give you an idea of the number you will be documenting. Keep in mind that some outbuildings may not contain animals at all, but that it is equally likely that other outbuildings may contain more animals than you would have expected.

There are many cases where an aerial map will not help you plan for the number of crime scenes you might encounter because all the animals are kept inside a residence on the property. Again, if you do not have insight from the early phases of your investigation, you can look to social media to try to gauge if the animals are kept in separate kennels or are loose in the residence. Neighbors might also have insight into how the suspect maintains the animals and the numbers present.

In every case it is a good rule of thumb to overestimate the number of animals and crime scenes you will be prepared to process rather than underestimate.

9.2.2.4 Time of Year

Given that every stall, cage, or kennel is a separate crime scene, and often documentation of such makes up the bulk of the evidence in your case, animal cruelty search warrants can take a long time to execute. Remember this while you are in the planning phase of your search warrant service because, depending on the time of year, you may have very few hours of natural light in the day to complete your evidence collection. It is dangerous to be loading livestock or collecting other species in the dark, and your evidence collection process will be impeded by the complication of darkness regardless of flood lights or other light sources. It is rare for a law enforcement agency to have the available resources to secure a search warrant scene overnight, so it is imperative that the person in charge of planning the execution of the warrant is doing so with the number of daylight hours in mind.

Another consideration related to time of year is the weather. From the nature of the personal protective equipment (PPE) for the warrant execution team to the method and means of animal transport, weather plays a critical role in search warrant service planning. In areas where mud can be an issue in fall and winter, there should be a plan for trailers and other large transport vehicles that will be responding to the scene. In parts of the country that experience extreme heat and humidity, the seized animals must be transported in a way that protects them from this danger and in a way that does not create additional conditions that a veterinarian will document upon initial exam so as to confuse the evidence related to the case.

Weather can also play a role in the evaluation of the evidence on scene. If the weather is cold, the bodies of deceased animals found on scene will have been preserved fairly well, but the warmer the temperature the faster the decomposition process will take place. It also becomes relevant in what you are documenting as evidence of the crime. It is not uncommon for water receptacles to have a frozen layer in the morning when a warrant is served, but that layer disappears within the first hour after the sun rises. That may not absolve an animal owner from neglect charges if animals are required under the law to have continued access to potable water, but it is something that a scene processor should include in their report and be able to testify about with confidence. If conditions of the site change over the course of the day, owing to changes in the weather, that is likely relevant to the case and should be noted. For example, if it starts raining and you notice the gutter drains directly into a horse stall creating standing water, this will be relevant information for the veterinarian to know when assessing the condition of the horse's feet.

9.2.2.5 Third-Party Animal Owners

There are several types of animal cruelty cases where third-party animal owners play a role, namely breeding and boarding facilities. A third-party owner is an individual, not the suspect(s), who may have an ownership interest in the victim animal(s) in a case. Any information that can be gathered about potential third-party animal owners during the initial investigation phase will reduce the number of challenges arising on the day of the search warrant service and decrease liability for all agencies involved as the investigation continues. Gathering this information during your initial interviews with the suspect will reduce the likelihood that a suspect will transfer ownership later to avoid criminal culpability; this is a particularly common phenomenon in equine neglect cases.

If you are aware of third-party owners, document their information ahead of time along with any identifying information related to the animal(s) they own or co-own who are in the suspect's custody. Make a plan for third-party owners who may respond to the scene of a search warrant execution, such that it does not disrupt your evidence collection process or the security of your scene. Decide ahead of time what documentation you are going to require establishing ownership. The type of documentation may vary depending on the species you are dealing with. You could require copies of contracts, veterinary records, or county licensing documents with the third party listed as the owner of that animal, or anything that connects that third party to a specific identifier on the animal, such as a tattoo, an ear tag, or a microchip.

9.2.2.6 Safety Plan

Search warrants are reliably unpredictable, and it goes without saying that there needs to be a safety plan in place. The safety plan should cover officer safety in serving the warrant and the plan for protecting the civilian agents operating under their direction on scene. Remember the high probability that processing the scene will take the better part of a day, if not every daylight hour; limited resources notwithstanding, do not at any point task a single officer with the impossible responsibility of protecting every nonsworn individual who is assisting with the animal handling or scene processing. It will take more civilians to assist with this warrant than most other criminal search warrants and it is law enforcement's duty to protect them while they are doing so.

You also need to plan to protect people from the animals themselves. Make sure you and others know how you will respond to a dog bite or a kick by a horse. If you are working with exotic species, have a plan of action in mind if someone is bitten or injured by those species where venom may be a factor.

Finally, have a safety plan in place for critically injured or ill animals. These animals will be identified in your initial walk-through and there needs to be a preconceived emergency plan for them. This is discussed in further detail in Sections 9.4.4, 9.5, 9.6.2.1, and Box 9.2.

9.3 Drafting of the Affidavit and Search Warrant

Even the most seasoned law enforcement officer might understandably balk when tasked with authoring an affidavit and search warrant in an animal cruelty case. Obviously, the basic structure and purpose are the same, but there are some nuances to animal crime warrants that are unique and important to incorporate into the format you are already familiar with using (see Appendix C for examples and templates of animal cruelty affidavits and warrants).

9.3.1 Introduction

Animal cruelty cases are probably not the most common cases for which your judges issue search warrants. As a result, they are likely less familiar with the anticruelty laws than they are with other state statutes. To address this, the first part of your affidavit can list the statute number and quote the wording of what constitutes the criminal conduct you are investigating and for which you are seeking to find supporting evidence.

9.3.2 Training and Experience

The "Training and Experience" section of the affidavit is where you can really shine. Resist the urge to cut and paste this section from your past warrants because you need to include all the reasons why you have the expertise to stand behind your statements in the affidavit. In some jurisdictions prosecutors even refer to this as your "hero statement" because it puts to paper that you are uniquely qualified, and maybe even overqualified, to understand the nuances of these crimes and the victim animals connected with them.

Do not discount *any* relevant training or experience you have had with animals or investigation of crimes involving animals. If you were ever a canine officer, that is important to include. If you grew up on a farm, that could become relevant, depending on the case at hand. Start documenting the number of animal calls you respond to because those statistics should be listed in this section. Review your training documentation and highlight courses you have taken that are relevant to animal cases. If you are deficient in training on the topic of animal crime investigation, then seek out ways to bolster this aspect of your skill set (see Appendix D for a list of online courses and certifications about animal behavior, veterinary forensics, and animal cruelty investigation).

9.3.3 Telling the Story

For the majority of animal cruelty cases, seeking a search warrant will not be the first phase of the investigation – meaning the affidavit is usually somewhat lengthy. When you are telling the judge, via the affidavit, what you have discovered during your investigation up to this point, be sure to organize the information in a way that makes it easy to follow. Typically, there are multiple witnesses and numerous visits to the suspect's property. Explain these chronologically and use separate headings for dates or names if you need to. Remember that this document becomes part of the public record and might be relied on by the animal care agency in the future in their pursuit of forfeiture of any seized animals. For these reasons it is important to be thorough in the information you are providing.

Even the most skilled writer cannot convey the details necessary for a third party to fully understand the significance of the existing evidence of the animal cruelty violation. Unless specifically directed not to do so by your prosecutor, you *must* include photos in the body of your affidavit. You also have the option of attaching them as an appendix and incorporating them into the affidavit that way,[7] but that is less effective than including them directly in the body of the document. This way the judge can read your description and then actually visualize and understand what you are trying to explain (Figure 9.1).

9.3.4   Articulate Probable Cause for the Crime(s)

Agencies may format their affidavits differently, but at some point, in the affidavit you must clearly articulate your probable cause for the crime(s) you are investigating and the evidence you expect to find and want to be able to seize. It can be helpful to list the items you would like to be able to seize first (see Section 9.3.5) and, using that list, make sure you are able to explain why you have probable cause for each item on the list.

You can rely on your training and experience, and you can rely on experts to substantiate your probable cause. The following examples[8] are statements you can make in the probable cause section of the affidavit after increasing your animal crime investigation statistics, or acquiring certification or training from any of the courses listed in Appendix D, from interviewing a named veterinarian (Box 9.1), or even from reading this book:

- I know, based on my training and experience, people who fail to provide for the minimum care of their animals as defined by statute often have items such as veterinary records that recommend or prescribe specific treatment that was not followed, or animal medications that have been prescribed but have not been administered to the animal.

Box 9.1   A Note to Veterinarians

Provide Expert Opinion to Law Enforcement

When law enforcement drafts a search warrant in a suspected animal cruelty case the veterinarian is an important contributor of information. In some cases, law enforcement may ask a veterinarian to review evidence including photos, witness statements, or animals prior to writing a warrant. In those cases, the veterinarian's role is to provide the expertise needed to assess evidence presented and offer evaluation of this evidence as well as ask additional questions if they arise. See Chapters 6 and 7 for additional information about the veterinarian's role and forensic examinations.

---

7 If you have the transcription of an interview you want to include or a veterinary report that you are relying on for your probable cause, then this is an appropriate method to include those documents.
8 Acknowledgment to the Oregon Humane Society for case materials provided and used in generating these examples.

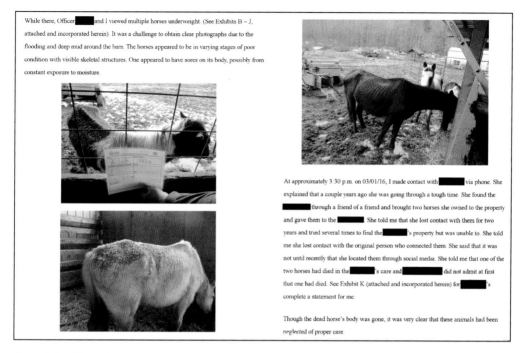

Figure 9.1 Photos incorporated directly into the body of your affidavit help convey the magnitude or severity of the situation. *Source:* Oregon Humane Society.

- I know, based on my training and experience in conducting animal neglect investigations, that people who keep a large number of animals on their property will often house them in vehicles, trailers, and any other structures available to them on the property.
- In my experience, veterinary records and medications are often found in vehicles or other outbuildings on a property containing a large number of animals.
- I know, based on my training and experience, that people who fail to provide the minimum care for their animals can have ample food supply but fail to feed the animal appropriate amounts of food to support health.
- Based on my training and experience, I also know that people who neglect one animal often have other animals in various stages of neglect, and that people who are unable to care for one species of animal on their property are often found to be neglecting all animal species within their control.
- Based on my training and experience, people who shelter or house many animals will bury, conceal, or burn deceased animals on site.
- Based on my interview with veterinarian Dr. Smith, I know that pregnant animals require specialized care and unborn animals can be negatively compromised at birth due to malnourishment and neglect experienced by the pregnant female prior to delivery.
- Based on my training and experience, animals who are victims of abuse and neglect often have a history of abuse and neglect and evidence of this can be found in the radiographs of the animal's body and by performing a thorough examination of the animal. The evidence of abuse or neglect may be in the form of broken bones in various stages of healing, or internal injuries not visible from the exterior of the body.

- Blood chemistry analysis often contains markers that indicate recent injury to tissues, comprehensive radiographs may identify recent as well as healed or healing fractures, and fecal and tissue samples may contain traces of blood or foreign materials, which are often seen in connection with physical injury and/or neglect.

Review the probable cause area of your affidavit being certain that it supports the area you are seeking to search and the evidence you expect to find and would like the authority to seize.

9.3.5 What to Request to Seize

The list of evidence you are requesting to seize will vary from case to case depending on the crime being investigated, the locations to be searched, and the species of victim animals. In an investigation into a failure to provide basic care, the food, medication, animals (dead, living, and unborn), veterinary records, and all items and documents associated with those categories are relevant to that investigation. It is important to educate yourself about the husbandry needs specific to each species on scene. The equipment, food, and medications necessary to maintain an equine in good health are going to be drastically different from those required for a reptile that needs very specific lighting and heat levels in order to survive (see Appendix B for a more comprehensive list of evidence potentially relevant to your animal cruelty investigation that you would want to include in your warrant).

In a physical abuse case, depending on how much you know about the reported incident, there may be particular things you are looking to seize or document in the setting of where the incident occurred. This would include evidence like carpet, flooring, blood spatter on the wall, toenails the animal may have lost in a struggle, scratch marks, weapons, restraints, cages, and fur.

Understand if you are requesting a search warrant for an animal fighting investigation, the evidence those cases are built on is consistent and specific. In some states the possession of the fighting paraphernalia is a crime in and of itself,[9] so it is imperative that you know what constitutes fighting paraphernalia. In a dogfighting case, you would want to include treadmills, medications, steroids, pit walls or flooring, blood samples, match books, restraints, magazines, bite sticks, and breeding records (see sample dogfighting warrant in Appendix C). In cockfighting warrants you need to be able to seize implements used to remove combs and waddles, steroids, medications, sparring blades, muffs, and evidence of bird conditioning (see sample cockfighting warrant in Appendix C). Speak with an expert on these types of investigations in order to ensure you will include all the evidence you are likely to come across.

Some pieces of evidence should almost always be included because they will be relevant regardless of the crime being investigated. The victim animal(s) are relevant evidence of the crime you are investigating. There may be a unique case in which is this not true, but that case is the anomaly not the rule. Include exams and labs associated with those victim animals in your items to seize. You must be able to have a veterinarian examine the victim animal(s) if that will produce additional evidence important to the investigation. Some states might construe a veterinary exam as an additional search [7] so you want to cover the evidence from these exams in your warrant if possible (see Appendix B for a list of evidence typically garnered from a veterinary exam that you might include

---

9 As of January 2021, 25 states criminalize possession of fighting paraphernalia: CA, FL, IL, IN, IA, KS, LA, MD, MI, MS, MO, NE, NH, NJ, NY, OK, OR, PA, SD, TN, TX, UT, VT, and WA.

in your search warrant). Deceased animals on the property could provide necessary insight into the suspect's conduct or pattern of neglect; you need to be able to seize these bodies if they will provide evidence relevant to your case.[10] Also include recently born and unborn animals in your items to seize in virtually every case. There are few animal offenses that would not either disproportionately impact an animal who is pregnant and/or cause lasting negative impact on an unborn and subsequently a newborn or juvenile animal Finally, given the integral role technology has come to play in our lives, nearly every criminal case would benefit from a forensic analysis of the technical devices associated with a suspect, such as cell phones, laptops, hard drives, or tablets.

9.3.6 Where to Request to Search

Animals and animal husbandry equipment can be located almost anywhere on a person's property; it is important to include all the areas you want to be able to search for evidence in your warrant.

9.3.6.1 Small Spaces

Whether you need to search for medications related to an animal neglect investigation, or steroids in an animal fighting investigation, or 150 cats in a one-bedroom apartment in an animal hoarding case, you need to be able to search in all areas of the residence and outbuildings, including tiny spaces in drawers or closets or cabinets. Be sure you are clear in your affidavit why you are likely to find evidence of the crime(s) you are investigating by searching these areas. The following is an example of a statement you can include in your affidavit to help explain why you need this authority to further your investigation:

> I know, based on my training and experience, animals contained in a residence with a large amount of debris and clutter can die of starvation, dehydration, and/or disease in multiple areas of a residence, including but not limited to: small spaces under or behind furniture, on top of shelves or tall furniture, areas in and around stuffed furniture, in any open container, behind bathroom fixtures, in closets, and any other area they are able to fit their body.[11] Based on my training and experience, I know people who have deceased animals in their possession will often keep them in freezers or refrigerators or bury them around the property.

9.3.6.2 Above and Below Ground

Finding deceased animals during an animal cruelty investigation is not uncommon and can provide significant information to an investigator when evaluated by an expert. It is important that you do not lose the opportunity to collect this information because you have not explained in your warrant why you are likely to find evidence both above and below ground on scene. Some perpetrators will attempt to hide deceased animal evidence by burying it on their property. People who hoard animals will often have a designated graveyard area of their property where they bury animals who die in their care. Paying to have a large animal properly rendered

---

10 Finding an elk body in a chest freezer of a suspect known to be a hunter or discovering a decomposing goat body that is not salvageable for a necropsy are examples of deceased animals you would not be likely to recover evidence from for your case and therefore would not be seeking to seize.

11 Acknowledgment to the Oregon Humane Society for case materials provided and used in generating these examples.

can be expensive, and it is not uncommon for people who neglect or abuse livestock to have animal remains buried on their premises. These remains may contain evidence of the animal cruelty you are investigating.

9.3.6.3 Outbuildings

Regardless of the animal crime you are investigating, there is a strong likelihood that you will find additional evidence of that crime in the outbuildings located on the property, in addition to the primary residence. If you are investigating neglect, outbuildings are areas where people would be likely to keep animal food, cleaning supplies, or the animals themselves. Having the authority to search outbuildings when investigating a breeding operation or an animal hoarding situation is extremely important. Animal breeders will operate their entire business from outbuildings on their property; it is where you are likely to find the victim animals and evidence of what care is or is not being provided. Individuals who hoard animals often run out of room in their home to house the animal population and, over time, they are forced to contain them in other outbuildings on their property. In these cases, the outbuilding may also be where the individual houses the deceased animals they are emotionally unable to part with. Farm animal owners, in addition to keeping their animals in barns on their property, frequently use outbuildings to house their animal husbandry supplies. It is crucial to include the authority to search outbuildings in warrants for the crime of animal fighting. Barns, sheds, and detached garages are ground zero for animal fighting events and large amounts of evidence would be lost if a warrant did not authorize investigators to search in those locations.

9.3.6.4 Vehicles

Much like outbuildings, vehicles can contain a wealth of evidence in animal cruelty cases and should be a location you request to search in your warrant. Whether a vehicle on a property is operational or not, it provides additional storage for animal food and caretaking supplies, feed store receipts, or veterinary records that have been left behind, and often even animals themselves or their DNA. Even if the crime you are investigating is not directly tied to a vehicle owned by the suspect, that does not mean it is not likely evidence of the crime will be found in that location. Take time in your affidavit to explain why you think you will find evidence in vehicles on scene. The following are examples of how you can make that connection in your affidavit:

- Based on my training and experience, I know evidence of animal neglect can be found on the premise where the animal is housed, within the animal owner's residence, curtilage, and transportation vehicles. Individuals who have animals in their custody and control often have items such as animal carriers, food, medications, medical records, feed bowls, and photographs of animals in their care, located in various areas of their residence, vehicles, and curtilage.

9.3.7 Who Will Participate

In the vast majority of animal cruelty search warrant executions, law enforcement will need significant assistance from non-law enforcement individuals. Make sure it is clear in your warrant you will be using animal handling experts, veterinary experts, and animal transporters to assist with the safe execution of the warrant. You would also include other government agencies that may be present and participating, such as code enforcement or department of human services.

Including these "civilian" agents in the warrant prevents future confusion or debate as to who was permitted to be on scene and assisting with the case.[12]

9.3.8 What Laws to Reference and How

Just as traditional law enforcement and prosecutors do not encounter animal cruelty cases on a regular basis, neither do judges, and it is important to remind them of the applicable laws. In the preamble of your affidavit you can insert the statutory language of the relevant animal crimes you are investigating. This gives the judge better context when reading the rest of your affidavit and increases their understanding of what evidence you are seeking to search for and seize.

It is also important to include statutory references to forfeiture or foreclosure laws implicated by your seizure of animals. If your state's forfeiture law includes an element that animals must be seized under a specific statute, then make clear that this statute is the authority you are making this request under. If there are certain crimes listed in your forfeiture law as eligible for this remedy, articulate that in your affidavit *and* your warrant documents. Make it abundantly clear that your seizure of animals falls under the circumstances that your state's forfeiture or foreclosure laws were designed to address. The following is an example of what that statement in your affidavit and warrant document might look like:

> I respectfully request that the Court specifically authorize the LOCAL HUMANE SOCIETY to impound all animals located on the premises under STATUTE AUTHORIZING SEIZURE, with the understanding that the LOCAL HUMANE SOCIETY may/will use other animal care providers as their agents to help fulfill their obligations under IMPOUNDED ANIMAL CARE STATUTE.

9.3.9 Prosecutor Role

While there may be formulaic warrants that you author in the course of your duties (i.e. driving under the influence of intoxicants [DUII] warrants) that may not be reviewed by a prosecutor prior to meeting with a judge, animal cruelty affidavits and warrants are very case specific and detailed and should be reviewed by a prosecutor prior to being put in front of a judge. This is an important step given the prosecutor who reviews the warrant is likely to be the prosecutor assigned to the case and to pursue forfeiture if a seizure of animals does occur. The prosecutor will have their own checklist in mind when reviewing your warrant that will act to strengthen the documents and decrease the vulnerability at or before trial.

9.3.10 Taking It to the Judge

Even if you are accustomed to bringing search warrants to judges in your jurisdiction, animal cruelty warrants may result in varying and unexpected reactions from reviewing judges. Be prepared

---

12 *State vs. Fay*, WL 7051326, (2020) – the court found that civilians assisting with the warrant execution did not violate the Fourth Amendment but "[I]t may be wise for officers to notify the issuing magistrate of the fact that civilians will assist in a warrant's execution, when it is possible to do so." https://www.animallaw.info/case/state-v-fay (accessed 9 August 2021).

to navigate these differing reactions respectfully. Some judges find the evidence presented to be extremely compelling and emotionally difficult to review. Other judges might be critical of the length of the documents, or the resources dedicated to these investigations. It is important for the author of the warrant to be deferential and respectful but confident enough to educate the judge about the information included and the reasons for including that information. Ultimately, this search warrant must stand up to attempts to excise, suppress, and controvert. If you are thorough, fair, and clear in your generation of the affidavit and the warrant it will be a solid foundation from which to build your case.

9.4 Before You Serve the Warrant

Serving any search warrant always involves planning ahead but serving search warrants in animal cruelty cases is likely to involve nontraditional partners and more nuanced considerations with respect to safety and evidence documentation and handling.

9.4.1 Aerial Maps

Together with the animal care experts and the veterinarian, law enforcement should review aerial maps of the property listed in the search warrant. From a public safety perspective this will be helpful to law enforcement in planning the approach to the property and areas vulnerable to nefarious activity. These aerial maps are easily available from free mapping programs found on the Internet.

9.4.2 Plan Your Process (Expect It to Change)

Another benefit of reviewing the aerial maps is their usefulness in planning for your process. If you are going to have to remove horses, for example, who are large and easily startled, you can make a plan, using the aerial maps, of the route for removing the victim horses, where the evidence documentation station should be located, and where the trailers will be able to fit in order to load the victim horses with the least amount of risk to their safety or others. You can identify outbuildings that need to be searched or areas that seem likely to contain buried animals or burned animal remains. Once you can visualize the property you can try to imagine how the search and seizure would logistically be carried out and in the safest way. Inevitably these plans will change with what you actually encounter on the scene, but you will be more nimbly able to adapt when you already have a strong familiarity with the layout of the property and an idea of how you want the process to flow. Visualizing the process ahead of time will also help ensure that your system will capture all of the information you need for your case. Thinking through the process ahead of time will guarantee that the animals will be photographed on scene, that the pond in the back 40 will be documented with photographs and video, that transport vehicles can move in and out in an orderly fashion, and that all members of the search warrant execution team can be kept safe by the officers while carrying out their duties on scene. Overall, this will ensure that the scene will be processed methodically.

9.4.3 The Little Things

With so many moving parts, it is often the most basic aspects of search warrant service preparation that get forgotten or left until the last minute. In order to avoid this phenomenon, create a search warrant packing list or checklist or use the one provided in Appendix B so you can rest assured you will not find yourself without something you need to do your job on scene. A key detail to include on your checklist is to charge the batteries on anything and everything that needs to be charged. At this time, you can consider how long you expect the warrant execution to take and whether or not you need to make a plan for additional battery charging. This stage in the warrant planning is also a good time to double check the settings on the cameras you will be using. If there is a time and date field, confirm that it has been updated since the last daylight savings event. You also want to check the settings for the file type and size on the cameras to make sure they work with the computer systems the law enforcement agency and prosecutor will be using and are familiar with. It is also important to have storage backups for cameras if you fill up an SD card on scene but still have photographs that need to be taken. If you cannot afford to have multiple backups, then make a plan for uploading the photos to a computer or flash drive on scene so you can continue to take photographs of the evidence and the scene without having to ration your available storage space.

With the need for civilians to assist with the execution of the warrant comes the need for multiple staging locations. Make sure to find a space that can accommodate an initial briefing on the morning of the warrant service that can be attended by all parties assisting on the scene and in a location where confidentiality is easy to maintain. Typically, these briefings would occur at the law enforcement precinct in a conference room or a law enforcement training facility. There also needs to be a designated staging area near the warrant service location where assisting civilians can wait while law enforcement enters the property and serves the warrant. Once the scene has been secured the processing team will respond to the property from this location. Examples of suitable staging areas are the parking lots of churches, fire departments, or schools. On occasion the staging area may just be the shoulder of a road near the warrant location. This is not ideal, however, because while law enforcement is in the process of serving the warrant the individuals waiting to assist are discussing their roles on scene, reviewing the warrant, collaborating, and fine tuning the plan for processing, and will benefit from an area that is large and safe enough to facilitate this use of time. The nature of transport vehicles is also a factor to consider when choosing a staging location.

9.4.4 Prepare for the Unexpected

Do not be thrown off by the unexpected. Regardless of how much time you put into planning your processes and strategies there will be events and circumstances you encounter on the scene that you have not accounted for; do not let this derail you. There are certain measures you can take to set yourself up to successfully manage surprises on the scene. Make a list of the closest animal supply stores, animal feed stores, and emergency veterinary clinics. If you are responding to a scene where livestock animals will potentially be found, make sure you have contact information on hand for a large-animal veterinarian. The lead law enforcement officer on the case should be openly communicating with the animal care agency about the number and nature of the animals expected and should be inquiring about the plan if more animals are discovered. Bring more PPE than you expect you will need, but do not use up valuable transport space by overpacking. Think ahead about designating someone as the runner if you encounter a need for more supplies or additional transport so that you can adapt quickly. Make everyone aware that the scene-processing plan is fluid, and they should be prepared to adapt given the circumstances found on scene. Assisting individuals need to understand the chain-of-command system on the scene and who they look to when unexpected situations arise. Empowering the team with that knowledge will allow them to meet these challenges in a calm and organized fashion, rather than becoming overwhelmed or frustrated.

9.4.5 Multijurisdictional Partnerships

The necessity to partner with multiple agencies across diverse disciplines to successfully serve a search warrant in an animal cruelty case is unavoidable. The law enforcement agencies bring expertise in the legal requirements of search and seizure, evidence collection protocols, interviewing techniques, and general scene safety, and as such can create a plan for those elements. Law enforcement needs to rely on other agencies and individuals to lend their expertise and resources to other aspects of the warrant service, such as placement of live animal evidence, storage of deceased or nonlive animal evidence, and response to unexpected species found on scene.

9.4.5.1 Placement of Animals

Regardless of the number of animals involved in a case, finding placement for the living evidence associated with the case – the animal(s) – can be the deciding factor in whether or not pursuing a search warrant is a viable option in the investigation of a criminal situation. Smaller, under-resourced counties may not have a county animal shelter and instead rely on local veterinarians to house the animals from their cases. In other counties, cases involving a significant number of animals may need to be placed in multiple nearby (or far) shelters. In either case, advanced communication and a baseline plan around where and with whom the animals will be placed needs to occur prior to serving the warrant. That is not to say plans will not change once you know exactly how many and what type of animals you are needing placement for, but because it is such a logistically intensive aspect of a successful warrant service, the partnerships need to be established prior to service.

9.4.5.2 Storage of Evidence

Depending on the case, you might need storage for deceased animals of varying sizes. If this is a possibility, look to partner with a university, with a veterinary school, or contact local shelters and animal clinics to determine what might be available to you on the day of the warrant service.

9.4.5.3 Unexpected Species

There are certain types of animal cruelty cases that tend to involve multiple species and unique species. If you are planning to serve a search warrant at a pet store, you should plan ahead for species you are not familiar with or not expecting. Cases involving a person who hoards animals can often include wildlife that have been domesticated by the suspect and, going into that warrant service, you should know who the wildlife rehabilitators are in your area and whether they are certified to care for and house these types of animals. It is ideal if you can partner with a veterinarian who has a broad range of experience with varying species and who will be able to triage the animals you find on scene, giving you time to connect with a specialty veterinarian for continued care and placement.

9.4.5.4 Clarity of Expectations

It is extremely important to be clear about what you expect these partners to provide on the scene and during the continued investigation. The average veterinary clinic or animal shelter is not going to have experience responding to a crime scene or managing evidence that has been removed from a crime scene. Law enforcement officers must have clear and timely communication around the needs of the case. You cannot assume that a veterinarian will conduct an exam and generate a report, or that an animal shelter understands not to adopt out or neuter an animal from a case. Equally, the veterinary and animal welfare entities must be clear to law enforcement about the feasibility of this assistance, the parameters of what they can offer, and any questions they have about any part of the process.

9.4.6 Confirm Veterinary and Animal Handler Experts

The sooner you can provide the veterinary and animal handler experts a description of their job on scene and post warrant execution, the better (Box 9.2). With this information, those entities can work together to come up with a plan that best helps them to safely and accurately assist on scene and afterward (see Appendix C for templates of job descriptions for civilian agents necessary for service of an animal cruelty search warrant). It would be helpful to provide an explanation of the incident command system at this time as well (see Appendix C for a template you can use to explain how incident command should work on a crime scene and who in your organization falls into what role in that command scheme).

9.4.7 Plan for Known Aggressive Animals

(See Section 9.2 "Prewarrant Considerations" at the beginning of this chapter for a review of why it is necessary to plan for known aggressive animals.)

9.4.8 Assess Need for Personal Protective Equipment

In addition to human waste and debris, search warrant executors will encounter all nature of animal feces, urine, ammonia, blood, parasites, and bacteria. In many cases the filth created by the animals will be multiple layers deep and found in small, unventilated rooms or areas.

Box 9.2   A Note to Veterinarians

Prepare to Assist with Warrant Service

A veterinarian who has agreed to assist a law enforcement agency with the execution of a search warrant should invest time preparing to fill the role that is expected of them. The veterinarian should prepare a list of items to take with them to the crime scene beyond the standard medical equipment of stethoscope, thermometer, and penlight (see Medical Exam Equipment Checklist in Appendix B). With the approval of the lead law enforcement agency, the veterinarian should also create a plan that includes referral to a local veterinary hospital for animals who are in immediate jeopardy or agonal. This plan might need to include prearrangements for payment and documentation. Always be aware that the impending warrant service is confidential and law enforcement should be aware of any proposed arrangements, including planning for transport and storage of deceased animals.

In all cases a briefing to discuss what is included in the warrant is held prior to the search. The veterinarian should inquire about the time and place of the briefing and plan to attend. Do not hesitate to ask to review what the warrant allows for in terms of permissible areas to search and what items to search for. Does it include animals, medications, records, computers, freezer, and refrigerator contents and so on? The veterinarian must know what is included so they are aware of what they are authorized to do on the scene. In some cases, an evidence collection team and other experts will be available to assist the veterinarian and in other cases the veterinarian may bring a veterinary assistant from their clinic. Prior to the warrant service the veterinarian and law enforcement should discuss who will be working the scene and what each person's role will be. Coordinating with other evidence collection professionals prior to starting the search saves missteps, avoids mistakes, and improves efficiency in what can be a long and detailed activity.

9.5   Preservice Briefing

Once you have drafted a thorough warrant, have received authority to serve it by a judge, and have engaged in all the preplanning possible, your warrant service day should begin with a briefing. This briefing should involve all entities who will be on the scene during the execution of the warrant. The location of the briefing should be a place where everyone can be present and confidential discussions can take place.

Law enforcement is accustomed to briefing before a warrant service to discuss the risk assessment, incident command roles, and an entry plan. However, many of the individuals who will be assisting you and whose expertise you are relying on likely do not participate in search warrant executions regularly or ever. Add agenda items to the briefing so that everyone involved is aware of important laws and considerations that are relevant to this event. It is law enforcement's job to educate the people who are assisting them so there are no missteps that might jeopardize the evidence collected during the execution of the warrant. Time spent underscoring some of these imperative reminders is necessary and should be accounted for in the schedule of the day.

This briefing is the ideal venue to explain the gravity of the situation to your processing team. The right to privacy in our homes (and in certain other areas of our lives) is enshrined in the Constitution. Search warrants are a legal way to penetrate that protection, granting certain individuals the authority to investigate a crime. This is *not* something that should be taken lightly, and the law does not take it lightly; any missteps can result in losing some or all of the evidence you find. If anyone assisting with the execution of the warrant accesses an area that is not covered by the warrant or removes property not included in the warrant, it could undermine the evidentiary value of all property removed under the authority of that warrant. Help them understand that you are forcing someone to let you on their property and into their home to search through rooms and containers that are personal to them. They must be professional and respectful at all times (see Appendix D for an outline of a preservice briefing in an animal case).

Read the warrant out loud to everyone during the preservice briefing. By reading the warrant you are ensuring that there is no misunderstanding of what areas are permissible to search and what you are allowed to seize. If you know of areas on the property that are not covered by the warrant, be sure to point out those areas. Similarly, if you know the warrant does not authorize you to search in small containers, make sure the processing team is aware of that parameter prior to entering the scene.

A reminder that is helpful to law enforcement and civilian partners alike is that the scene is a crime scene, and you should treat it as such. If you would not allow third parties to walk around and through a crime scene on a drug warrant or a warrant in a homicide case, then you should not permit it on this warrant. Making it clear that the animals themselves are evidence is a critical component of this. Law enforcement and scene processors should refrain from taking selfies with the animals or kissing, hugging, feeding, or moving them. Unless your organization specifically allows cell phones to be used to document the evidence and the scene in a warrant service, then all participants should be told not to use cell phones outside of communication with approved parties.

Humor can be a coping mechanism when individuals are confronted with distressing or stressful circumstances. Therefore, during a preservice briefing, the facilitator should caution against joking or laughing while at the scene. Photography and videography are on-going throughout the execution, as well as a possibility of media presence, and joking and laughing can be misinterpreted or painted in a bad light. Members of the media listen to police scanners and learn where search warrants are being carried out. Owing to the public interest in animal cruelty cases, it is not uncommon for members of the media to show up to the scene. Make certain anyone assisting in the search warrant knows who the point of contact to the media is and that they should not engage with the media while they are carrying out their duties on the scene.

With the opportunity of having everyone in the room at the same time, take time to make sure the roles on the scene are clear.[13] Use a whiteboard or a visual aid to lay out the incident command points of contact and go around the room and confirm every person can articulate their role in the process and can identify the person to whom they report. During this part of the briefing, you can clarify who is permitted to talk with or approach the suspect. Typically, this will be a very short list of people. In turn, make sure those people know what to do if the responding veterinarian has questions for the suspect about a particular animal or in responding to an emergency situation occurring on the scene with an animal.

Finally, make sure to review the safety plan. This plan extends beyond officer safety in serving the warrant and covers the plan for ensuring the safety of the civilian partners on the scene, for as long as they are on the scene. Part of this plan should also include the plan for any safety risks posed by the animals to the people on scene.

9.6 Serving the Warrant

After your preservice briefing, everyone should depart from the briefing location and convene at the designated staging area near the location listed on the warrant. At this point, the law enforcement officers assigned to assist with serving the warrant and securing the scene will proceed to the warrant location. It is worthwhile to note that several law enforcement personnel should be stationed with the civilian assisting partners at the staging area while the warrant is served. This is for safety reasons as well as ease of communication with the scene.

9.6.1 Serving the Warrant

The officer who authored the warrant should be the individual to serve the warrant, along with additional law enforcement officers, for safety reasons. Traditional law enforcement agencies will have detailed protocols on serving a warrant to an individual. Of course, department policy should be adhered to in all cases. There are a few reminders worth underscoring. It is this moment where your planning with respect to any guard dogs gets put to the test. If you encounter the guard dogs that you expected, do not lose yourself in the adrenaline of the situation and forget that you have a plan in place. If you encounter guard dogs you did not expect, you should have a plan for that as well.[14]

Once you have safely reached the main access point to the residence or building, be sure to engage in a practice known as "knock and announce." Unless a search warrant authorizes otherwise, law enforcement is required to knock at the entryway to the property and announce that they are law enforcement there to serve a search warrant [8]. Part of serving the warrant includes securing the scene. On these search warrants law enforcement *must* be overly thorough in this endeavor, keeping in mind that the scene-processing team is not composed of

---

13 See Appendix C for job descriptions of on scene roles.
14 See Section 9.2 on "Prewarrant Considerations."

sworn officers equipped with firearms and defensive tactics training. Veterinarians and animal handlers and evidence technicians will be accessing every authorized area in the warrant and will not always be accompanied by a law enforcement officer. Secure the scene to the greatest extent possible and then make the call to the staging area to begin the next phase – executing the search warrant.

9.6.2 Scene Processing

Depending on the nature of the scene and the animals involved, once it is secure you may choose to stagger the people who are responding to the scene from the staging area. You could first approve a small group of individuals to engage in the initial steps of the warrant execution and call in the larger group of scene processors after the initial steps are completed. There are advantages, however, to calling the entire scene-processing group to the scene, which allows time for discussions about adjustments to premade plans and for set-up to occur while a select few engage in the initial walk-through phase.

9.6.2.1 Initial Walk-Through

One of the first things the lead officer on the case needs to do, after the scene has been secured, is take the lead veterinarian on a walk-through of the scene. The walk-through with the veterinarian is multifunctional. In order for the officer to understand what evidence is subject to seizure and what is not, the officer needs the expertise of the veterinarian. In doing the walk-through of the scene, the veterinarian should be taking copious notes, or dictating to a scribe or recording device, to facilitate an accurate report, and so the officer can properly interpret the scene. The initial walk-through is a time when the veterinarian can respond to any emergency situations involving suffering, sick, or injured animals. If there is an emergency situation involving an animal and the veterinarian identifies it as such, do not delay medical assistance to that animal. The evidence-processing/documenting team should be called over immediately to document the condition and location of the animal, but the medical well-being of the animal is paramount.

A person from the assisting animal care agency should also accompany the lead officer and the veterinarian on the initial walk-through. It is relevant for the organization that will be capturing, identifying, and housing the animals to visualize the layout with respect to where the animals are located and hear the veterinarian's initial assessment. This walk-through will also inform any changes that need to be made to the original evidence-processing plan (Box 9.3).

Box 9.3   Case Example

In this case example, the warrant execution team arrived on scene prepared to seize up to 40 dogs and puppies from a substandard rescue organization's warehouse. The initial walk-through revealed that the warehouse contained over 150 dogs and puppies. The witness who had reported the conditions inside the warehouse that led to the search warrant had entered the warehouse on a day when most of the dogs were offsite at adoption events. After the initial walk-through the execution team arranged for additional handlers, transport vehicles, and carriers to be dispatched to the scene.

9.6.2.2 Veterinarian's Role: Initial Walk-Through

During the initial walk-through of the scene the veterinarian will identify emergent medical cases, help assess the workload, and fine-tune the plan for processing the animal evidence. During this walk-through, the veterinarian will be discussing with the lead law enforcement agent any observations they make that are relevant to the statutes and evidence listed in the warrant. Collection and recording of information during the warrant search is a required part of the veterinarian's duty and is the final goal beyond assisting the animals and people involved. Assigning an assistant to help scribe, photograph, or record video facilitates the collection of information and helps to ensure that even large volumes of information are recorded efficiently and accurately. Documentation must include live evidence (animals), deceased animals, and all animal-related materials. The veterinarian must be thorough in the details they record – time, date, temperature, and all relevant environmental findings, such as:

- Inventory of food and water available (including type and quantities and feed samples)
- Fecal samples
- Medications
- Observations about housing:
  - Space
  - Exposure to elements, danger, or stress
  - Size
  - Shape
  - Indoor or outdoor
  - Temperature
  - Sanitation
  - Access to food and water
  - Bedding
- Exercise notes and any relevant behavior and training information.

The veterinarian should document how they received the information they are documenting. Did they interview the owner, or did an officer tell them, or did they garner it from someone else's medical records? Were they on scene and observed these items?

> Example: Upon entering the warehouse, I noted that 11 cats and 15 kittens were housed in traditional travel kennels that measured approximately 14 by 20 inches and approximately 10 inches tall. No food, water, or bedding was found in any of the six carriers examined. All kennels were of the same make and model. Each kennel floor was covered in feces and urine, which was also found on the paws and ventral (belly side) of the abdomens of each of the animals. Photos of the kennels and an inventory of animals/kennel accompany this report.

9.7 Start Documenting the Scene

9.7.1 Temperature

Upon accessing the scene, document the temperature outside and in buildings housing animals. Temperature can factor into assessments of adequate shelter, bedding, and water. Given that the temperature is likely to change it is worthwhile to document it as the scene processing is carried out over the course of the day.

9.7.2 Map

Assign someone to draw a map of the property or, alternatively, adapt an aerial drawing to show the layout you are witnessing the day of the warrant execution. The map should also reflect the customized location identifiers you will be assigning to each building or area housing animals and, if possible, the units within that area being used to house animals. This map will be referenced multiple times during the warrant execution, several times after you have left the scene, and potentially during trial. Make sure that it is legible and as clear as possible. Use graph paper if you are going to draw a map. Adapting an aerial map is not ideal but preferable to a hand-drawn map that is poorly done and difficult to understand (Figure 9.2).

9.7.3 Initial Scene Video

The initial scene video should be a priority once you have accessed the property. This video is important because your warrant process may take a long time depending on the number of animals and/or their temperament. The video will capture the scene the way it was when you first entered the property. It can help refute claims that the animals' kennels became filled with feces over the course of the day, or that the warrant service team damaged some aspect of the property, or that an animal sustained an injury during the course of the warrant process. Body camera footage is not an adequate substitute for the initial scene video.

Ideally this video is taken as one long recording without interruption so it is clear you are capturing everything. There are rare circumstances in which the scene layout allows for this, but best efforts should be made to stop and start as little as possible. Be sure to include the address and other identifying markers of the property so it is clear that the property matches the one described in the warrant. It can also be helpful if the videographer states their name and the date at the beginning of each video. This identifies who can authenticate the footage later and can resolve any questions arising out of inaccurate date and time stamps attached to the footage.

Take your time when recording the property. Multiple individuals will be reviewing this footage at various stages in the case, and you want to provide a useful resource that does not inspire motion sickness in the audience. Walk slowly and pause frequently to give the camera time to focus. This video takes a long time to create, but other processes can begin simultaneously, so do not feel rushed to complete it.

Educate yourself about the audio features of the video-recording tool you are using before you need to use it on scene. For a couple of reasons, it is important to know whether audio will be picked up when you are recording. You do not want any chatter recorded on your video that could be misinterpreted or misconstrued later. Make sure to announce yourself when you enter an area with other individuals present and let them know you are recording. Another consideration is the laws in your state about recording the suspect without their knowledge. Make sure you are aware if you are picking up the suspect's statements in the audio of your video and understand what disclosure requirements your state has about that situation.

9.8 System for Evidence Documentation and Processing

Every location and case are going to be different and thus your plan for evidence documentation and processing may adapt to accommodate those differences, but there are fundamentals of the process that should be consistent through every animal cruelty search warrant you execute.

(a)

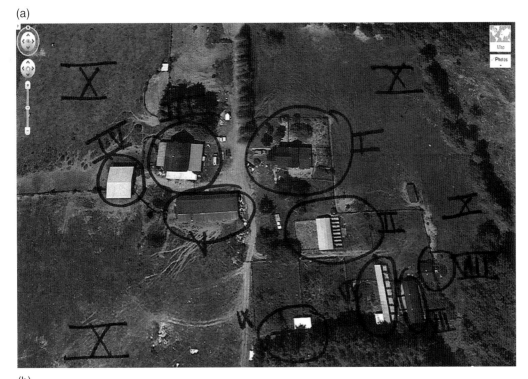

(b)

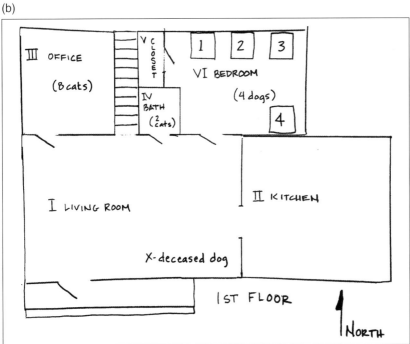

Figure 9.2 Depending on the size of the property, using an aerial map instead of a hand-drawn map may be preferable, though a hand-drawn map allows for inclusion of more details about the location. *Source:* Oregon Humane Society.

9.8.1   Document Conditions

In many animal cruelty cases, the location where the animal(s) are housed onsite is directly related to the alleged criminal violation, so do not rush the documentation of the conditions. While someone is taking the scene video, another person should be taking general photos of the scene and of the areas and items the veterinarian has indicated are relevant to the animals' condition.

9.8.2   Separate Crime Scenes

Any enclosures or areas where animals are kept should be treated as individual crime scenes. For example, if you open the door to an outbuilding on the property and discover eight dog runs containing multiple dogs in each run, then each of those eight enclosures should be given a separate identifier and not lumped in with "Outbuilding I" as a singular crime scene or area. This is important is because what is provided to the animals in each area can be drastically different. For example, the dogs in the eighth enclosure are aggressive such that the suspect did not want to enter to clean out the enclosure and just dumped the food over the wall onto the floor to feed them, whereas the dogs in the second enclosure are friendly and their area has clearly been cleaned more frequently.

If possible, attach the assigned unique identifier to each enclosure or area so everyone processing the scene refers to the area in the same way. One method of labeling the separate enclosures or kennels is with a small hang tag that indicates the larger crime scene (e.g. "Outbuilding I") and then the smaller enclosure within that outbuilding (e.g. "Unit 1") (Figure 9.3).

In cases where the animals have free rein to move around an entire building or residence, then that whole location becomes the crime scene because all the resources (or lack thereof) in that location are what has been available to that population of animals, and it is where they have been residing.

Once the areas are labeled, take photos of the animals in each enclosure. If you can get the crime scene designation in the photo with the animals that is one option, otherwise take a photo of the location identifier and then a photo (or photos) of the animals contained therein (Figure 9.4).

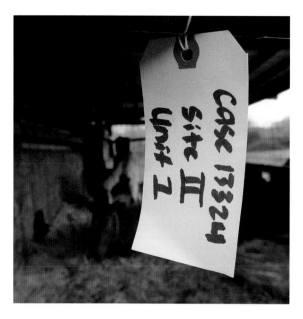

Figure 9.3   Once this identifier is attached, each photo or video series taken of this area should capture the information on the tag so it can be referenced in the future in connection with the animals housed there. *Source:* Oregon Humane Society.

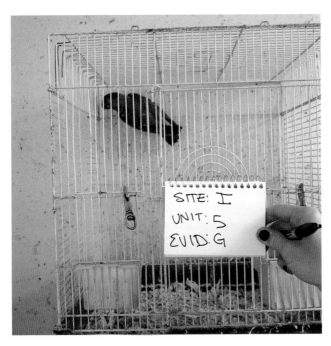

Figure 9.4 Identifying the animal and including the habitat in the photo provides documentation of the violation(s), with the victim animal uniquely identified before the evidence has left the scene. This can become extremely valuable to the case if there are future issues with chain of custody resulting in evidence suppression. *Source:* Oregon Humane Society.

Once the animals have been removed from the enclosure, assign someone to go back to each area and thoroughly document the conditions inside each enclosure. Take pictures from the four corners of the enclosure, if possible, and any areas relevant to the cruelty violations being investigated.

9.9 Processing the Animals

Once the documentation of the animals in the conditions you found them in is completed, removal of the animals can begin. The exception to this is if the veterinarian previously identified an animal in need of emergency medical care, in which case that animal should have been attended to immediately. Law enforcement officers should always defer to the animal-handling experts on the order and method of removing animals.

9.9.1 Veterinarian's Role: Animal Processing on Scene

Once the walk-through is complete the veterinarian should participate in the determination of a safe and secure area to set up the onsite process of evidence collection and physical exam.

Consider lighting, interference of sound, temperature, and access to other experts in working the scene. For example, if you are processing cats from a hoarding scene, you may need a lighted area set up inside a garage to provide coverage and prevent escape of animals. If you are processing a scene with 25 large and vocal dogs, setting up in an area in which the noise is buffered enough to allow good communication between people would be best.

Once a work area is set up, the veterinarian will meet with the individuals they will be working with, clarify the process, and each person's role and responsibilities. On scene examinations must be as consistent as possible and for that reason may be truncated. If only critical parts of the exam will be done on scene, the veterinarian will complete a more comprehensive exam later, but within 24 hours of the search warrant execution, if possible. For consistency and to prevent confusion, use the same form for both exams and be clear about what procedures are done in each circumstance. For instance, when processing rabbits from a hoarding case the veterinarian may determine that signalment including sex and approximate age will be collected on the scene so that the animals can be appropriately separated, and the full exam will be done the next day at a shelter or veterinary hospital. The form should include a specific area to indicate the next steps and a color-coding system that helps prioritize medical needs and/or categorize behavioral observations immediately.

> Example of animal processing on scene: Each dog will be leashed and walked to the examination station. The veterinary assistants will identify and collar each dog. The evidence tech and assistant will take identifying photos of each dog. Once these steps are complete the veterinarian will do an onsite exam that includes the following parameters: collect signalment (age, breed, sex, description), scan for microchip, record animal ID number from collar.

9.9.2 Order of Removal

It is important to be thoughtful about how the animals are removed and transported from the scene. There are several factors the individual appointed as the logistics coordinator should be taking into consideration when making the plan for animal removal. You want to consider factors related to the animals themselves, such as temperament and vulnerability with respect to age or medical conditions. It is also important to factor in the resources available to you in the way of handlers, transportation vehicles, and transport kennels. If animals will be transported to different animal care facilities, you must consider the distance the animals will have to travel, and the impact weather could have on that journey. Capturing animals in waning light or after dark drastically increases the difficulty of that endeavor and a logistics coordinator should always be aware of how many daylight hours remain in contrast with how many animals remain. For example, it might make sense to load and transport the horses on scene who are familiar with being handled first instead of spending many initial hours attempting to capture and load the more fearful horses first.

9.9.3 Process of Removal

Using a methodical process to remove the animals ensures few mistakes and reliable evidence. Due to unpredictable factors like temperament or illness you may have to deviate from your ideal plan for removal. Generally speaking, your evidence processing station should be located close to where the animals are being removed so handlers can stop at the station with the animal to complete the necessary documentation. The handler should take note of the area the animal was

---

Box 9.4 Tip

Many organizations choose to assign a letter or combination of letters to each animal as a unique identifier. The animal can then be given a name beginning with that letter, which makes it easy for caretakers to remember the animal's evidentiary identifier.

---

removed from and inform the evidence technicians of that location. Then the animal should be assigned a unique evidence identifier (Box 9.4) and have his/her photo taken with an evidence placard indicating the location on scene and the ID assigned. Depending on the species and temperament, this is the point where you would affix something to the animal, a paper collar for example, that displays their unique identifier. Ideally, the paper evidence placard used for that animal's photo can be taped or adhered to their transport kennel so staff on the receiving end can easily identify and document them.

When you have animals whose temperaments or medical condition prevent them from being processed in the typical manner, do your best to uphold as many aspects of that process as you can. If an animal had to be captured and put directly into a carrier, then take a photo of the animal in the carrier. Instead of attaching the collar to the animal, you can attach it to the carrier. Always make sure the evidence technicians know when an animal is removed from the scene so they can account for that removal. It is vitally important to take at least one identifying photo on the scene of every animal removed. The crime scene is not the time to engage in extensive veterinary exams and full photo documentation of the animal you are removing, but an identifying photo should be a static part of your process.

9.10 Forms

Documentation is the backbone of evidence collection and chain of custody. The following outlines several forms that can be helpful and utilized during the execution of a search warrant in an animal cruelty case. You do not have to use all these forms in order to process a scene successfully and thoroughly. In fact, do not employ a documentation process that is either so cumbersome or complicated that it results in frequent mistakes or inconsistent use on the scene, which in turn creates a vulnerability in your case. Templates for these forms can be found in Appendix B.

9.10.1 Property in Custody Form

This is a standard form used in traditional law enforcement to document any property you are taking into custody belonging to the suspect. Generally, these forms are not created with live animal evidence in mind. Decide how you are going to categorize and identify the animals on the form prior to going on the scene. Also, remember the items connected with the animal – collars, for example – are also property that you need to include. If the animal is of a certain species, you might be removing the animal in the habitat it is currently being housed in, and the habitat should therefore be entered on the Property in Custody form as well. For example, if you are seizing a bearded dragon and the aquarium he was housed in on the scene, you would include the bearded dragon and the aquarium on the Property in Custody form and list the items contained in the aquarium such as a water/food dish or attached light fixture.

9.10.2 Camera Log

If scene processors are going to be sharing cameras it can be helpful to have a camera log located at the evidence-processing station where the cameras are signed in and out. This is helpful for authentication purposes if the case ends up going to trial. It is also helpful when the witnesses are generating their statements to know what photographs or video they took on scene that day. Alternative options would include specific processors assigned to a single camera or designated SD cards for cameras. It is generally not a good idea to use a personal or agency-issued cell phone when documenting a crime scene during a search warrant. Doing so could result in that phone being catalogued as evidence for the case, and evidence photographs become commingled with personal photographs.

9.10.3 Habitat Evaluation Form

When the investigation involves how animals have been housed or maintained, then extra effort should be made to thoroughly document that on scene. In addition to the photographs of the enclosures housing animals – both before and after the animals are removed – you can have an animal husbandry expert fill out a Habitat Evaluation form noting what is present in the enclosure for the animal in the way of food, water, bedding, size, light source, and how clean it looks and smells. This can capture information you may accidentally miss in photographs or video (Figure 9.5).

(b)

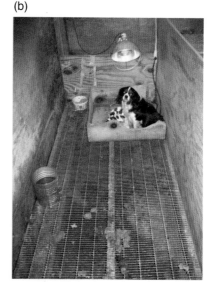

(a)

SITE:	II	RUN / CAGE / YARD / (OTHER) Pen
UNIT:	11	DIMENSIONS (APPROXIMATE): ~3' x 8'
# ANIMALS:	6	FLOORING MATERIAL: wire
FOOD:	(YES) / NO	OBSERVATIONS: Full food bowl
WATER:	(YES) / NO	OBSERVATIONS: Old tin can, clear water
BEDDING:	YES / (NO)	OBSERVATIONS: Potato's in a wood box with a metal heating pad.
SHELTER:	# 0	OBSERVATIONS: No additional shelter
FECES:	(YES) / NO	OBSERVATIONS: Copious amounts of fecal matter, ~6-7 bowel movements piled on the wire.
URINE:	(YES) / NO	OBSERVATIONS: Pools of urine under kennel.

Figure 9.5   Using a habitat evaluation form ensures that the scene processing team is collecting all the relevant information for each enclosure and helps to capture aspects that photos or videos cannot, such as ammonia level, dampness, or temperature. *Source:* Oregon Humane Society.

9.10.4 Transport Inventory

The transport inventory serves two purposes. First, it substantiates a link in the chain of custody; and, second, it confirms that every animal who was loaded into the vehicle also came out of the vehicle. These inventory sheets serve to be even more helpful when the animals are going to different animal care facilities or foster homes because they create a clear record of which animals were sent where.

9.10.5 Notice Language

Some state forfeiture or foreclosure statutes require that the suspect be given notice of those remedies available to the state and animal caregivers on the day the animals are removed from the suspect's custody. Providing the suspect with a printout of the language in the statute does not require any questioning, but the officer who delivers this information to the suspect should mention doing so in their crime report to create a record that the notice was provided. If other officers or witnesses were present, they should also include this detail in their reports or statements. Check with your prosecutor ahead of time to inquire whether any notice requirement might pertain to the animals in the case for which you are serving the warrant (see Chapter 15 for additional information on forfeiture and foreclosure).

9.10.6 Confidentiality Forms

Many of animal cruelty cases, it takes several people to execute a search warrant safely, efficiently, and effectively. Most of these people will not be traditional law enforcement officers who are familiar with the confidentiality requirements of the investigation. By bringing confidentiality forms for the scene processors who are civilians you are both educating them about the importance of this and documenting their agreement to comply. Passing out these agreements and getting them signed during the initial briefing is ideal because all the parties will be present. It is difficult to accomplish this paperwork and be thorough while the scene is being processed. Designate someone as the person who will collect the completed forms and provide them to the lead officer and/or the prosecutor as part of the discovery in the case.

9.10.7 Relinquishment Forms

When you seize animals with a search warrant, they still belong to the suspect, but on occasion the suspect will be interested and willing to voluntarily relinquish their ownership interest in the animals or a portion of the animals on the day the search warrant is executed. Of course, law enforcement officers must always adhere to the strict rules that apply when a suspect has invoked their right to counsel or their right to remain silent. If the situation enables a conversation about ownership of the animals, the lead officer on the case needs to use that opportunity for the benefit of the animals, the animal care agency, and the suspect.

The suspect's decision to relinquish ownership of the animals should not weigh on their guilt or innocence with respect to the cruelty violation being investigated. As such, you should not make deals or exchanges pertaining to the criminal charges in exchange for the surrender. Find out from the animal care agency how much it costs to care for an animal each day, and let the suspect know that is the charge the suspect will incur per animal daily to provide for the continued care of their property. If you are an animal care entity, make sure you have this information ready to provide to the law enforcement officers on the scene.

If the suspect decides to relinquish some or all of the animals the day of the search warrant, you want to be ready to effectuate that in a way that will hold up to future scrutiny. Make sure you are identifying who is the legal owner of the property (i.e. the animals) and describe as specifically as possible which animals are being relinquished. You can identify them by their unique evidence identifier and/or physical markings or colorings or where they were housed on the scene. There should be no discrepancy about which animals are being surrendered. Depending on the case, it may also be important to include unborn offspring in the relinquishment paperwork. These cases would include those where animals are visibly pregnant, or when there are numerous offspring of any age at the scene, or when there are animals of both sexes found housed together on the scene. See Appendix B and C for example relinquishment forms and templates.

9.10.8 Scene Access Log

The scene access log may be a form that traditional law enforcement is accustomed to using, but, if not, consider providing one for use at search warrants in which you participate. The individual posted at the access point to the scene should maintain this log. When people enter or leave the scene, they must document that movement on this form. Any search warrant execution can attract onlookers and your chain of custody could become vulnerable if a third party claims to have accessed the scene when it should have been secure. Treat this crime scene like any other crime scene you are processing and do not allow access to unauthorized people.

9.10.9 Evidence Placards

Using an evidence placard helps clarify the image in the photos from the crime scene. The placard should include the date and the case number, at the very least. It should also include the unique evidence identifier assigned to the piece of evidence. Again, do not choose to include too much information so that it significantly slows down your process or creates unnecessary confusion; for example, if the evidence placard calls a horse "brown" and the veterinarian refers to it as a "dark bay." Preprinting evidence placards with the date and case number in advance of executing the warrant is an option that can save time, but index cards can also work well on the scene and for affixing to carriers. For cases involving large animals, you may need a bigger placard attached to the end of a pole in order to safely get it in the photograph with the animal.

9.10.10 Chain of Custody Forms

Once the animal(s) leave the property the chain of custody begins. Be sure to have several chain of custody forms on hand at the search warrant execution to ensure consistency among animal caregivers in documenting the chain of custody.

9.11 Discovering Evidence of Other Crimes

During the search warrant execution evidence of another or multiple other crimes may be discovered. The person who discovers what they believe to be evidence of a crime not listed in the warrant should immediately alert the incident commander. At this point the prosecutor should be notified and determine how to proceed.

9.12   The First 24 Hours After the Search Warrant Execution

Serving and executing a search warrant in an animal cruelty case often takes the better part of a day and is mentally and physically taxing on the individuals assisting. In these cases, the conclusion of the warrant service marks the beginning of more long days for the foreseeable future. In addition to the veterinary exams, documentation, and animal care that need to take place right away, there is time-sensitive paperwork that must be promptly addressed.

9.12.1   Veterinarian's Role: Immediately Post Warrant Service

When animals and evidence are transported from the scene, if possible, the veterinarian should travel to the shelter/location where the animals are headed. This enables the veterinarian or their assistant to verify that all animals examined onsite arrived at the location and were secured at the sheltering site. That information becomes part of the veterinary report.

Next the lead veterinarian formulates a plan for the animals that includes what additional examination requirements, diagnostic testing, treatment, enrichment, and overall animal care processes are necessary for the animals. Coordinating the follow-up, educating those responsible for the plan, and assigning continued record keeping responsibilities are critical next steps for the lead veterinarian. The findings on the scene provide insight for the veterinarian to help establish the team, resources, and plans for care of large or small populations of animals, while at the same time meeting the critical individual needs of each animal.

9.12.2   The Paperwork

9.12.2.1   Warrant Return
Law enforcement officers should complete the warrant return without delay. You can include various appendices to the warrant return such as the Property in Custody forms and a sample of the photographs you took on scene. The photo appendix is important to affirm to the judge that you did, in fact, find the evidence you expected to find. The photos can also inform initial charging discussions the prosecutor may be having. Once the warrant return has occurred, the warrant becomes public record, and the law enforcement agency should notify the partners as the media may acquire a copy of the documents.

9.12.2.2   Chain of Custody Documentation in Place
As soon as the animals leave the scene, the chain of custody documentation should be in place for them. Once they have arrived at the facility where they will be housed, it is a good idea for someone to double check that the chain of custody documentation is in place and that it matches the evidence animal to whom it relates. It is also an important time to make sure the staff filling out the chain of custody paperwork have been adequately trained on how to use it, what to do with the completed forms, and where to find additional forms. The lead law enforcement officer should inquire about the chain of custody plan for the animals and sometimes may need to work

collaboratively with the animal care agency to develop a system that will work for the purpose of the case, without sacrificing the care and well-being of the animals.

9.12.2.3   Paperwork Generated by the Warrant Service

All the thorough documentation you created on scene by utilizing all or some of the forms mentioned earlier in the chapter will have gone to waste if they are not scanned or otherwise preserved in the case file. As soon as possible, it is prudent to create copies in addition to saving the documentation produced on the scene. The copies should also be saved in the hardcopy of the case file to provide a backup should anything happen to the originals. Designate someone to ensure this step happens and who can take the necessary steps to ensure it gets produced in discovery for the case if/when necessary.

9.12.2.4   Notice About Reports

The lead law enforcement officer needs to notify the civilian scene-processing team and other husbandry and veterinary experts if the officer would like them to produce a witness statement about the search warrant execution or a report about the animals. Explain to the witness what is expected from these statements or reports and the deadline to provide them (see Chapter 12 for more detailed guidance on report writing in animal cruelty cases).

Everyone who participated in the search warrant execution should produce a witness statement. This statement will help the prosecutor know who to call as a witness for various aspects of the case, and it will serve to refresh your memory if the day of trial actually occurs. Often, when these cases do go to trial, it is over a year since the search warrant was served. In order to recall important details from that day you must write them in a statement, and you must do so close in time to when the warrant was executed so the recollection is clear.

9.12.2.5   The Animals

The animals seized under the search warrant need to be examined as soon as possible by a veterinarian (see Chapter 13 for detailed guidance on Protective Custody animals). The prosecutor and the lead law enforcement officer on the case should establish a point of contact at the animal care agency to use on an on-going basis as the investigation continues and as the animals are forensically evaluated and then held as evidence. Immediately begin a system for tracking the costs associated with the care and treatment of the animals, in order to provide that information for restitution and preconviction forfeiture purposes.

9.12.2.6   Media Plan

The media tends to be interested in animal cruelty cases, and agencies and organizations should expect and plan for a media response (see Chapter 14 for more detailed guidance on media and fundraising).

References

1 Constitution of the United States, Amendment 4 (USA), (1791).

2 *Illinois vs. Rodriguez* (1990) 110 S. Ct. 2793.

3 Garner, B.A. (ed.) (2019). *Black's Law Dictionary Standard*, 11e, 325. St. Paul, MN: Thomson Reuters.

4 *State v. Dicke* (2014) 258, Or. App 678.

5 National Animal Care & Control Association (2014). NACA guidelines. https://www.nacanet.org/wp-content/uploads/2019/03/NACA_Guidelines.pdf. (accessed 30 May 2021).

6 Animal Behavior Associates, Inc. (n.d.). TASERS® for animals? https://animalbehaviorassociates. com/tasers-for-animals (accessed 30 May 2021).

7 *State vs. Newcomb*, 359, Or. 756, (2016).

8 *Wilson vs. Arkansas*, 514 US 927, 936, (1995).

10

Evidence Collection

Emily Lewis

Evidence collection in an animal cruelty case can be as simple as seizing and packaging a receipt from a feed store or as complicated as seizing an unsocial pregnant Chihuahua. This chapter will take an in-depth look at evidence collection in criminal animal cruelty investigations. Building on the foundation of basic animal husbandry laid out in Chapter 2, this chapter will establish what could be considered evidence, how that evidence should be attained and packaged, and the various ways to document the evidence. Given that the conundrum of living evidence can result in a reluctance to investigate these cases in the first place, this chapter also seeks to alleviate any hesitation by providing guidance on the measures that can be taken to adhere to proper evidence handling protocols, while doing so humanely when dealing with living beings.

10.1 What is Evidence?

Evidence is a broad term used to refer to "something that tends to prove or disprove the existence of an alleged fact" [1]. For the purposes of this book, we are focusing on evidence relevant to animal cruelty cases and the measures that can be taken to promote its usefulness at trial. Evidence can be a document, a tangible item, recordings, or testimony.

10.2 How Evidence in Animal Cruelty Cases Differs from Traditional Property Crimes

In many ways evidence collected in animal cruelty investigations does not differ from traditional property or person crimes, but in other obvious ways it is drastically different. That stark contrast can be attributed to the presence of living and nonliving evidence in animal cruelty investigations.

10.2.1 Nonliving Evidence

Using the language of the law that has allegedly been violated is important in determining what would be evidence in that animal cruelty investigation. If the law contains terms or phrases that are vague or subjective, then law enforcement, prosecutors, and veterinarians need to discuss what the terms mean both in the context of the case law of the jurisdiction, accepted practices within the community, and in the veterinary medical field.

Animal Cruelty Investigations: A Collaborative Approach from Victim to Verdict™, First Edition.
Edited by Kris Otteman, Linda Fielder, and Emily Lewis.
© 2022 John Wiley & Sons, Inc. Published 2022 by John Wiley & Sons, Inc.
Companion website: www.wiley.com/go/otteman/victimtoverdict

10.2.1.1 Paperwork

Paperwork is a relevant piece of evidence for almost every animal cruelty violation. In neglect and abuse cases veterinary records provide a timeline, can prove a mental state, can reveal additional victims, and establish ownership. Paperwork is a significant piece of evidence in animal fighting cases. Documentation of matches, breeding and trading arrangements, or rules of the game are extremely relevant. Do not overlook receipts as another form of paperwork relevant to an animal cruelty investigation. Receipts from a feed store or pet shop for animal care products or from a renderer in a livestock case can go a long way in piecing together a timeline and confirming or undermining statements made by suspects and witnesses. Finally, paperwork can become the backbone of large-scale breeder or animal rescue cases. Establishing how long an animal is under the care and control of the suspect is crucial to those cases, as well as determining what other parties may be able to provide additional information to investigators. It is also important to note that documenting the lack of paperwork (i.e. veterinary records, adoption contracts, feed invoices) is also relevant evidence to the case (Figure 10.1).

10.2.1.2 Medication

Medication is an obvious piece of evidence in an animal cruelty case. If an animal is suffering from a chronic condition, such as an ear infection, and the suspect has no medication for that condition, that is compelling evidence. If the suspect has a prescription medication onsite but the bottle is full and never administered, that is compelling evidence. Medications, steroids, and hormones are commonly found at the scene of an animal fighting location and are important pieces of the puzzle when investigating these crimes. In some states even the possession of such paraphernalia is a crime.[1] Another important factor to consider when deciding to seize or just photograph medications on the scene is

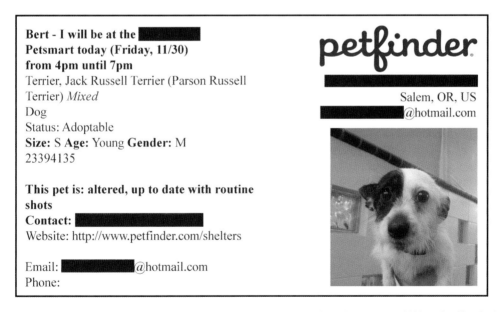

Figure 10.1 When investigating a rescue, collecting paperwork like this helps establish a timeline for how long the animal has been in the care of the suspect. *Source:* Oregon Humane Society.

---

1 As of January 2021, 25 states criminalize possession of fighting paraphernalia: CA, FL, IL, IN, IA, KS, LA, MD, MI, MS, MO, NE, NH, NH, NY, OK, OR, PA, SD, TN, TX, UT, VT, and WA.

whether the medication is for a life-threatening condition, seizures for example, and it is likely you will need to provide the animal with that medication before the animal can see a veterinarian for that condition. It is extremely important to consult with a veterinarian or have a veterinarian on the scene and involved in evaluating the medications found during an investigation.

10.2.1.3 Husbandry Supplies

Rarely does a photo of an animal being kept in poor conditions sustain a neglect charge on its own. Without documentation of the presence or absence of species-appropriate husbandry supplies it becomes very difficult for a prosecutor to meet their burden in proving the case. Again, law enforcement *must* partner with experts to understand what the husbandry needs are for the species they are investigating in order to evaluate adequately the reported violation.

10.2.1.4 Habitats

In many neglect investigations, the habitat an animal is residing in is relevant evidence. From the water source to the nature of the bedding provided, the whole habitat is important to the forensic veterinary evaluation. Of course, depending on the size and species of the animal, you may not realistically be able to seize an entire habitat. In those cases, be sure to document the enclosure or area through other means so any medical conditions can be evaluated in that context. Experts will be helpful to law enforcement in this arena as well, to indicate what aspects of the habitats are tied directly to the health and welfare of the animal(s) at issue. For example, reptiles require, among other things, very specific heat and light accommodations (Figure 10.2).

10.2.1.5 Electronics

Electronics play a rapidly expanding role in people's lives; do not ignore them as a source of viable and relevant evidence in animal cruelty investigations. If you have the processing resources and the probable cause to believe evidence will be found on a suspect's phone or computer, consider collecting them as evidence. If you are unfamiliar with processing this type of evidence or do not have the resources to facilitate the forensics necessary to extract the evidence, then it is not advisable to seize these items. In collecting electronics as evidence, you are representing that you will process them as such. It is worthwhile to look for flash drives or other electronic storage devices, particularly in cases involving large-scale breeders or rescues and in animal fighting investigations.

(a)   (b)

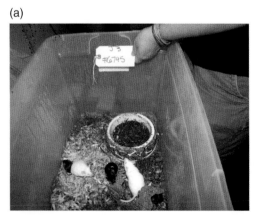 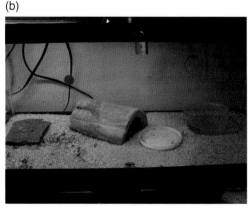

Figure 10.2   (a and b) Connecting ulcerated feet to a urine-soaked enclosure, or bone disease to inadequate light sources, provides necessary evidence in a case and could make the difference between offense levels in some states. *Source:* Oregon Humane Society.

10.2.1.6 Deceased Animals

The body of a deceased animal found on the scene can be extremely valuable evidence to a case or it can have almost no evidentiary value. The veterinarian assisting in a case may not be able to ascertain any relevant or useful information from an animal who has been deceased for an extended period of time. If the body is discovered in a freezer and appears to have been stored there close in time to when death occurred, it is likely a veterinarian would be able to garner information from that body that could be helpful to an investigation. If you do not have the resources to remove and store a large animal body, like a horse for example, then consult with your expert veterinarian and take the photos, videos, and any samples they suggest as an alternative to removing the entire body. Often the area surrounding a dead animal can provide significant information to a veterinarian with respect to how the animal died (see Chapter 11). When deciding to seize a dead animal as evidence, consider what that animal will add to the case with respect to proving or disproving the violation that has been reported. Do you know how long the suspect had that animal? Will you be able to determine a cause of death? Are you able to identify that animal specifically? If you can determine the cause of death, will you also be able to pinpoint on or around when death occurred?

10.2.1.7 Where and How to Look for Relevant Nonliving Evidence

Sometimes nonliving evidence in animal cruelty investigations is located in areas you would not expect. First, if the situation is appropriate, consider asking the suspect where to locate particular items like vet records or medications. In scenarios where the suspect is not receptive to these questions or you are not permitted to question the suspect, you must be thorough in your search for nonliving evidence. As mentioned in Chapter 9, records, receipts, and other animal husbandry supplies can be found in outbuildings and vehicles around the property. Animal medications are frequently found on nightstands, coffee tables, and in the medicine cabinet of the bathroom. Occasionally vet records or notes can be found at the bottom of purses, posted on the refrigerator, or in the kennel with the animal. Be sure to check all freezer locations on the scene for remains of deceased animals, in addition to recently disturbed earth or burn piles on the property (Figure 10.3).

10.2.2 Living Evidence

Not only is the animal itself evidence, but it is also categorized as "property" under the law. This makes the animal victim a unique type of evidence because the evidence animal is property but is also alive and has sentience.

10.2.2.1 Which Animals Are Evidence?

We have established that the animals subject to an animal cruelty violation are considered evidence. It becomes more complicated when the suspect possesses additional animals who are either not victims of the violation currently being investigated, or, for any number of reasons, do not appear in the moment to be suffering from neglect, despite residing in the same circumstances as the clearly victimized animals.

Always return to the language of the search warrant, the language of the statutes you are investigating, and the opinions of the experts when a question of authority to seize a particular piece of evidence arises. If there is a species of animal not addressed in your search warrant and that animal is perhaps housed in a different location on the property – an indoor cat you discover during a search warrant about neglected horses, for example – then you likely do not have the authority to seize that animal. A search warrant in an animal cruelty case is not a blanket pass to seize every animal on a property.

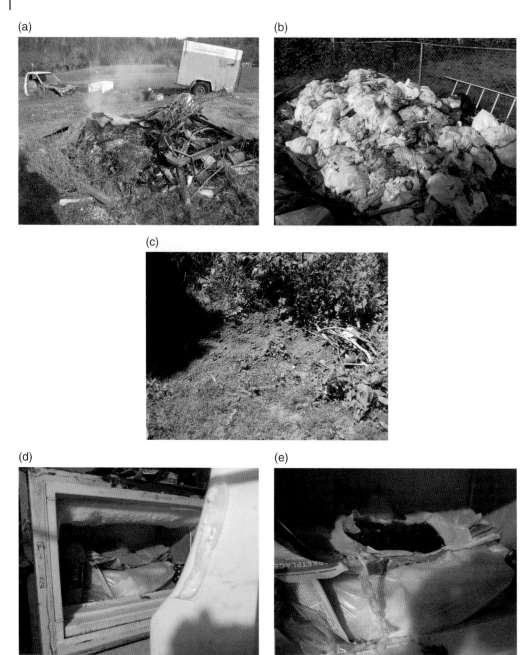

Figure 10.3 (a–e) All of these areas may contain animal remains or other evidence of animal cruelty. A plastic bag in the freezer shown in (d) contained the remains of the cat pictured in (e). Before you search in these areas, review the warrant document to confirm you have the authority to do so. *Source:* Oregon Humane Society.

That being said, it is possible that you will discover additional animals of varying species who are also evidence of an animal cruelty violation. Therefore, it is important to include "any other neglected or abused animals" in your search warrant as part of the list of evidence to be seized. If you discover animals who are victims of a completely separate crime than those discussed in your affidavit, it would be best practice to contact your prosecutor to determine whether or not you lock down the scene and amend the warrant with the new information.

The decision around what animals to seize gets more complicated when you encounter animals of disparate body conditions living in the same or similar environments. These are the scenarios in which the veterinary expert on the scene is extremely valuable. Keep in mind it is ultimately the lead officer on the case who will take responsibility for which animals were seized, but the officer should do so through thoughtful discussion with a veterinarian and in review of the language of the relevant statutes. An animal may be a perfect weight, but if the state law requires a certain level of sanitation be met, or if the other evidence indicates there is no food available to provide to the animals, then there is still cause to seize that animal. In animal hoarding cases the population of animals will develop a hierarchy when competing for resources, which will lead to varying body conditions in the population. A veterinarian will be able to explain this phenomenon and the reality that the hierarchy will continue to reproduce itself, such that any animals left behind will continue to be prevented from accessing what few resources are available. A veterinarian will also help you understand the amount of food and other resources necessary to care for the population of animals found at the scene, and this can help in the decision of which animals need to be seized.

10.2.2.2 Options if Not Seizing All the Animals

If certain animals are not seized, it does not mean that you abandon your oversight of their care. If you do not have the probable cause to seize an animal at the scene, but the amount of food remaining and the chronic failure to provide care to other animals on the property create concern for the remaining animals, there are some actions you can take. If the veterinarian tells you the amount of food on the scene is enough to feed those animals for two days, let the suspect know you will be following up after that time to confirm that additional food has been procured. If there are medical issues in the early stages of development with any of the animals, have the veterinarian generate a treatment plan the suspect needs to implement, and then follow up to confirm that it was implemented or addressed. Finally, if an officer is concerned about a suspect's ability to care for animals going forward, they can talk with the prosecutor about the terms of the release order and the stipulation that the suspect not possess animals in the interim of trial or the resolution of the case.

10.2.3 Where and How to Look for Live Animal Evidence

Even though animals are living pieces of evidence, it can still be very difficult to locate the animal evidence at a scene. Common challenges include items and debris preventing access to areas housing animals, intentional hiding of animals by the suspect, or unconventional layout of outbuildings and kennels (Figure 10.4).

When you are responding to an animal hoarding case or a location with a lot of debris for animals to hide in and around, the best tools you have are patience and remaining calm. Try to use as few animal handlers as possible in order to reduce the stress level for the animals, with the hope they will reveal their location. Let the expert handlers guide where that species of animal is likely to hide and use caution when capturing a cornered and/or panicked animal. An individual who hoards animals as well as items creates an environment that will take all day to process thoroughly. Make sure to keep an eye out for carriers, cages, or vivariums and be sure to check inside each one you find. Behind and under furniture are common areas for scared animals to hide. Remember that some animals can get into cupboards, on top of appliances, and in closets. The panicked nature of the animals and the necessity to ensure the safety of the

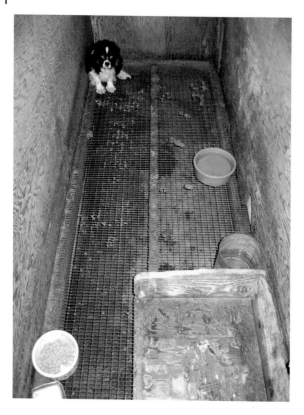

Figure 10.4 This enclosure, and several others like it, were discovered in a closed off room attached to the back of a barn. The layout of the building and entry and exit points concealed this room from crime scene processors until well into the search warrant execution. A review of an aerial map of the property revealed its existence prior to closing the scene, but it could easily have been overlooked if scene processors had not been diligent in reviewing the layout of the outbuildings. *Source:* Oregon Humane Society.

handlers, means that mutiple attempts to capture an animal may be required before they can safely be secured in a carrier or processed through the evidence staging area (Figure 10.5).

Whether you are investigating animal hoarding, a bad actor animal breeder or rescuer, or a small-scale animal neglect case, there is always a possibility – a likelihood in some cases – that the suspect will intentionally hide animals. Be aware this is a possibility and that it might mean the animals have been moved to another location with an acquaintance of the suspect. A thorough search of the property and the buildings is very important and must include looking in rooms, containers, and vehicles, if you have the authority to do so.

If a suspect has many animals in their custody, it is common for the holding areas, kennels, and runs to be added on to structures in a haphazard or disjointed way. Individuals looking for live animal evidence can easily overlook an entire room or area if the structure is arranged in such a way to mask the presence of that area. If you are aware of this possibility going into a scene, you are less likely to leave evidence animals behind.

10.3 How to Package the Evidence

Not all evidence can be packaged in the same way and that becomes abundantly clear in animal cruelty cases. Obviously, a living animal cannot be packaged in the traditional sense of the word at all, but the integrity of most other evidence in these cases relies on proper packaging. There are overarching concepts that apply to packaging evidence regardless of the nature of the evidence: the date it was packaged, who was the last person to package it, where it was originally located and by who, and finally some aspect of the packaging that indicates it has not been tampered with.

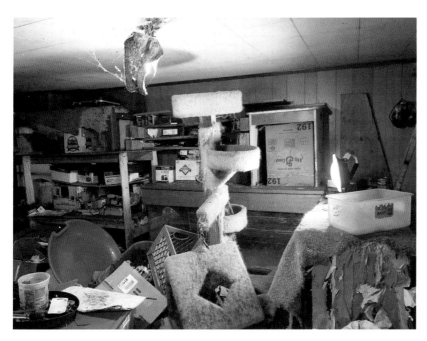

Figure 10.5   In hoarding cases locating and capturing animals can be complicated by the amount of clutter and objects where animals can hide. In this case, handlers worked to locate and place over 30 cats in carriers without noticing what appeared to be an empty and darkened aquarium against a wall. Investigators later discovered a 6′ boa in the home. *Source:* Oregon Humane Society.

10.3.1   What Is Chain of Custody?

The chain of custody is the thread that tracks a piece of evidence and who it encounters, from where it was found at the scene of a crime, to the point it is being offered as evidence of that crime. Each time the evidence is moved, or the custodian of the evidence changes, that creates another link in the chain. If each link in the chain is well documented, then that piece of evidence can be given a lot of weight in court, i.e. it would be difficult to argue that it had been tampered with. If there are gaps in the chain, that piece of evidence might be less persuasive in court if it can be admitted as a piece of evidence at all.

Throughout this book, and with the chain of custody in particular, we reiterate that it is important for all professionals working on animal cruelty cases to remember that the animal, even though it is a piece of evidence, is still a living, sentient being that requires care and treatment to prevent its suffering. A break in the chain of custody does not extinguish the evidentiary value of a living animal, and lifesaving care or emergency treatment must never be withheld in an effort to preserve a link in the chain of custody.

10.3.2   Nonliving Evidence

10.3.2.1   Paperwork

As referenced in Chapter 9, a significant amount of evidence can be found in the paperwork in the suspect's custody. This is an example of evidence that mirrors that of traditional crimes which law enforcement investigate and, as such, any officer on the scene will be familiar with how to package paperwork evidence. The primary consideration for packaging this evidence is to preserve its integrity by enclosing it in a waterproof and tamperproof receptacle. Include as much information as possible, such as where it was found, who found it, the date, the case number, the time it was found, who packaged it, and any other relevant information. Be aware this evidence will likely have to be referenced in the future as the investigation continues and have a process in place to preserve the information from the initial packaging, as well as who has accessed and packaged the paperwork since that time. This applies to paperwork evidence relevant to animal cruelty investigations such as veterinary records, receipts, phone bills, sale records, adoption contracts, litter records, breeding records, ownership documents, calendars, invoices, post-it notes, and transfer records.

10.3.2.2 Food Samples

In certain cases, it will be important to seize samples of the animals' food from the scene in addition to documenting the food through video, photographs, and witness statements. Before you seize food samples, consider why you are doing so and whether having a physical sample of the food furthers the investigation and the potential charges. If it does and you are sending it to a lab to get the nutrient breakdown, for example, then be sure you are procuring the sample and packaging it in a way that sets it up well for that purpose (Figure 10.6).

10.3.2.3 Water Samples

Water is a standard element of required care for animals in every state. In many cases, lack of potable water can be demonstrated through photo and video evidence, i.e. there is no water, the water is frozen, or the water is so contaminated with debris and filth it is clearly not drinkable. There may be a case where it is necessary to test the water that is available to the animals. Make sure you establish where you will have the water samples tested and understand the packaging and/or shipping requirements (see Appendix D for labs that offer water sample testing). Establish this resource prior to removing water from a scene for sampling.

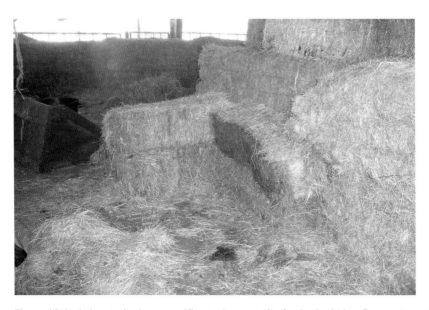

Figure 10.6 Laboratories have specific requirements for feed submission. Be sure to understand how samples must be collected, stored, and shipped in order to make sure they are able to be processed, and that the analyses are accurate. The samples of the hay taken for this case were not taken in the manner preferred by the laboratory and the resulting testimony from the technician was detrimental to the case. *Source:* Oregon Humane Society.

10.3.2.4 Tissue Samples

The animal's body can also be considered the "scene" of a crime, such that removal of anything from the body creates a separate piece of evidence and initiates a new chain of custody for that piece of evidence. The chain of custody for these items needs to include the unique evidence identifier of the animal it was removed from. Both living and deceased animals can have samples removed from them. During forensic evaluation and medical treatment living animals produce additional evidence, such as blood or tissue samples, that are extracted for further analysis. In the course of medical treatment items such as hair mats, nail or hoof trimmings, and teeth may be removed, and these items will also become separate pieces of evidence. When performing a forensic necropsy the veterinarian may remove samples from tissue and organs for further analysis. These samples are then suspended in formalin or other medium, as indicated by the diagnostic laboratory that will perform the pathology. Once the samples have been sent to the lab and tested the lab results become the evidence. It should not be detrimental to the evidentiary value of the tissue that the process of forensically evaluating it renders it unreturnable in its original form, as long as the chain of custody is documented throughout the process.

10.3.2.5 Fecal Samples

A lot of evidence can be gathered through analysis of a victim animal's fecal material. In addition to the numerous parasites that can be confirmed, fecal tests can also indicate whether an animal ingested nonnutritive material, usually in an effort to feel full when they are suffering from starvation, or if there is internal bleeding, or disease.

Fecal samples can be removed from the scene where an animal was housed or can be collected from the animal, once it has been taken into custody. They should be refrigerated and submitted for analysis as quickly as possible. Samples from the scene can indicate the presence of parasites and the risk to the population of animals. Samples taken in connection with a specific animal are directly relevant to the potential charges relating to that animal. In either case, the broad concepts of evidence collection and packaging apply: document when the sample was taken, from where, and by whom. Like tissue samples, once the sample has been tested, that piece of evidence becomes the lab results and the chain of custody will follow the sample through the testing and result process.

10.3.2.6 Medication

In most cases, animal medications are relevant to an animal cruelty investigation and need to be seized and/or documented. It is important to package the medication in a way that will not cause it to spill or leak, because the amount of medication and the condition you found it in are part of what constitutes its evidentiary value. Be sure to consult with your veterinarian about what environment the medications must be stored in to preserve their condition. Also keep in mind at some point the medication may need to be counted, measured, or photographed after it has been seized and placed in Protective Custody.

10.3.2.6.1 Medication for an Existing Life-Threatening Condition

It is very important to determine as soon as possible whether an animal you are seizing also has medication at the scene for a life-threatening condition. An example of this would be an animal who has seizures or is suffering from diabetes and is currently on medication to manage that issue, or any animal who is being treated with antibiotics or painkillers for a critical illness. Veterinarians need to be on the lookout for these types of medications and feel empowered to speak up if one is located. Instead of transferring the live animal and the medication seized as evidence to separate locations, the medicine and associated chain of custody forms must follow the animal. The chain of custody for the medicine needs to include documentation of when, how much, and who administered it to the animal.

10.3.2.7 Mats

Preserved mats from a severely ungroomed animal can be compelling evidence in an animal neglect case. After you have documented the matted animal with photographs, if the mats are dry when you remove them you can consider packaging them in a plastic bag. If the mats have any amount of moisture in them, package them in a paper bag and continue to replace the packaging as the evidence soaks through the bag or begins to dry out. As with any evidence removed from a victim animal, the animal evidence identifier for the animal needs to be included in the information on the packaging of the mats from that animal.

10.3.2.8 Restraints (Collars, Leashes, Halters, Ropes)

Restraints are seized as evidence, particularly in an investigation into the sexual assault of an animal, embedded collar or halter case, abandonment cases, and starvation cases. When these are forensically evaluated after they are initially seized, they may even produce additional evidence in the form of blood, hair, nails, and DNA. Again, if the restraint is at all damp, package it in a paper evidence bag to give it the opportunity to dry out, before transferring it to another type of evidence packaging option. Any evidence that is removed from the restraint during the forensic evaluation is given a separate evidence identifier and separate chain of custody forms that include the evidence identifier for the restraint and/or the animal the restraint was removed from.

10.3.2.9 DNA

10.3.2.9.1 Human

Veterinarians and traditional law enforcement need to partner on cases where forensic veterinary exams are likely to discover potential human DNA. Traditional law enforcement will have procedures in place for how these samples need to be extracted and where they can be sent for evaluation. Prior to removing fibers or swabbing beneath claws on an animal in an effort to locate human DNA, veterinarians should have a conversation with the law enforcement partner in that case.

10.3.2.9.2 Animal

In the majority of cases, animal DNA testing is not going to be necessary to prove the animal cruelty violation, but it is good to understand the resources available when a case outcome does rely on that information. In 2010, the University of California, Davis Veterinary Genetic Laboratory became the location for "Canine CODIS," a dog DNA database focused on linking animal fighting rings and perpetrators [2]. UC Davis Veterinary Genetic Laboratory also processes animal DNA in furtherance of animal cruelty cases where it would be relevant, such as theft of a companion animal, identifying remains, distinguishing between predation and physical abuse, and linking a suspect to an animal cruelty crime scene or event [3]. Their website is very specific about the sampling and packaging requirements and must be reviewed prior to engaging in the process. It is important to note that DNA testing in these cases can be a very expensive endeavor. Consider whether it is necessary to prove the violation you are alleging and explore options for financial assistance if it is a necessary step in your investigation (see Appendix D for resources for financial assistance and animal DNA testing laboratories).

10.3.2.10 Animal Remains

Just as the living animals can be evidence in a case, so too can deceased animals. On the scene be sure to consult with your lead veterinarian to determine whether seizing the body of an animal would further your investigation. Often a dead animal on the scene is too decomposed and an exam would not garner much useful information. If there is a large animal deceased on the scene, again consult with the responding veterinarian or contact a partner veterinarian. In many cases documenting the deceased animal's positioning and surrounding areas and seizing certain samples from the body can be enough for the veterinarian to evaluate the death, without having to seize a 1000+ lb animal and preserve it until trial. If you seize an animal at the scene, put the body in a plastic body bag and label it as you would all other evidence you seize from the scene. Some jurisdictions may require you to label this bag with a biohazard indicator.

Unless a necropsy can be performed within 24 hours of receiving the body, the body must be refrigerated until necropsy, and can remain in the body bag until then. If refrigeration is not an option, then freezing is acceptable; however, some tissue changes and testing can be altered or compromised with freezing. Remains can safely be refrigerated for prolonged periods of time (weeks) until exam if needed with little further decomposition. In both instances, the best way to package and preserve an animal body long term is in a body bag in a refrigerator or freezer environment. The location itself should be a secure area if it is walk-in freezer storage, or have restricted access, if it is a stand-alone unit. Affix a tag to the body bag with the identifying information listed and the chain of custody forms available to track the body if it is being moved for necropsy or photography. If an animal body is thawing in preparation for a necropsy, be sure to place something underneath it to prevent any liquids from contaminating other evidence or areas. If a necropsy is conducted, do not dispose of the remains at the conclusion of the exam. Repackage the remains into the body bag and secure them in the refrigerator or freezer area until the lead officer or prosecutor on the case gives you different instructions. Keep in mind in some cases the defense may enlist another veterinarian to examine the remains, or in some cases remains may be returned to a family member for burial or cremation.

Depending on how large an animal body is, it can be very difficult or expensive to preserve the body in a refrigerator or freezer until trial. It is worthwhile to inquire with the lead officer or prosecutor on a case about dispositioning deceased animals that are being held pending resolution in a case. The prosecutor can give the defense an opportunity to examine the body, and if all the evidence has been gathered with all parties having an opportunity to review/examine it, then the body should be approved for disposition and not have to be held in storage until trial.

10.3.2.11 Animal Organs, Bones, Body Parts

Preserving animal organs or body parts follows the same parameters as preserving the body as a whole. Animal bones can be dried and then packaged and retained outside of cold storage. Maintaining the chain of custody throughout the drying process is important.

10.3.3 Living Evidence

10.3.3.1 Labeling and Evidence Identifiers

Evidence animals need to be uniquely identified and labeled with that identifier for chain of custody and charging purposes. The tendency can be to assign the evidence animal a number as their unique identifier. This can become problematic when the animals are then given names by their caretakers and the animal needs to be tracked using two different unique identifiers (e.g. the numerical ID and the newly bestowed name). This issue can be resolved by assigning unique evidence *letters* to the animals on the scene rather than numbers. The animal is then assigned a name that begins with its evidence letter. This allows staff to refer to the evidence animal by name but preserves the unique evidence identifier from the scene within that name (Figure 10.7).

(a)

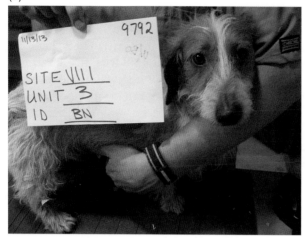

(b)

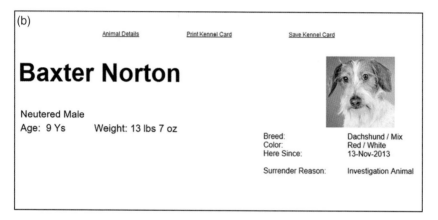

Animal Details   Print Kennel Card   Save Kennel Card

Baxter Norton

Neutered Male
Age: 9 Ys   Weight: 13 lbs 7 oz

Breed: Dachshund / Mix
Color: Red / White
Here Since: 13-Nov-2013

Surrender Reason: Investigation Animal

Figure 10.7 (a and b) The dog in this case was assigned the unique evidence identifier of "BN" and was given the name "Baxter Norton" to match his evidence identifier. *Source:* Oregon Humane Society.

Depending on the temperament and species, labeling the evidence animals can be easy or it can be almost impossible. The identifier is intended to be temporary, as seized animals are property belonging to the defendant, and unless necessary for medical reasons or chain of custody, the animals should not be permanently altered in any way (microchipping, tattoo, branding, etc.) while being held in Protective Custody. Dogs and cats can be labeled with temporary collars listing their evidence identifier. Horses and livestock can sometimes be labeled using a livestock crayon directly on their shoulder or rump. It is also possible to braid an evidence label into a horse's mane as a labeling option with more longevity. Leg bands can be used to label poultry and birds. Herds of livestock that are bred to look identical present a challenge to labeling and might need a more permanent identifier such as an ear tag. In some cases, scene processing might involve the use of a chute in order to adequately process and identify the animals (Figures 10.8).

Small animals, such as rabbits, pose another problem for labeling with a unique identifier. With these types of animals, try to use a marker and write the identifier on the inside of their ear. Be creative if you need to, but it is worth the time to come up with a solution. The need to identify and distinguish each animal from the scene is crucial in each case, and there must be a plan in place for this component of the evidence process prior to responding to a scene to remove animals.

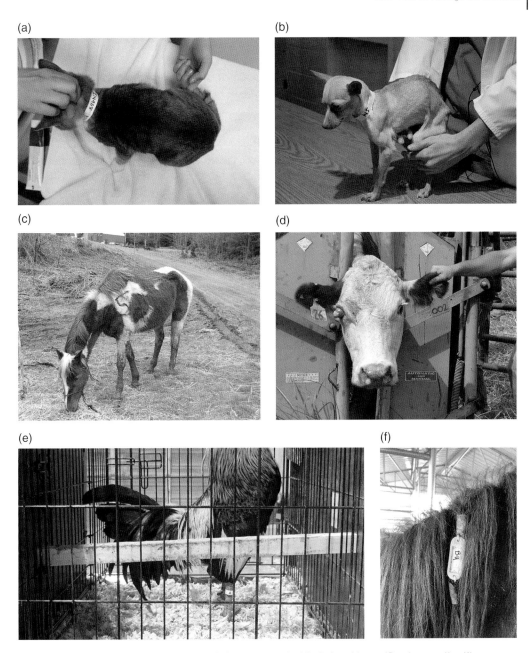

Figure 10.8 (a–f) Some animals can easily be connected with their evidence ID using a collar, like cats and dogs. Livestock animals can be more difficult to label, requiring more creative solutions like braiding a key ring into a horse's mane and securing it with a zip tie. Leg bands for identifying birds are readily available online or at local feed stores. *Source:* Oregon Humane Society.

10.3.3.2 Photographing on the Scene

There are two types of photographs you need to take of evidence animals on the scene – photos that clearly depict how they appeared as you found them in the environment and then an identifying photo with a placard that lists their unique evidence identifier. Photographing the animals as you found them when you arrived on the scene is important evidence for the investigation. These are the photos that will be especially compelling when you later pair them with the veterinarian's evaluation of the animals (Figure 10.9).

They can also capture behaviors and postures that are relevant to the examining veterinarian and the case. Depending on the set-up of the enclosures or the area the animals are being housed in, it can be difficult to get clear photos of every animal in this way. Do your best to capture the animals and their environment (Figure 10.10).

If there is redundancy built into your scene-processing procedures, then you will always be able to link a victim animal to where they were kept on the property and have clear photos of what that specific area looked like, even if you were not able to clearly capture that in a single photo. For example, each animal's evidence placard will list their evidence identifier and the location in which they were housed on the scene. If you take photos of each area that housed animals after the

(a)

(b)

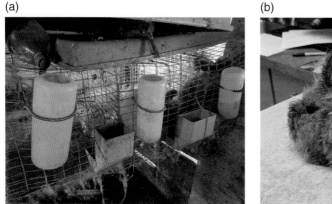
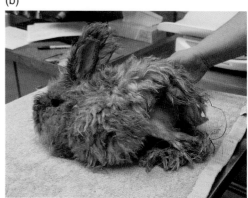

Figure 10.9   (a and b) The gray rabbit in the cage can be viewed in the environment that may have contributed to the medical issues he was later diagnosed with during his forensic exam. *Source:* Oregon Humane Society.

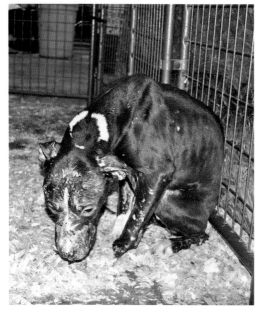

Figure 10.10   This dog's posture and demeanor provided the veterinarian in this case additional information about the dynamics with the other dogs she was housed with, which likely contributed to the condition she was found in. *Source:* Oregon Humane Society.

animals have been removed, you can connect those photos to the animals housed in that area, based on the location represented on their evidence placard (Figure 10.11).

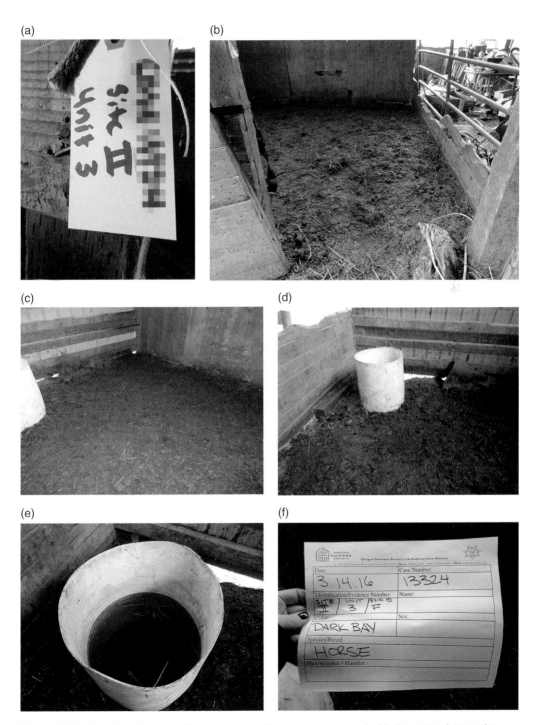

Figure 10.11 (a–h) In this series of photos the location is clearly marked with the name given to the outbuilding, "Site II," and also the enclosure within that outbuilding, "Unit 3." The evidence placard for the horse housed in that enclosure references those identifiers, which connects the horse to that location and those conditions on the scene. *Source:* Oregon Humane Society.

(g)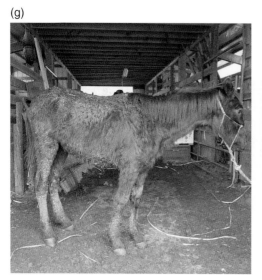

(h)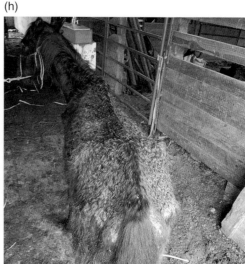

Figure 10.11   (Continued)

Once you have determined which animals were housed in which areas, you can denote those areas on the initial scene video and initial scene photographs, even further linking the specific animal to their location on the property. The location the animals were found on the scene will also be recorded in the Property in Custody (PIC) paperwork and any inventory forms kept by the evidence technicians during the scene processing.

It is extremely important to get a photo of the animal identified with its unique evidence letter (or number) prior to leaving the scene. Once the evidence animal departs from the scene, the chain of custody for that animal begins to develop. Knowing how difficult it can be to maintain a pristine or traditional chain of custody for a living animal, it will strengthen your case to have photos of every single animal from the location before there is any vulnerability in the chain of custody that could be exploited later at trial. If the temperament or species of the animal prevents you from taking an evidence photo with a placard at the evidence-processing area, then be creative about how you can get the photo with the evidence identifier. For example, if cats living in an animal hoarding situation need to be captured and crated inside the residence, then bring the carrier to the evidence-processing area and take a clear photo of the placard and in the very next photo take the picture of the cat through the front of the carrier as best you can (Figure 10.12).

If you have a pasture containing difficult-to-handle livestock, you can employ the same strategy: take a photo of the placard and then focus the camera on the animal in the pasture and take its photo before the stress of loading onto the trailer makes it too difficult.

(See Chapter 9 for the context of photographing the live evidence in your scene processing procedures.)

10.3.3.3   Property in Custody Form

Traditional law enforcement officers are accustomed to using a PIC form in their cases, but most of those forms are not created with living animal evidence in mind. This means that you will have to be creative on the scene with making sure you are filling out all the areas on the form in a way that is consistent and adequately represents the piece of evidence you are listing. Try not to be too specific with breed designations or advanced color descriptions of the animals on this list, because

(b)

(a)

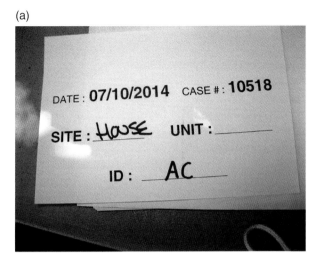
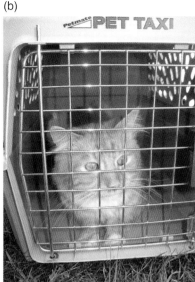

Figure 10.12 (a) The evidence placard associated with this cat was photographed first to identify that this orange tabby was located in the house uncontained (i.e. not in a unit), and has been assigned the evidence identifier "AC." Then the photo that follows (b) captures the cat and connects her to the information on the placard before she is transported away from the scene. Always do your best to get at least one identifying photo of each seized animal before they leave the property. *Source:* Oregon Humane Society.

veterinarians and other experts will be generating reports later that may use different terms in referring to the same animal, which can cause unnecessary confusion. For example, list cats as "adult," "juvenile," or "kitten" rather than estimating their ages in years and months. Also, be aware if the animal you are listing is presented to you with additional items of evidence attached to them, for example wearing a collar, or a harness, or living inside of an aquarium. Think in advance about how you are going to document that on the version of the PIC form you have available to you.

10.3.3.4 Chain of Custody

It takes training and effort to maintain an ironclad chain of custody for a living animal piece of evidence. If the individuals caring for and medically treating the evidence animals understand why it is so important, they are more likely to adhere to the policies and procedures in place to carry it out successfully. The prosecutor must be able to demonstrate the animal being referred to in court is the same animal who was seized as evidence on the day it came into the care of law enforcement, a veterinarian, or an animal shelter. In order to prove that is the case, a prosecutor will need to be able to trace who has interacted with that animal since that day. If the prosecutor struggles to meet this requirement, it can result in some or all the evidence related to that animal (exams, lab results, photographs, behavior assessments) becoming inadmissible at trial.

One way of preserving the chain of custody for an evidence animal is through hardcopy chain of custody forms. These forms act as a sign in/out for anyone interacting with the animal (see Appendix B for templates of these forms that you can use). Make the process as simple and convenient as possible to increase the likelihood that staff and volunteers will take the time to adhere to it. Include provisions in your policies and procedures for collecting this paperwork on a regular basis and include it in the case file (Figure 10.13).

**PROTECTIVE CUSTODY
ANIMAL SIGN OUT/IN**

NAME: █████			SHELTERBUDDY AID: ████████		
OHS CASE # ████████		EVIDENCE ITEM# 16074- 231330		EVIDENCE REPORT # 377	

ALL WRITING MUST BE LEGIBLE

Date	Time In	Reason	Time Out	Initials
4/29/19	4:25pm	Feeding, exam, PT outside	4:35pm	EF
4/30/19	7:38am	Feeding, outside, PT, exam	7:58a	KL
4-30-19	10:19 aM	TLC	10:23 aM	KEN
4/30/19	12:30p	Feeding, outside, PT	12:55p	KL
4/30/19	4:15pm	outside, weight	4:47p	EF
4/30/19	5:06pm	Feeding, outside, exam	5:14p	KL
5/1/19	7:55am	Feeding, outside PT, exam	8:12a	KL
5/1/19	8:30am	Socialization	8:35am	DG/JW
5/1/19	11:50 am	Socialization/offer water	11:55am	ADM
5/1/19	12:25p	feeding outside	12:32p	KL
5/1/19	4:05p	feeding, outside	4:15	KL
5/1/19	5:12	outside, water	5:21	EF
5/2/19	7:28a	feeding outside, exam, PT	7:48a	KL
5/2/19	850	Socialization	855	ADM
5/2/19	12:30	feeding outside	12:45	KL
5/2/19	12:45	outside, PT, weight	1:30	EF
5/2/19	453	Socialization	459	ADM

Figure 10.13   This form tracks the chain of custody for a live animal. Every instance the animal was fed, walked, provided enrichment, examined, or otherwise engaged with by any person was tracked on this sheet that was connected to the secured area the animal was housed in. *Source:* Oregon Humane Society.

A way to bolster the chain of custody documentation is to house the evidence animals in a secure location. This can be a designated, secure area of a shelter, it can be a secured warehouse facility, or it can be a single kennel that is locked with a padlock only authorized personnel are able to access (Figure 10.14).

If you are housing livestock animals who are evidence, you can add additional security to a pasture or barn to ensure animals are not being removed or tampered with. Consider adding cameras that could support your written chain of custody documentation. When you are thinking creatively in advance about where and how you can securely house the evidence animals, it is helpful to pair that thinking with listing the vulnerabilities of that location, and how you can address those.

Many traditional property rooms that house stagnant evidence use specialized software to electronically tag and track the evidence. Again, these systems have been developed without thinking extensively about the concept of living animal evidence. The software, and the technology and equipment necessary to implement its use, can be expensive but ultimately can create a more user-friendly and detailed tracking of evidence in your custody (see Appendix D for a list of companies commonly used by law enforcement for this purpose). It is worth noting that all chain of custody methods rely on the users' consistency and adherence to policy and procedures. The strength of the chain of custody is not enhanced or reduced by the method an agency chooses to document it – it is determined by the individuals creating the chain. A well-utilized paper system or a creative

(a)

(b)

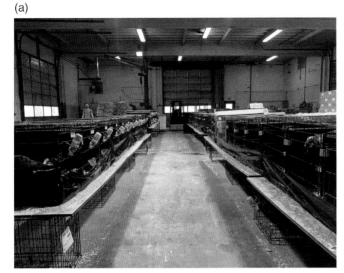
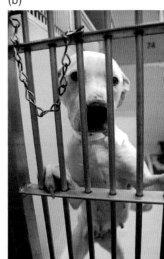

Figure 10.14   It can be easier to track chain of custody and monitor a population of protective custody animals when they are housed in a secure warehouse away from other animals. This is especially true if you are working with a unique group of animals like the fighting roosters pictured in the warehouse in (a). However, running an entirely separate facility creates a significant drain on resources. If Protective Custody animals are housed in a shelter alongside animals that are available for adoption, like the dog in (b), additional measures need to be taken to ensure their security, such as the chain and lock combination shown here. *Source:* Oregon Humane Society.

utilization of an existing shelter software or database can be equally as effective as an electronic tracking system typically used by law enforcement.

10.3.3.5   When an Evidence Animal Requires an Emergency Response

Given that these investigations by and large involve an injured or ill animal, in some cases that victim evidence animal will be in critical condition. Animals must not suffer neglect while in your care, evidentiary status notwithstanding. Provide swift and adequate treatment as needed. The chain of custody is important during all veterinary exams of evidence animals, but it must never result in withholding the administration of lifesaving care and treatment to a victim animal.

There are many ways to connect the links in the chain of custody. Draft your policies to reflect a scenario in which, if an animal needs emergency, lifesaving care, the chain of custody will be documented through witness statements and veterinary records so as not to hinder the necessary medical care to the suffering animal.

10.3.3.6   Pregnant Evidence Animals

Inanimate evidence does not multiply after being taken into custody, but animals can and will do that. If a pregnant animal gives birth, you do not treat the offspring as the same piece of evidence as the animal who gave birth, because they are a completely separate living beings at that point. Once a pregnant evidence animal gives birth, each offspring is treated as another animal in Protective Custody in that case. That means each offspring receives a unique evidence identifier and dedicated chain of custody forms. It is important to notify the prosecutor and the lead law enforcement officer on the case when this occurs (see Chapter 13 for Protective Custody foster options for evidence animals born in care).

10.3.3.7 Evidence Animals That Cannot Be Touched or Handled

Some cases involve evidence animals that are dangerous or difficult to handle. Animals who that are untrained, feral, venomous, frightened, protecting young, or wild make the application of the basic principles of evidence collection and tracking very difficult, if not impossible. The safety of the individuals processing the scene and caring for the evidence animals in Protective Custody is of paramount concern. The safety of the animals themselves is also a significant factor to consider. Always equip yourself with the best animal handling experts at your disposal for the species you expect to encounter. Learn about these resources prior to needing them.

If you are on the scene and unable to capture an evidence animal safely, there are alternatives that can be considered. One option is to leave the animal(s) in the care of the owner with specific directions on what care needs to be provided and the timeline by which it needs to be provided. If the animal needs food, water, or over-the-counter medication and the scene response team has those resources available, the officer and veterinarian can collaborate on the decision of what to provide to the owner. Provide these instructions in writing, with a copy to the provider, and make a note of this in your report. Another option that some agencies may employ is the use of sedation or anesthesia. In some cases, sedating a dangerous or otherwise unhandleable animal is the most humane and safe option for capture and transport. The use of chemical capture methods requires the proper equipment and licensing, and must be planned and performed by a veterinarian or other professional certified in administering these drugs. Depending on the species and how cooperative the owner is, another option is leaving live capture traps for these animals. Without exception, these traps need to be checked with strict regularity if this option is employed.

In most cases, if you enlist trusted expert handlers and serve a warrant as early as possible to give yourself enough time, you will likely be able to safely capture even behaviorally difficult animals. This is an example of a time you would have to be creative in obtaining an on-scene photo of the animals with their evidence identifier. Ultimately it may not be possible, but the effort should be made. For example, you may have to photograph a fearful cat after they have been captured and put into a carrier. Take a photo of the evidence placard and then take a photo of the cat through an opening in the carrier. If it is too dangerous to photograph a horse while it is being led by a handler, then take a photo of the evidence placard with the unique identifier and then photograph the horse while it is loose in the pasture or after it has already been loaded, through a gap in the trailer wall (Figure 10.15).

On the scene, flag the carriers or transport vehicles with these particular animals so the individuals intaking the animals are aware and can take precautions. Make a plan in advance with the intake team that you will use an obvious signal, like brightly colored duct tape affixed to the carriers or across the trailer door, to provide a clear indication to use extra caution as the animals contained inside present a behavior risk. This added visual cue can reduce the risk of accident or injury when these animals arrive at the next phase of their processing.

The veterinary exams of these animals are likely to be different from those of animals that are easier to handle. It is important for the veterinarian to be consistent in the exams of the difficult animals and explain in the final veterinary report why the exam process was different for that population of evidence animals (see Appendix B for a veterinary exam form that includes a behavior score and notes about handling).

Instead of these evidence animals receiving less human interaction because they are likely dangerous, they need more attention given to their behavioral enrichment (see Chapter 13 for more information about enrichment for Protective Custody animals). The day these animals are removed from a property may be the first day they have ever seen another human, been treated by a

Figure 10.15 Attaching the evidence placard to the end of this pole permitted the scene-processing team to document this agitated stallion at the scene without putting themselves or the horse in danger. *Source:* Oregon Humane Society.

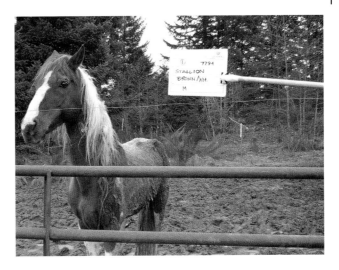

veterinarian, or had experience of riding in a vehicle; any one of which would be a terrifying experience for them. As they become more comfortable with their surroundings, confident in their interactions, and healthier, many of the animals initially thought to be unsocial or aggressive may prove to be resilient and affectionate companions. Give the animals a chance to come around after the traumatic experience of being processed in an animal cruelty case before you give them a label that could be detrimental to their future placement.

10.3.3.8 Aquatic Evidence Animals

The general principles of live animal evidence collection and preservation apply regardless of the species. If a case involves aquatic evidence animals, make the best effort you can to document and identify them individually on the scene. Enlist veterinary and animal husbandry experts prior to taking these animals into custody so they can receive the necessary forensic exams and be provided the proper care while in Protective Custody. Connect the chain of custody forms with their habitat, in a way that documents who is interacting with them and when.

10.3.3.9 When an Evidence Animal Bites

Inevitably an evidence animal is going to bite or otherwise injure (scratch, gore, sting, kick) a staff member or a volunteer who is interacting with them. This does not change anything about their evidentiary status. It is worthwhile to evaluate the circumstances of the bite, to rule out the possibility it was motivated by a response to pain from an injury or illness. Otherwise, any organization that is working with – either caring for or medically treating – Protective Custody animals needs to have policies and procedures in place for responding to a bite incident. The policies will include referral to any Public Health Administration or Occupational Safety and Health Administration (OHSA) requirements for employers, employees and volunteers, as well as state requirements for reporting the incident, quarantine of the animal, and documentation in the animal's medical notes. Staff routinely engaged in veterinary medicine and animal handling should consider a prophylactic rabies vaccine, especially in areas of known rabies transmission.

10.3.3.10 Euthanizing Evidence Animals

Given the nature of living evidence, it is likely at some point an evidence animal will pass away or must be humanely euthanized while it is still under Protective Custody; that is the nature of this evidence. If there is an emergency situation, such as a badly abused cat who presents as a part of a cruelty investigation, or an animal becomes hopelessly sick or injured while in care, a veterinarian must be consulted to determine the need to act immediately to provide humane euthanasia if no other treatment options are viable. Do not withhold humane euthanasia to an actively dying animal, based on its status as evidence. In the event a shelter is housing an evidence animal that requires euthanasia by trained and licensed nonveterinary staff, the same requirements for documentation and decision making hold true. Consult a veterinarian in these cases, whenever possible without prolonging an animal's suffering.

In some cases, an evidence animal's medical condition has progressed such that the quality of life and prognosis for recovery do not offer a humane situation for that animal. An example of this would be a cat with leukemia that has progressed, and palliative care does not keep the animal in a reasonable amount of comfort. Acute emergencies may occur, such as canine bloat, that even with veterinary intervention may result in the demise of the dog. In any case that you have time, prior to the action of euthanasia, attempt to alert the prosecutor and/or lead law enforcement officer on the case, but again do not unnecessarily prolong the suffering of the animal and take immediate action when necessary.

Document these scenarios well and make that documentation part of your chain of custody paperwork and your discovery to the prosecutor. Include what time the animal was found, by whom, and what steps were taken to render aid and/or determine that euthanasia was appropriate. Do not dispose of the body until authorized to do so by the prosecutor. Package and label the body and store it in a cooler, if one is available, until a decision is made regarding necropsy. The veterinarian and prosecutor will discuss whether a necropsy in the case of a euthanasia, unattended, or unexpected death of an evidence animal would contribute important information to the case.

10.4 What to Do with Evidence Until Trial

10.4.1 Nonliving Evidence

10.4.1.1 Evaluation and Documentation After Seizure

To further your investigation into the alleged crime, after nonliving evidence is seized, put a plan in place for evaluating and further documenting that evidence. Count and compare medication to veterinary receipts and timelines. Review transfer records and adoption contracts and compare them to the animals seized from the scene. This information can be included in the veterinarian's report along with a timeline that explains, in the best manner possible, injuries and illnesses the veterinarian discovers. Laptops and cell phones need to be taken to a lab or facility that can forensically evaluate them and report on the content. Depending on whether the suspect is in custody, some of this evaluation and documentation needs to happen very quickly and can influence the charging decision of the prosecutor. When a person is being held in custody (i.e. jail), there are strict timeframes that expedite the charging process to ensure that an individual is not kept against their will for a prolonged period of time.

10.4.1.2 Defendant's Access

At some point the defendant may file a motion to view and evaluate the evidence. This motion will typically be granted. If there is nonliving evidence located somewhere other than a traditional property room, the prosecutor and/or lead law enforcement officer must play an active role in orchestrating when and how the defendant interacts with that evidence. This responsibility should not fall to the veterinarians or animal care agencies, who do not have the expertise or experience to navigate that encounter without outside assistance. This process should mirror, to the extent possible, the existing process in place at the law enforcement agency for defense viewing of evidence and should be documented in the chain of custody paperwork.

10.4.2   Live Evidence

10.4.2.1   Duties and Expectations for Holding Live Evidence

When agreeing to be the caretaker for evidence animals, an organization and the individuals responsible are committing to meeting specific expectations and duties. All participating entities and individuals must discuss these expectations and duties prior to the intake of the evidence animals so there is no confusion. Providing role clarity and details about everyone's responsibility will prevent mistakes and errors that could have a negative effect on the investigation and outcome of the case. Holding live evidence means that every effort will be made to maintain the chain of custody; that the animals will receive proper husbandry and adequate veterinary care for their species and physical conditions; that any documentation produced in relation to the animals while they are being held will be preserved and disclosed to the prosecutor and lead law enforcement agency on the case; and, finally, that the animals will be held in Protective Custody until their status as evidence changes.

10.4.2.2   Is All Paperwork Associated with Ongoing Care of the Animal Evidence?

The process of multiple individuals caring for a population of animals produces a lot of documentation, such as medication logs, veterinary treatment records, cleaning, exercise, and movement records. All this documentation is part of the case record for as long as the animal retains its status as evidence. Prohibit staff and volunteers from taking unofficial photos of the animals who are being held as evidence, and make sure they understand that any photographs they do take must be submitted to the case file. Behavior notes or medical treatment notes also will become part of the case file. Even emails sent to other staff members referencing the care, improvement, decline, or behavior of the animals can be considered evidence in the case that is required to be produced to the prosecutor. Thus, planning ahead and training the individuals involved in caring for the animals about how to properly document the animals' care and progress, such that it is not occurring through personal emails or text messages, facilitate the process of accurately gathering this information when necessary.

10.4.2.3   Is Recovery Considered Evidence?

The charges and subsequent prosecution of an animal cruelty case will rely on the evidence relating to the condition or circumstance of the animal at the time the alleged crime was committed. A judge may not deem the condition or circumstances of the animal since it was removed from the defendant's custody and control relevant to the case. If there is not documentation of recovery, for example if the animal was never seized or located, it does not negate the charge and the existing evidence of the crime that was committed. There may be cases where the documentation of recovery of a victim animal who sustained an injury or suffered from illness or emaciation can be considered relevant evidence in the case. However, some prosecutors may hesitate to introduce evidence of a recovered animal in a trial because it can give jury members or judges comfort about the status of the animal, which can translate into leniency in their review of the facts of the case.

10.4.2.4   Third-Party Owners

In investigations into breeders, boarding facilities, or animal rescues there are often third-party owners of the evidence animals. Have a plan for responding to these individuals going into the investigation. When animals are seized in a case, they are evidence, and the forensic exam conducted in the first 24 hours provides additional crucial evidence to the case. Do not disposition a seized evidence animal to a third-party owner prior to undergoing all the forensic documentation and exam necessary for the case.

If the Protective Custody animal has been documented, examined, and is not in a critical medical condition, then the agency holding the animal must collaborate with the prosecutor and/or law enforcement agency about the plan for dispositioning the owned animals to the third-party owners. There may be stipulations around this endeavor, such as a signed agreement to make the animal available as needed in the investigation, or a stipulation not to return the animal to the custody or control of the defendant.

10.4.2.5   Defendant's Access

A defendant has a right to view and evaluate the evidence, but when that evidence is also the victim of the crime the parameters around what kind of access a defendant gets may differ. Typically, the defendant will enlist an agent to view the evidence on their behalf, either a veterinarian or their lawyer. As with the nonliving evidence, the prosecutor and the lead law enforcement agency must be involved with the logistics of how this access is carried out. It is best practice for anyone who participates in the visit to the evidence animals to generate a report about what happened and what was said or discussed at that time. Although it may be logistically difficult to facilitate, particularly when evidence animals are being held in Protective Custody foster care, it can often be helpful to the resolution of a case for a defendant to have a party they trust view the animals and the way they are being kept and treated.

10.5   Evidence at Trial

10.5.1   Nonliving Evidence

The trial is the reason so many precautions are taken when it comes to safeguarding and tracking the evidence in criminal cases. Prosecutors have an extremely high volume of cases and often cannot begin their preparation until the week of or the week before trial in many animal cruelty cases. Throughout the course of the case through the criminal justice system, it is important to keep in regular contact with the prosecutor assigned to the case. Once the prosecutor feels confident the case will be going to trial in the short term, it is helpful for the animal care agency and/or the lead law enforcement agency to remind the prosecutor what evidence is being held pending the outcome of that proceeding. To demonstrate the odor to the judge or jury the prosecutor may want to admit the bag of shaved mats into evidence at trial instead of a photo. The prosecutor could request the bottle of medication seized from the scene or the collar found on the victim animal. The chain of custody documentation must follow the item to and from court.

10.5.2   Living Evidence

On rare occasions the living animal who is the subject of the case is subpoenaed into the trial as evidence. Before this happens, there are several arguments the prosecutor needs to make in an effort to prevent this circumstance. First, the animal is the victim of the crime and the psychological impact not only of being subjected to the unfamiliar courthouse but also of being confronted with their abuser should not be discounted. Second, the actual presence of the animal must be relevant in order to be admitted as evidence. The prosecutor must push back to determine what is gained by subjecting the living animal to this experience rather than using photography and videography to demonstrate the relevant evidence to the judge or jury.

If live animals are required to be present at the trial, then accommodations must be met. If a judge decides that it is relevant and necessary for the victim animals to be present at the trial, the animal care agency is within their rights to request a plan for entry through courthouse security, times, and locations the animal(s) may relieve itself, and who will accompany the animal in the courtroom. As with the nonliving evidence, make sure to maintain the chain of custody to and from the courtroom.

10.6 Evidence After Trial

The conclusion of the trial does not equate to immediate disposition of the evidence being held for that case. There are various factors that agencies holding evidence must consider and grapple with when dispositioning evidence, both nonliving and living.

10.6.1 Nonliving Evidence

10.6.1.1 Timeframes for Retention

Depending on the nature of the crime and the evidence, there are statutory mandates on how long an agency must retain the evidence. For example, records related to a case involving a homicide are likely to have longer retention time periods than records from a lower-level misdemeanor charge. If you are a veterinary clinic or animal care agency in possession of records related to a criminal investigation without the means to preserve those records, make sure the law enforcement entity investigating the case has the full complement of those records in order to meet their obligation under the law.

State laws will likely accommodate requests to dispose of biological evidence prior to the final adjudication of the case or before the statutory retention period. Typically, early disposal of evidence would require notification and approval by the prosecutor and adequate notice to the defendant. If a veterinary clinic or an animal shelter is holding biological evidence related to a previously closed or adjudicated case, a representative can, and should, contact the law enforcement agency assigned to the case to determine appropriate next steps.

(See Appendix D for examples of state laws regarding retention and disposition of evidence.)

10.6.1.2 Notice to Defendants

Many state statutes require notice to the defendant prior to disposition of evidence in their case. Generally, this would consist of a certified letter sent to their last known address indicating what evidence is being dispositioned and explaining what action they need to take if they would like to reclaim the item(s). If you do not have a safe and secure location to return evidence to individuals, it is your responsibility to provide an alternative method for returning the items and documenting the return. Typically, if the previous owner of the evidence does not claim the evidence within a certain timeframe (specified in your notice), the evidence will automatically be dispositioned.

10.6.1.3 Disposal Methods

If evidence has been released for disposal, the items must be disposed of safely and in accordance with state law. Biological evidence must be disposed of in an approved method for that item. Animal shelters that are equipped with a crematorium can utilize that equipment for disposal of released evidence. Records must be destroyed in a way that ensures confidentiality and upholds protection of criminal justice information in accordance with that state's laws.

10.6.1.4 Use at Shelter or Donation to Shelter

When dispositioning evidence from an animal cruelty case, some items, such as kennels or cages, may be suitable for use in an animal shelter or with an animal rescue. Releasing an item to inventory or donation is only a viable option when the retention time has expired, and the original owner of the item has opted not to reclaim the item. In order to include this as a disposition option, an agency must include criteria in their evidence policies regarding what requirements must be met, including the nature and quality of the item. The following is an example of how this would be covered in a policy manual:

> In an effort to reduce unnecessary waste, when an item of evidence is unclaimed by an owner and no longer needs to be retained for purposes of a criminal case, it can be incorporated into the shelter inventory if:

- It is of a quality that meets the needs and requirements of the shelter.
- Agency Supervisor provides approval in writing.

10.6.2 Living Evidence

You want to do your best to honor the principles of evidence disposition in how you treat the animals involved in a case but remember you are adapting them to living beings. Think about how you can apply inanimate property evidence principles of disposition to this living evidence. Ask yourself, what are the underlying important principles or concepts to uphold and how can those be adapted humanely to living evidence?

10.6.2.1 Third-Party Owners

In some cases, the animal care agency may be required to maintain the victim animal through the conclusion of the trial, despite documented third-party ownership. When the case has concluded at the trial level, it is an appropriate time to approach the prosecutor or the lead law enforcement agency with a request to disposition the evidence to that third party, if the defendant's ownership has been forfeited. Even if there are reservations about the ability of that third party to provide proper care for the animal, it is unlikely there is a legal means to prevent the return of the animal to an individual with existing ownership rights to that animal. It is important to remember in that situation, the case involved only the defendant and not the third party.

10.6.2.2 Adoptions

If the conclusion of the trial phase of a case results in forfeiture of the animals to the animal care agency, then proper disposition of those animals can occur through adoptions to new homes. Making the animal(s) available for adoption could carry with it varying degrees of risk. Defendants can move to appeal both a preconviction forfeiture and a trial verdict, but must give notice of intent to do so on strict timeframes. Defendants can also file a motion to stay, which, if granted, prevents the parties from moving forward with the outcome of a preconviction forfeiture or the execution of a sentence until the appeal has been heard and decided on. Communicate with the prosecutor assigned to the case to understand the status of ownership of the victim animals and, if possible, discuss with counsel the level of risk your organization is willing to take on in moving forward with adoptions immediately after a forfeiture proceeding or a verdict at trial.

There are other factors to consider in post-trial adoptions as well. Some states have laws that directly contemplate the court vesting ownership in someone other than a shelter.[2] It is important to consider whether or not to include any specialized language or clauses in the adoption contracts of victim animals (see examples in Appendix C). Some states specifically criminalize the act of adopting a victim animal and returning it to the defendant,[3] and this could be underscored in an adoption contract in those states. If the adoption agency has ownership of the victim animals, they are within their rights to include special requirements for adopters of those animals. Animals are resilient and remarkable in their ability to recover from severe trauma, but in an effort to spare them that fate a second time, it is the responsibility of their caretakers to make best, legally sound, efforts to ensure their future safety.

10.6.3 Conclusion

Evidence collection, documentation, and presentation to the court may seem like an arduous and impossible task; one that is fraught with pitfalls and potential for mistakes. However, it is the evidence and the handling of this evidence – whether inanimate or living – that carry the story of the affected animal and preserve the integrity of the system, from the events that led to the animal's status as evidence, to presentation in front of a judge or jury who ultimately determine the outcome of the case. When the fundamentals of good process, documentation, and follow-up are paired with solid reporting, everyone involved in evidence collection can rest assured that they have done an excellent job in their part of a criminal animal cruelty case.

References

1 Garner, B.A. (ed.) (2019). *Black's Law Dictionary Standard*, 11e, 697–698. St. Paul, MN: Thomson Reuters.
2 University of California Davis (n.d.). Using a CODIS (Combined DNA Index System) to fight dog fighting. https://vgl.ucdavis.edu/forensics/canine-codis (accessed 30 May 2021).
3 University of California Davis (n.d.). Pioneering animal forensic science through collaborative research and evidence-based science, establishing best practices, and providing expert testimony. https://vgl.ucdavis.edu/forensics (accessed 30 May 2021).

---

2 Arkansas, "appropriate place of custody," Arkansas Code Annotated, title 5, subtitle 6, chapter 62, subchapter 1, s 5-62-106(d) 2009 (AR); Connecticut "any person found to be suitable or worthy of such responsibility by the court," Connecticut General Statutes Annotated, title 22, chapter 435, s 22-329a(g), 29-108e(d) 1995 (CT); Indiana, "the State Veterinarian can make recommendation to court regarding disposition of forfeited animal that are in the animal's best interests, and court shall give substantial weight to that recommendation," Annotated Indiana Code, title 35, article 46, chapter 3, s 35-46-3-6 1987 (IN); Oregon, "the agency may give preference to placing forfeited animal with family or friend who did not contribute to the cruelty," Oregon Revised Statutes Annotated, title 16, chapter 167, s 167.348 1995 (OR); Rhode Island, "any person found to be suitable or worthy of such responsibility by the court," General Laws of Rhode Island Annotated, title 4, chapter 1.2, s 4-1.2-5(1) 2019 (RI); South Dakota, "Suitable caretaker or facility as prescribed in rule by the board," South Dakota Codified Laws, title 40, chapter 40-1, s 40-1-34 1991 (SD); Vermont, "other individual deemed appropriate by the court," Vermont Statutes Annotated, Crimes and Criminal Procedure, title 13, Pt 1, chapter 8, subchapter 1, s 353(c) 1989 (VT).
3 Oregon is an example: Oregon Revised Statutes Annotated, title 16, chapter 167, s 167.349 2009 (OR).

11

Veterinary Forensic Necropsy
Kris Otteman and Zarah Hedge

Veterinarians are trained to perform traditional postmortem (after death) examinations. The technical term that describes this procedure in veterinary medicine is *necropsy*. Depending on the type of veterinary practice – general, specialized, shelter, or university – the necropsy procedure may be something done often, occasionally, or always referred to an outside expert. The necropsy serves the same purpose as an autopsy in the human field: to confirm or determine cause and/or manner of death.

11.1   How a Forensic Necropsy is Different

Necropsy in a traditional veterinary case might be used to confirm and explore a clinical diagnosis, such as cancer, or to determine if an undiagnosed incident, such as a ruptured spleen, was the cause of an animal's death. When a veterinarian performs a necropsy to aid an animal cruelty investigation, the procedure becomes "forensic." In a forensic necropsy, the veterinarian uses medical and scientific methods to collect information that may be used as evidence in a legal case. Causes of death such as starvation, blunt force trauma, gunshot, and hyperthermia may be confirmed or ruled out through forensic necropsy. The process includes examination of the animal's body including the internal organs and tissues, performing and interpreting X-rays, as well as conducting histopathology and other laboratory tests. The forensic necropsy is conducted in a consistent, thorough, and objective manner. It is the responsibility of the veterinarian to gather all the information possible and to use this information to draw conclusions about the cause and manner of death. The veterinarian is not in the position to determine guilt or innocence, but functions in the important role of presenting facts and findings that are essential to the investigation.

11.2   The Importance of the Forensic Necropsy

Investigators should not disregard a deceased animal before seeking a veterinarian's advice. Critical evidence can be gleaned from badly decomposed remains, or even dry bones, in some cases. Even in cases where the cause of death is clear, or those with a confession in hand, the

Animal Cruelty Investigations: A Collaborative Approach from Victim to Verdict^{TM}, First Edition.
Edited by Kris Otteman, Linda Fielder, and Emily Lewis.
© 2022 John Wiley & Sons, Inc. Published 2022 by John Wiley & Sons, Inc.
Companion website: www.wiley.com/go/otteman/victimtoverdict

forensic necropsy serves to provide additional or confirmatory evidence that may impact the charges or the outcome of the case. For example, a deceased dog is found with gunshot wounds to the head and chest. The neighbor has admitted to shooting the dog because it had entered his backyard and was charging at him. The veterinarian performs a forensic necropsy at the request of the investigating law enforcement agency. The veterinarian examines the wounds externally and internally and can establish the trajectory as well as the bullet's entrance and exit points. These findings show that the dog was shot from behind, meaning it was actually moving away from the neighbor when it was shot – evidence that casts considerable doubt on the narrative provided to the investigator and may, therefore, change the outcome of the case.

Forensic necropsies can also provide answers to particular questions that arise during an investigation. For example, without a necropsy an arson investigator cannot know if a cat was killed before the fire was set or if its death was attributed to being confined in the home with the smoke and fire. Prosecutors may request necropsies as a means of determining what charges to file in a case like the one above. In some cases, the additional information or questions posed by the officer or prosecutor may focus or direct the veterinarian to a specific part of the necropsy.

Investigators, prosecutors, and animal control agencies should all establish a working relationship with a veterinarian who is willing to perform forensic necropsies for criminal cases. The veterinarian must understand and adhere to consistent protocols, keep detailed notes, generate thorough reports, and agree to testify to their findings in court. As with any case that benefits from the help of an expert, it is much easier to find the right expertise before you need it rather than wait until an emergency arises.

11.3   Necropsy at the Owner's Request

An animal owner's request for a traditional cause-of-death necropsy can evolve into a forensic necropsy. Whether the initial decision to conduct a necropsy stems from a veterinarian's recommendation in order to confirm a diagnosis or an owner's request in an effort to find closure after the death of their pet, either can result in findings that prompt a more thorough forensic necropsy and criminal investigation.

An example of this would be a dog who suddenly suffered multiple seizures and collapsed after visiting the dog park, was rushed to an emergency hospital, but died before care could be initiated. In this case a traditional necropsy would rule out a diagnosis like heat stroke or an underlying end-stage disease. In speaking with the owner, the veterinarian learns that several recent reports of poisoning had been linked to the same dog park the owner had visited. The veterinarian, with the owner's permission, may investigate the cause of death by completing a forensic necropsy including examination of the stomach and intestinal contents for evidence of poisoning and collection of samples for possible identification of a toxic substance. The veterinarian, suspecting criminal activity, would then contact law enforcement.

11.4   Packaging and Storing Remains Prior to Necropsy

Ideally, forensic necropsies are performed shortly after or the same day as the death of the animal. This is not always practical or possible, and so the method of packaging and storing the body is very important. Because the examination of tissues (skin, muscle, organs) is the foundation of necropsy procedures, maintaining the vitality of those tissues is critical. Refrigeration is always preferable over freezing, when possible. The remains are evidence and must be identified and packaged as such so their chain of custody and security is memorialized. Chapter 10 of this book contains detailed information about properly identifying, packaging, and storing remains awaiting necropsy as well as long-term storage after the procedure.

11.5   Forensic Necropsy Equipment and Protocols

As the field of veterinary forensics expands, numerous universities, scientific organizations, and veterinary specialists have developed and published recommended forensic necropsy protocols. Forensic necropsies are performed in state-of-the-art animal crime labs and university teaching hospitals, as well as in single-doctor practices, animal shelters with medical services, and even in the field at the crime scene. They can include very sophisticated analysis such as electron micros-copy and DNA analysis, or they can be performed with a basic surgery pack and radiology set-up. While state-of-the-art equipment may be necessary to provide very specific evidence in some cases, most cases benefit from and are conclusive as a result of a thorough and detailed gross (visual) examination of the victim animal. Do not be tempted to dismiss the impact necropsy can make in the investigation of a cruelty case, and understand that a skilled clinician with modest equipment and access to laboratory services can provide more evidence in most cases than specialized diag-nostic equipment. This chapter provides an array of recommendations and steps veterinarians should consider, and is intended to support, not supplant, previously published protocols. If you are providing forensic veterinary necropsies to aid in the investigation of cruelty cases, consider using the forms and processes provided here or create necropsy protocols that are particular to your practice and follow those protocols precisely.

11.6   Case History

Before beginning a forensic necropsy, the veterinarian requests, reads, and analyzes all materials that are available from the investigation. This includes previous medical records, the initial report to law enforcement, and witness statements that led to law enforcement requesting a necropsy. This does not create bias but rather informs the doctor to consider the circumstances and to con-clude, when possible, the chain of events and outcomes. Creating a timeline of known or sus-pected key events prior to beginning the necropsy and a list of open questions that need to be answered can guide the veterinarian in their process. Determining and documenting what did and did not cause injury, illness, or death in the animal informs the investigator regarding next steps and eventually the prosecutor if criminal charges are brought.

11.7   Preparing to Perform the Necropsy

11.7.1   The Importance of an Assistant

As with any surgical procedure, an assistant can be a second or third pair of helping hands to the veterinarian. In performing a forensic necropsy, it can be difficult for a lone veterinarian to per-form the procedure, make notes, place placards and measuring scales, take photographs, and

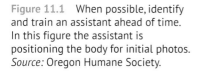

Figure 11.1 When possible, identify and train an assistant ahead of time. In this figure the assistant is positioning the body for initial photos. *Source:* Oregon Humane Society.

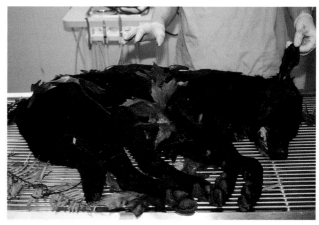

collect and package samples and evidence simultaneously. A technician, assistant, or fellow veterinarian who can act as a scribe, photographer, and general helper provides the assistance and assurance you need to be certain the evidence identified during the procedure is correctly recorded, collected, processed, and stored. If you find yourself performing a necropsy without assistance, take your time in performing each necessary step of the process to be certain all aspects of the procedure are completed according to your protocol. If possible, identify staff who may be available to assist and provide basic training on the overall process proactively (Figure 11.1).

11.7.2 Crime Scene Evaluation

Information observed, collected, and analyzed from a crime scene is very important to a forensic necropsy in most cases. Be prepared to assist at a crime scene, visit a scene during processing, or review information and evidence collected at the scene by other investigators, veterinarians, or evidence technicians. By considering all of the information available and related to what happened at the scene, the necropsy is better informed, and you can conclude details that may otherwise be left as open questions. Photos, scene diagrams, and accelerants taken from the scene of an arson fire may assist in processing samples to determine if the animal died before, during, or after the fire. Antibiotics and steroid injectable drugs collected at a "game cock" farm prompt the veterinarian to investigate the injuries and deaths of poultry collected with the possibility of cockfighting in mind (Figures 11.2 and 11.3).

11.7.3 Photography

Photographs become evidence and also illustrate the veterinarian's findings during necropsy. The investigators, attorneys, judges, and jury will all need to understand your findings, and photographs are the best way to ensure comprehension. Make sure the camera you use can take clear, close-range photos or, if it is not able to, avoid taking photos at close range. Make sure the date and time stamp feature is set to the correct date and time. Insert a data storage card that is clear and has ample memory. While photographing evidence, never delete a photo in the series, even if it is blurry or is a photo of the inside of your coat pocket. Missing photo files can look suspect in a criminal case packet. Take photographs throughout the necropsy and include views

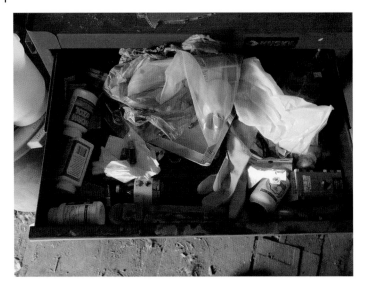

Figure 11.2 Supplies and equipment found in the animal's environment provide clues that are invaluable to understanding the overall conditions in which the animal has lived. *Source:* Oregon Humane Society.

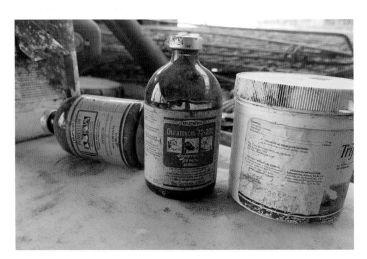

Figure 11.3 These medications discovered on scene support the probability that the deceased birds were used for cockfighting. *Source:* Oregon Humane Society.

that demonstrate key findings such as scars, wounds, bruising, and internal bleeding. Place a measuring scale next to wounds to show size. As mentioned in Chapter 7, use the three-point (far, mid, and close-up) technique of photography to clearly document the position, aspect, extent, and other attributes of the finding you are documenting. It can be helpful to create a log of photos that lists what each photo demonstrates, as a reference for report writing. Always use a camera; do not use a personal cell phone. For more information on photographing evidence, see Chapter 9.

11.7.4 Video

Videography is not commonly used to illustrate findings in necropsy procedures; however, use of video to document a specific finding in a necropsy is warranted if this is the best way to illustrate the finding. When video is utilized, include the concepts of proper identification and perspective, and only have audio on if you intend for the audio to be part of your report. Verify the correct date and time on all camera equipment prior to use.

11.7.5   Medical Notes, Forms, and Templates

Working from a form or template can help ensure all procedural steps are followed and recorded. A voice recorder or dictation software may be helpful, especially when performing necropsies without assistance. Prepare for documentation ahead of time by selecting appropriate forms, and have charts and references available that will facilitate thorough and orderly documentation. If possible, become familiar with the forms ahead of time and use the same system with all cases to ensure consistency. Handwritten notes, computer-typed notes, and recordings are all acceptable means of documentation that can be utilized when compiling the final necropsy report.

A necropsy form listing all major areas of evaluation is helpful to ensure nothing is forgotten. The use of body scar or wound charts aids in documenting scars and wounds present on the body, which is useful in many cases, including suspected animal fighting and nonaccidental injury cases. Body condition score charts for the specific species should be utilized and a body condition score recorded during the external exam. Other charts, such as dental charts, are useful for capturing organized and correct documentation.

11.7.6   Necropsy Tools and Equipment

Prior to beginning the forensic necropsy, it is important that you have all the necessary specific equipment to perform the procedure. Put together a necropsy kit with appropriate instruments for the species and size of the animal to be necropsied (see Appendix B for a Medical Exam Equipment Checklist). This may include surgical instruments, such as a scalpel blade and forceps, to enable the veterinarian to enter and evaluate internal organs, scissors or garden shears to cut into the thoracic cavity, and a hand saw, hatchet, or Stryker saw to enter the skull. Large and small scales should be available during the necropsy to allow for documentation of weight of the animal and animal tissues. Trajectory rods or similar tools may be useful for tracing the path of a projectile, such as a bullet. The kit should also include various measurement tools, including a scalpel handle with measurement on one side, measuring tape, and rulers. Other equipment to have on hand includes various sizes of plastic ziplock bags, paper bags, various sized jars with formalin fixative, microscope slides, syringes and needles, and synthetic swabs on plastic shafts. Other testing equipment may be needed depending on the type of samples and testing that are needed for the specific necropsy.

11.7.7   Forensic Necropsy

For further information on the topics in this section, see [1].

11.7.7.1   Step 1 Initial Exam of Remains and Accompanying Materials
Prior to handling the remains and any other items that are included with the remains, proper personal protective equipment should be donned. Handling and performing a necropsy can potentially expose individuals to various infectious and zoonotic diseases, and protective equipment such as gloves, gowns, boots, coveralls or scrubs, face and respiratory protection may be needed.

Maintain appropriate chain of custody records for remains and samples throughout and after the necropsy procedure by documenting how the animal was received, stored, moved, and by whom. Record what is known about time of death and conditions, and where the animal was prior to receipt, including information about storage conditions and location.

Assign a veterinarian to complete the exam and other individuals such as technicians, veterinary students, or law enforcement personnel who will carry out duties including scribe, photography, sample collection, radiography, or other needed assistance. These individuals work under the direction and authority of the veterinarian in charge of the procedure. Record the names and duties of all individuals involved or assisting (Box 11.1).

Include the following steps as appropriate to the case:

- Complete an evidence placard including unique case number and/or animal identifier and animal description (weight, sex, species, breed, approximate age, date, and time).
- Photograph the packaging undisturbed (Figures 11.4–11.6).
- Photograph the documents and materials included with the package.
- Photograph in an "opened state" including:
  - Right and left lateral recumbency
  - Dorsal and ventral
  - Cranial and caudal views
- Record the weight of the remains without packaging or other items and take a photo of the scale used for this purpose.
- Scan for a microchip and look for tattoos and/or ear tipping, or other tags or identifiers, and record that information found on the placard, in the notes, and with a photograph.
- Document and take photos of all items presented with the body, such as halters, tags, collars, bandages, and leg bands.

Box 11.1   Example

Veterinary technician Sally Smith completed radiographs of the remains and assisted throughout the necropsy as both scribe and general assistant. Detective Joe Jones from the Pleasantville Police Department served as photographer.

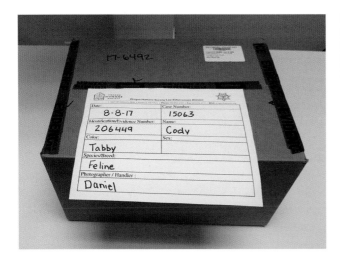

Figure 11.4   Start taking photographs upon receipt of the remains and continue throughout the process. *Source:* Oregon Humane Society.

Figure 11.5 Collect far, mid, and close-uprange photos in sequence to show animal identification and overall appearance. *Source:* Oregon Humane Society.

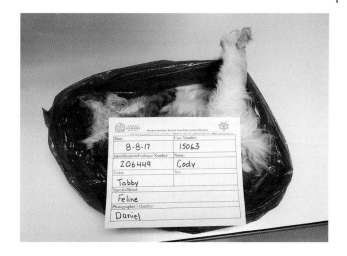

Figure 11.6 Photos verify important procedures and demonstrate chain of custody. *Source:* Oregon Humane Society.

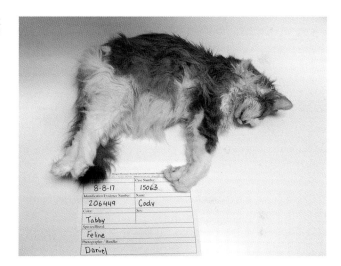

- Search for and collect trace evidence on the body.
- If samples for DNA analysis of animal remains are necessary, note the sample's origin, such as blood, fur, or tissue and label it clearly with an evidence identifier.
- If collection of samples for DNA analysis from an inanimate object is warranted, use caution to avoid cross contamination with other samples and use an evidence identifier and source description (for example, knife blade, #23456).
- Change gloves between types of evidence as appropriate to avoid cross-contamination (Box 11.2).

11.7.7.2 Step 2 Diagnostic Imaging

Full-body radiography of the deceased victim is recommended, prior to all forensic necropsies, as this additional diagnostic step confirms suspected findings and may unveil unknown or otherwise difficult-to-find evidence. Previously healed fractures of ribs or other bones, projectiles, or ingested

---

Box 11.2 Example

DNA from dog with bites and stab wounds and DNA from sample of blood and on handle of knife could be used to identify victim, dog bite aggressor (dog bites), and human assailant (knife), and to confirm that blood on knife is from victim dog.

---

materials that could be overlooked or unseen, such as foil, are found with imaging. Diagnostic imaging should be performed when decomposition obscures or causes loss of identifying features and/or there is evidence of trauma in animals. Taking standard overall full-body views is sufficient for initial imaging.

Guidelines for imaging include:

- Full-body radiographs and specific additional views of areas of concern. Plan ahead based on case history for special views or techniques, such as use of probes, that may assist in final determination and illustration of findings.
- Record the name of the technician performing imaging and include it in the report.
- Ensure that all radiographs are properly labeled, including date and animal ID, and the location where they were taken (hospital identification).
- Diagnostic imaging should be performed in all cases of nonaccidental injury, gunshot injuries, charred remains, and decomposed remains.

11.7.7.3 Step 3 Plan for Diagnostics

Veterinarians performing forensic necropsies must have access to a diagnostic laboratory that can provide histology and a facility that can provide diagnostic imaging. Access to a radiologist or other expert to assist in concluding diagnostic imaging findings is helpful in some cases.

Toxicology is a vast field of analysis, thus narrowing the suspected toxins and planning ahead to collaborate with the laboratory of choice to determine sample collection and preservation is essential. Most common sampling for toxicology includes blood, plasma, stomach contents, liver, and kidney.

The histology, chemistry, toxicology, or other reports should include identification of the laboratory and individuals who performed the tests, the source of the sample (canine, liver, animal ID, and case ID), the type of test or screen performed, the method used, results of the test, and interpretation to the extent possible (normal, abnormal, toxic level). It is beneficial to contact the laboratory in advance of requesting specialized testing to ensure samples are collected and stored properly for the testing that is needed. Oftentimes, storage containers or swabs that would be needed for the specific test can be ordered in advance from the laboratory.

Microscopic Findings

Histopathology should be considered in many cases, especially those without obvious cause of death after gross necropsy or to confirm diagnosis. Careful consideration of what to sample and how to preserve samples prevents loss of integrity of the sample. In many cases, it is prudent to collect standard samples from organs and preserve the tissues in formalin, properly labeled and securely stored in case histopathology is necessary in the future. Saving samples for toxicology may require larger volumes of specific organs that are preserved by refrigeration and are perishable. Plan ahead by contacting the lab once potential toxins are identified so that the process proceeds quickly and efficiently (Box 11.3).

Box 11.3   Example

All samples must be collected, labeled, packaged, and preserved with both the integrity of the sample preservation and the protection of the chain of custody in mind.

   Example: Sections of left and right kidneys and liver were collected during the necropsy of Sparkie (patient ID 123456, case number 21-2468) and placed in laboratory-provided plastic containers with formalin. The containers were labeled, laboratory request form for histopathology, case history, and chain of custody forms are completed and included in the package to be shipped to Oregon Veterinary Diagnostic Laboratory.

11.7.7.4   Step 4 External Exam

Perform the external examination in a manner similar to that of a live animal, and record detailed findings by use of a scribe, notes, or recording device. Document and photograph the body condition score of the animal. If available, use a species-specific body condition score system and include that system in the documentation. Details surrounding muscle mass and external fat stores should be included, along with the body condition score. Verify the sex of the animal if possible from external examination. Document and photograph presence of tattoos, spay/neuter scar, or other surgical scars and medical shaving. Evaluate and photograph the eyes, ears, nails, claws, hooves, and/or beak as needed to demonstrate their condition. Dentition, external parasites, and fecal and/or urine scald should be evaluated and documented [2].

   Estimating the time since death, or postmortem interval (PMI), can be important in forensic cases. However, it is important to understand that estimating time of death accurately is challenging as it is widely dependent on many factors, including both internal and external environmental factors, species, and time since death (accuracy declines as the timeline increases) [3]. No one method can reliably estimate time of death [2]. Algor mortis, the cooling of the body after death, has been used to estimate time of death, but studies have found that animals cool at different temperatures, making extrapolation between species difficult [2]. Document if the body is in rigor mortis and if livor mortis is present; include the specific location(s). Rigor mortis results when muscle contracts after death as a result of depletion of the normal chemicals produced by the body. Muscles remain contracted until decomposition begins. Rigor mortis typically occurs between 2 and 6 hours after death and persists for 36 hours, but this is subject to different factors including environmental and antemortem internal temperature of the animal [2]. If the body was frozen prior to postmortem exam, it will affect some findings, and the ability to record rigor mortis. Livor mortis occurs as a result of the effect of gravity on the fluids in the body after death. Blood and other fluid will pool on the dependent or downward side of the body once the heart stops. Lividity can provide insight as to the position the animal was in during the time immediately postmortem. In comparison, livor mortis in humans sets in 30 minutes to 2 hours postmortem, and fixed livor between 8 and 12 hours [2]. The level of decomposition in the body, the presence of insects, whether postmortem scavenging occurred, and other postmortem changes should also be documented. Describe odors, such as those found with decomposition, external substances, feces, and urine, and note whether there is urine scalding or staining, pressure wounds, or fecal material present on the coat.

   Document external wounds, scars, and injuries prior to removal of hair, feathers, or debris. The scars/wounds are measured and documented on a scar/wound body chart as well as described in the necropsy record. The injuries should be described by type, size, location, shape, pattern, and any other important feature. Photographs of scars and wounds should be taken at various distances (close-up, midrange, and far away) as part of evidence collection. Hair can be clipped around wounds or to evaluate for areas of bruising that are not readily seen, due to the presence of the hair coat. Use a photo scale and take a minimum of one photograph per finding, including a faraway photo to illustrate the wounds or injury position on the body, a midrange photo, and a close-up of each wound. Examples include wounds, bites, lacerations, urine staining, pressure wounds, bruising, or evidence of scavenging. Use a photo scale to show the size of findings in photos. Look for and document the degree of decomposition, rigor, presence or absence of parasites, and any other findings.

11.7.7.5 Step 5 Internal Exam

If possible, the necropsy should be performed in a designated area that has running water, good ventilation, and can be cleaned and disinfected (or rinsed in the case of a field necropsy site). Follow a stepwise approach and thorough evaluation of internal contents and organs to prevent missing a step or forgetting to document or collect crucial information. If possible, position the animal on the dorsum or left side (horse's right side). The skin should be dissected, followed by the muscle layer and deeper tissues, to evaluate and expose bruising and/or other external injuries. Document and photograph any abnormalities. A routine necropsy procedure can be followed but may be altered based on the specific case and initial exam findings. A photo scale and markers can be used to demonstrate size and location of injuries or abnormalities for photography and documentation. Probes, wires, or other trajectory tools may be beneficial in evaluating gunshot wound trajectory, vascular injury, or other abnormalities to the organs or tissues. Collect relevant samples of organs, blood, urine, feces, or gastrointestinal tract contents [1].

Oral Cavity, Ears, Integument, and Subcutaneous Exam

- Document the condition of the dentition and oral cavity including lesions, foreign material injury, or disease (Figure 11.7).
- Document damage to the teeth including broken or loose teeth as a result of disease or injury.
- Examine the ears including the pinna (ear flap) and external ear canal. Document findings of parasites, hemorrhage, or bruising.
- Document and describe injuries to all subcutaneous tissues including bruising, petechiae, or hemorrhage.

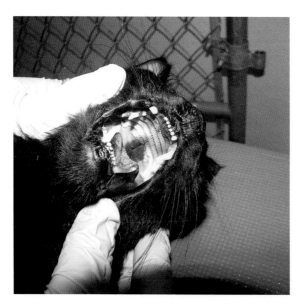

Figure 11.7 Use photography to illustrate and document specific findings. In this case, broken teeth, soft tissue injuries to palate, and mucosa above incisors are all visible. Radiographs of this feline skull will mirror the written and photographic findings as they reveal fractures of facial bones. *Source:* Oregon Humane Society.

Neck
- Examine the neck area including soft tissue, and the airway including the larynx and trachea.
- Dissect the dorsal and or ventral neck in cases of occult injury or suspected neck trauma, or to further investigate radiographic findings or other necropsy findings.

Thorax and Abdomen
- Examine organs as found.
- Describe evidence of surgery.
- Describe adhesions, foreign body, abnormal fluid, accumulation of blood (clotted or not), penetrations, and hernias.
- Remove, dissect, and describe abnormalities of organs, and list organs examined and found to be normal.
- Collect samples for microscope evaluation as warranted based on your findings and opinion.

Head
- Examine the eyes and surrounding tissues including the conjunctiva, sclera, globe, and palpebral tissues. Make note of any scleral hemorrhage or discoloration and intraocular hemorrhage or discoloration.
- Examine the head and remove hair and skin to access potential trauma to head and neck regions. Dissect, as necessary.
- Remove and examine the brain when findings and history warrant this. Document epidural, subdural, or subarachnoid hemorrhage or other findings.
- Document abnormalities with photographs.
- Examine and document fractures or damage to cranium and all osseous structures.

Extremities
Examine extremities including the tail, limbs, pads, hooves, nails, and skin, and document injuries including wounds as in other parts of the body. Look for toenail damage for evidence of shredding of claws or abrasions to pads; examine the base of the tail in canines and felines for evidence of tail fracture or subcutaneous hemorrhage as a result of tail entrapment or pull. Examine the feet, hocks, hip bones, and other prominent areas for pressure wounds due to kenneling, or abrasions from collars, chains, or other physical elements.

Bruising
- Examine for bruising of skin, muscle, or internal organs, which occurs in some cases of blunt or sharp force trauma or with some metabolic or toxic diseases or events. Evaluate the skin carefully and document bruising using photography and measurements (Figure 11.8). Shaving the coat reveals margins and the extent of skin bruises. Consider coat and skin color when inspecting potentially bruised areas as dark fur and pigment of skin can make it more difficult to visualize the bruise. Look for subcutaneous, muscle, and internal bruising, bleeding, and damage associated with any superficial (skin) bruise that is found. Use the same methods of documentation of all bruising and hemorrhage found in all layers.
- Evaluate the time and extent of bruising relative to cause of death. Bruising develops with continued circulation of blood, thus occurs premortem.

Fractures
- Diagnostic imaging will reveal most fractures; however, some very small fractures may not be revealed by routine radiographic imaging. Confirm fractures visualized with imaging by gross necropsy and photography when necessary.

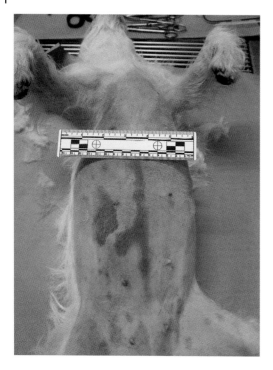

Figure 11.8 Hemorrhage into skin, tissues under the skin, and muscle results in color change and patterns. Use photographs, written description, and photo scale to document findings. In this case external findings aligned with internal injuries of a lacerated liver and broken ribs. *Source:* Oregon Humane Society.

- Subluxation or microfractures of important and even vital joints may cause death and are not seen with traditional radiographs. Necropsy and careful dissection may reveal findings such as subluxation of the cervical spine. Examine, photograph, and describe tissues around the fracture site.
- Determining the estimated timeline when fractures occurred may also be important but can be difficult owing to a variety of internal and external factors, as well as differences between species, that affect bone repair. Normal healing time is 8–12 weeks for most bones; however, if the fracture is unstable, it will prolong healing and may lead to delayed union, nonunion, or mal-union of fractures [4].
- "A rough estimate of healing time includes:
  - Grossly unstable fracture with hematoma only (0–24 hours)
  - Unstable fracture with histological evidence of undifferentiated mesenchymal cells and neovascularization (24–48 hours)
  - Unstable fracture with earliest evidence of woven bone (36 hours)
  - Stable fracture with evidence of primary callus of bone and hyaline cartilage (4–6 weeks)
  - Stable fracture with evidence of woven bone progressing to lamellar bone (months–years)" [5].
- Histology of bone fractures can be useful in identifying the healing stage of the bones involved.

Gunshot Wounds and Projectile/Penetrating Injuries

- Diagnostic imaging findings assist in guiding necropsy decisions made by the veterinarian when investigating a projectile injury to an animal. Evidence of projectiles may be found in remains, depending on the caliber of a projectile, size of the animal, and distance. If a projectile passes through an animal, the entry and exit wounds may help reveal the type of projectile, distance, and the position of the animal at the time of the event. Entry wounds are typically smaller and better delineated than exit wounds, which can vary in dimensions depending on the size, shape, and caliber of the projectile (bullet, pellet, arrow, etc. [Figure 11.9]).

- Describe all injuries and abnormalities, measure wound size, and locate wounds.
- Document the location of wounds found in the skin of extremities, abdomen, neck, thorax, head, or limbs by finding two reference points and measuring using a photo scale. Document the wounds based upon the anatomic region such as head, thorax, etc (Figure 11.10).
- Look for and describe the presence of gunshot-related findings including soot, burns, stippling of hair or skin, searing, abrasion ring, muzzle imprint, or lacerations.
- If projectiles are retrieved from remains, photograph with a scale, and document the type of projectile found if known, or if unable to identify, indicate so.
- Evaluate for pre- and postmortem hemorrhage in proximity to these wounds.

Figure 11.9 Full-body imaging provides the examiner with information about the size and shape of objects such as pellets, bullets, shot, or other materials, and reveals information about their approximate location. *Source:* Oregon Humane Society.

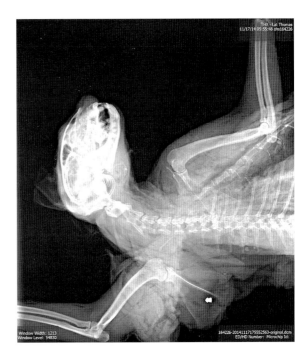

Figure 11.10 The use of a linear object can help trace the trajectory of penetrating wounds. In this photo a small circular entry wound on top of the head is traced to the exit wound, which is larger and resulted in a small amount of hemorrhage. These findings were consistent with a gunshot wound to the top of the head, exiting the body at the chest and into the ground below the cat. *Source:* Oregon Humane Society.

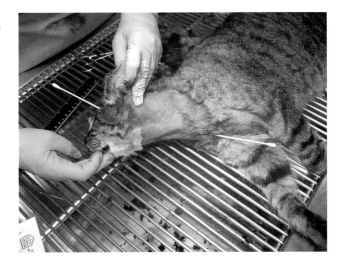

Sharp Force Injury

- Sharp force injuries are characterized by sharp margins of the wounds (Figure 11.11).
- Keep in mind that blunt force trauma delivered over bone or with a large implement can spread force in such a manner as to appear like a sharp force injury. Look at the margins of the wound carefully for sharp cutting of hair or skin vs. a "smashed and split" appearance.
- Describe the wound(s) in terms of size, shape, and location.
- Measure the depth and estimate the direction and track of wounds such as stabs (Figure 11.12).
- Examine and evaluate damage to subcutaneous tissues including bone, organ, muscle, and fat.
- Evaluate for pre- and postmortem hemorrhage around these wounds.
- Radiographic imaging provides documentation and evidence of the presence of projectiles, which in some cases are difficult to locate and recover from remains.
- Recover (when possible) and preserve foreign bodies of evidentiary value (arrow, bullet, pellet, shot, or knife).

Blunt Force Injury

- Describe all external (skin bruising and damage), subcutaneous, and muscle damage.
- Describe all internal (bone, organs, soft tissue) damage.
- Correlate external and superficial damage to internal damage if relevant (Box 11.4).

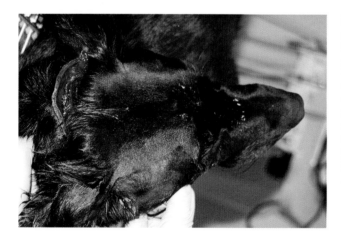

Figure 11.11 Describe and photograph the appearance of wound margins and associated bleeding. This photo illustrates a clean wound margin with sharp edges. The depth of the wound extends into the vertebral column and is representative of one fatal blow to the dog. By documenting the wound from the external to internal perspectives, the story about what happened unfolds step by step. *Source:* Oregon Humane Society.

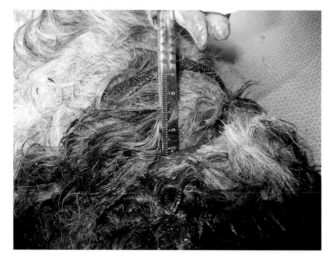

Figure 11.12 Collect measurements of wound dimensions prior to disrupting the overall presentation of the injury and repeat these measurements when needed as the necropsy or exam proceeds. *Source:* Oregon Humane Society.

Box 11.4   Example

Deep bruise to skin on ventral abdomen in 40 lb dog that extends from last rib on left side to inguinal area cranial to caudal and from midline to halfway between spinal column and ventral midline is seen on external exam and well-demarcated margins are seen after clipping the area to remove hair. Upon opening the abdomen, free blood was found pooling in the abdomen and the left lobes of the liver are severely damaged. The force of the external trauma carried into the abdomen lacerating and crushing the liver, causing internal bleeding and ultimately the death of this dog.

Puncture Wounds

- Describe the size and shape of the puncture and note the pattern and distance between punctures. For example, canine bite marks may have a pattern of two punctures that are aligned and could be repeated in various areas.
- Describe the location on the body anatomically and by using two reference points and diagrams or charts.

Injuries with Patterns

- May include gunshot pellets, bite wounds, chemical, or heat burns.
- Describe, measure, and photograph the injury and pattern size and shape.
- Describe the location of the injury.
- If samples are taken for DNA or chemicals such as accelerants, make a note of where on the body the samples were collected.
- If bite wounds are sampled for DNA, make a note and photograph which bite wounds were sampled.

Burns

- Consider the type of burn and sample and document accordingly describing the appearance, size, shape, extent, depth, smell, distribution, and impact of the burn (Figure 11.13).
- These may include heat, chemical, or electrical burns.

Drowning

- Evaluate skin, pads, and extremities overall for evidence of water saturation and wrinkling.
- Evaluate the upper and lower airway for the presence of edema and color.
- Collect samples of trachea and lung for histopathology.
- Examine the stomach contents for water and sample, if deemed appropriate.

Suspected Sexual Abuse

- Look for evidence of penetration of vulva or rectum such as bruising or fluid deposition around the external area.
- Collect nail clippings or scrapings for analysis of trace evidence including fur, fiber, and DNA.
- Search for biological stains including urine, semen, and blood using an alternative light source.
- Collect samples from susceptible areas including the oral cavity, rectum, prepuce, or vagina. Consider low volume flushing or swabbing techniques.

(a)

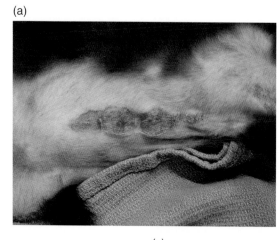

(b)   (c)

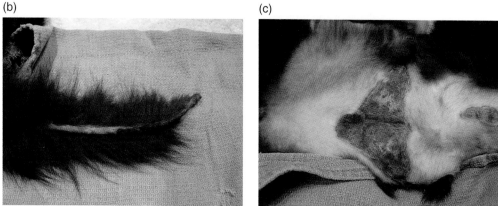

Figure 11.13   (a–c) The shape and appearance of wounds from thermal and chemical burns may provide clues about how and when the injuries occurred. *Source:* Oregon Humane Society.

Starvation/Emaciation

- Describe and document evidence of body condition including presence or absence of body fat in key areas: omental (intra-abdominal), perirenal, intercostal, and pericardial.
- Document estimation of body condition score and the scale used.
- Document the amount and elements of the contents of the gastrointestinal tract including the stomach and large and small bowel. Note what is found: food, feces, foreign bodies, liquid, dirt, debris (pica), blood, or other characteristics.
- Collect fecal samples and gastrointestinal contents, as necessary.
- Bone marrow collection and analysis for fat content has been used for further documentation of starvation [6]. If necessary, sample the femur and locate a laboratory that can do this analysis. Normal ranges for bone marrow fat content have been established for canine, equine, and bovine species [6].

Strangulation

Types of strangulation may include hanging, ligature, or manual compression. Each of these types of strangulation may result in specific injuries. Observe for ligature marks or compression damage and bruising to skin, subcutaneous, and deep muscle of the neck, head, or other affected areas. Describe the findings accordingly. When possible, document ligature length, type, and composition, and save as evidence.

- Describe pre- or postmortem hemorrhage and bruising including the depth and extent of these findings.
- Look for and describe petechial changes in the face, conjunctiva, periorbital tissues, sclerae, and upper trunk of the body.
- Look for injury to the ribs, intercostal muscles, and thoracic contents.
- Examine and collect samples as deemed appropriate of lung, cardiac tissue, trachea, and laryngeal areas.

11.7.7.6 Step 6 Storage of Remains after Necropsy

Disposition of Remains

Upon completion of the necropsy, place abdominal and thoracic contents that are not collected for further evaluation into the appropriate cavity and close the body. Suturing is not necessary or recommended. Wrap and tag the remains including all of the assigned identifiers (case number and animal ID). Place the remains in secure cold storage and complete the chain of custody form indicating this has been done. Final disposition of remains must be approved by law enforcement and/ or a prosecutor or owner or all three, depending upon the circumstances of the case. In order to determine the appropriate outcome, start by asking the investigator for guidance and direction. If a determination for disposition such as cremation or other release of remains is made, document this communication in writing. Keep in mind that it is possible that another veterinarian may be called to review the remains and the report if the case proceeds through the legal process, or another expert is called in for any reason.

For More Information

The necropsy process may depend upon the type of injury or cause of death suspected. Additional guidance for specific cases can be found in Appendix A.

11.8   The Necropsy Report

The necropsy report is the place to bring together all your findings and explain to the reader what they tell you about the circumstances of the animal's death. All necropsy reports must be written in technical and professional format and include layman's terms when possible, to supplement medical terminology and improve understanding and readability by nonveterinarians. By using a consistent format and outline for the report, the readability improves and the report writing task itself is less onerous. See resources in Appendices B and C.

11.8.1   Heading

The heading provides a snapshot by which the reader can ascertain key identifying information about the case, the victim, and the veterinarian. This section includes the veterinarian's name and contact information, the date and time the procedure was performed, the investigating agency, lead agent's name, the case number, and animal evidence ID. This information can be provided in fillable fields and checkboxes. Include spaces for microchip or tag ID and a description of the animal. Using a letterhead is a helpful way to provide information for the clinic or agency and veterinarian.

11.8.2 Introduction and Narrative Section

The narrative explains, in the veterinarian's words, how the information and the animal came to them and what steps they took to prepare or review information in advance of performing the necropsy (Box 11.5).

You may use this area to discuss additional records and reports received, and highlight facts that may be relevant to your findings in the forensic necropsy. If you were the veterinarian on the scene when this animal was discovered, alive or deceased, this is the section of the report where you can discuss your observations from the scene. If you were provided previous veterinary records for the animal, this is the section to highlight noteworthy aspects of those records.

11.8.3 Findings Section

The findings section of the necropsy report is scientific and fact based, describing what procedures were done, what tests were ordered or completed, and what observations you made during each procedure. Document what you found, what you did not find, and any unexpected findings. Photographs in this section help to show what you are explaining. Label the photograph and include arrows or circles, if necessary, to clarify for the reader the area of the photograph you are referencing.

The findings section is much like a medical record and will include medical terminology. It will be read, however, by professionals in the field of criminal justice and law, and so you will want to be certain that each of your findings also includes an explanation in layman's terms. Similarly, explain laboratory results beyond noting that the results were abnormal – explain what the findings mean (Box 11.6).

It is reasonable in this section to make use of your veterinary training and practical experience in relating your findings. As long as your statements are true (never exaggerate), it can be helpful to the reader to understand your reactions or learn how you are comparing this specimen or victim to a normal animal (Box 11.7).

Box 11.5   Example

I received a hand-delivered copy of incident report # 2013-12249, written by Officer Smith, Badge # 12345, and a flash drive of photos from the scene. I read the report, reviewed the photos, and opened a case within our agency, case # 98765.

Box 11.6   Example

I noted that the CK (creatine kinase) values in the chemistry profile were markedly elevated. This is an abnormal finding in a healthy adult dog. Elevated CK can be an indicator of recent acute muscle injury. A normal canine CK range is 22–198 U/l (units per liter) and the CK value for this sample was 1201.

Box 11.7   Example

I could smell the overwhelming stench of ammonia from 15 ft away, before I entered the exam room. I saw that the cat's body was wet, and the white fur was stained brown with what appeared to be feces and urine. The cat's back paw pads and haunches were ulcerated, and I could visualize muscle and tendon in the left hock wound. The staining of saturation was visible from the animal's feet up to its neck. I have not ever seen a cat so saturated with its own excrement.

11.8.4   Summary Section

The summary section of the report makes the connections between the findings from the forensic necropsy and the other information available to you about the case, which should be referenced in the narrative section. If you took samples during the forensic necropsy, you can mention that those results are pending and how the results will factor into your opinion.

Overall, the focus of this section is to connect the environment or facts of the investigation to what you found on the animal. For example, if the suspect told the officer that the cat fell down the stairs but one of your findings is a split palate, the summary section is where you state your opinion that a split palate results from significant impact to the face and is extremely unlikely to result from falling down stairs. Using this example, this is the point where you introduce your expertise in animal behavior to explain that a cat rarely, if ever, falls down stairs without the influence of an outside force. Think of the summary section as building the foundation for your overall conclusions that will follow in the next section.

If specific elements of an exam were not completed, include the reason and consequences as well as the justification for this in this section of the report.

11.8.5   Conclusion Section and Final Veterinary Opinion

The conclusion section differs from the summary section in that you are making concrete statements about what all this information means. The conclusion is where you include information about important rule outs, such as being hit by a car, predation, or disease. If there is a barrier to making a conclusion, discuss what that is, if it can be overcome, and how. This is the section where you can opine about the timeline of the death and the level of pain and suffering, and where you paint the picture for the reader of what happened in this animal's final weeks, days, hours, minutes, and seconds of living. End this section with a strong, succinct statement that embodies your final conclusion(s) (Boxes 11.8 and 11.9).

While forensic necropsy provides valuable evidence in most investigations, there may be instances when it is impossible to glean additional evidence in this manner. In cases where the evidence has been altered or lost to time, decomposition, or other conditions outside your control, be sure to create a narrative, record your findings and summary, and use the conclusion section to explain this to the reader.

11.8.6   Referencing the Law

The veterinarian's ability to articulate findings in an animal case, whether it is a live animal exam or a necropsy, can propel a case from inactivity or avoidance into an active investigation and prosecution. Because these cases are less frequently adjudicated than more common criminal matters

---

Box 11.8   Examples

Example: Decomposition of the cat was advanced to the degree that only skeletal remains were available for exam and a cause of death could not be determined. The time of death based on the location and state of the remains is estimated to be greater than four to six months.

Example: Upon examination of the animal and all of the available medical records, client history, and law enforcement reports, it appears that the animal died of a severe sudden metabolic event that is not consistent with external trauma or injury. Based on these findings, the laboratory results that are pending for toxicology are essential and likely the final step in either concluding a cause of death or in concluding that I am not able to determine a specific cause.

Example: The most recent injuries found are consistent with blunt force trauma and it is unlikely that they were caused by an automobile accident owing to the lack of damage to skin or extremities. It is unlikely that these injuries were caused by another animal, owing to the lack of bite wounds or damage consistent with this type of incident. Medical records and radiographs document three separate events in which the dog was injured prior to her death. Rib and head fractures such as this indicate a repetitive injury pattern that is consistent with repetitive nonaccidental injury. The location and type of injures are consistent with blunt force trauma consistent with kicking, punching, or throwing an animal this size.

Box 11.9   Examples

Specific findings and timeline:
- The dog was injured sometime on approximately December 2, 2012 and sustained broken ribs and thoracic trauma.
- Radiographs (X-rays) taken on December 29, 2012 confirm healing rib fractures (approximately four weeks old) and acute (new – within days) rib fractures and a severe head injury with acute fractures of the skull and facial bones.
- Physical exam and radiographs on February 15, 2012 confirm healing fractures consistent with injuries sustained both 6 and 10 weeks ago.

---

pertaining to humans, local prosecutors often appreciate a veterinarian who not only helps them rule in or out that a crime has occurred, but also puts the findings in context with the relevant animal protection laws. Consider drawing a conclusion in your report that clearly articulates what the findings may mean in the context of the language of the animal cruelty statutes in the state. This is not an effort to act as judge or jury but rather to bring to light the relevant law that the prosecutor may consider (Box 11.10).

11.8.7   Signature and Attachments

Do not forget to include your signature and contact information at the end of your report. Investigators and prosecutors need this information for follow-up and to issue subpoenas if the case goes to trial. It is also important to mention any related attachments or other materials that are referenced in the report. This can be a simple statement such as "photos of the necropsy and a copy of the radiographs and final lab results are provided as an attachment to this report."

> **Box 11.10 Example**
>
> In summary, the forensic necropsy (autopsy) findings are consistent with death by asphyxiation with no evidence of disease or other causes of death found. Shredded claw nails on the front paws of this cat may indicate an effort to hang on and get away from the event and healed rib fractures seen on x-ray may indicate previous non-accidental injury. Killing in the manner of strangulation/asphyxiation is inhumane, tortuous, and results in a very painful, stressful, and prolonged death for the cat. A person commits the crime of aggravated animal abuse in the first degree (ORS 167.322) if they maliciously kill an animal.

11.9 Next Steps

After you conclude the forensic necropsy, one of your next steps is to provide your report to the investigating entity along with a list of remaining questions that would further enable you to evaluate your necropsy findings. Include any open questions as a separate document or in the narrative as appropriate. Each case offers the opportunity to consider what else would assist the investigation, based on the veterinarian's expert insight into the findings of the forensic necropsy and related reports.

11.10 An Important Reminder

A major hurdle in animal cruelty investigations can be finding a veterinarian who is willing and accessible for the purpose of completing a forensic necropsy. Without access to these skills and the commitment by the veterinary profession to contribute to this cause, the animal victim, and in some cases a human victim, are voiceless and justice is not served. The veterinarian provides the expertise to support the truth in these cases, which not only serves justice but dispatches cases that in fact are not criminal after the facts are exposed.

References

1 International Veterinary Forensic Sciences Association. (2020). Veterinary forensic postmortem examination standards. https://www.ivfsa.org/wp-content/uploads/2020/12/IVFSA-Veterinary-Forensic-Postmortem-Exam-Standards_Approved-2020_with-authors.pdf (accessed 16 August 2021).

2 Brooks, J.W. (2016). Postmortem changes in animal carcasses and estimation of the postmortem interval. *Vet. Pathol.* 53 (5) https://journals.sagepub.com/doi/pdf/10.1177/0300985816629720.

3 Brooks, J.W. and Sutton, L. (2018). Postmortem changes and estimating the postmortem interval. In: *Veterinary Forensic Pathology*, vol. 1 (ed. J. Brooks), 43–63. Cham: Springer International Publishing.

4 Kapler, M. and Dycus, D. (2016). A practitioner's guide to fracture management. Part 2: Selection of fixation technique and external coaptation. https://todaysveterinarypractice.com/wp-content/uploads/sites/4/2016/06/T1509F02.pdf (accessed 16 August 2021)

5 Ressel, L., Hetzel, U., and Ricci, E. (2016). Blunt force trauma in veterinary forensic pathology. *Vet. Pathol.* 53 (5): 21.

6 Rogers, E. and Stern, A.W. (eds.) (2021). *Veterinary Forensics: Investigation, Evidence Collection, and Expert Testimony*. London: CRC Press.

12

Report Writing
Emily Lewis

12.1 Introduction

Every effort to conduct a flawless animal cruelty investigation can be undermined if the individuals involved do not document that investigation through detailed and timely reports.

Generating reports and statements in a case can be intimidating and time consuming, but they are a necessary component of participating in investigations. These statements and reports serve a variety of functions, not the least of which is to preserve your experience for your own reference later when you are called upon to answer questions about that experience. It is well worth prioritizing this task and devoting time and thought to these documents.

12.2 General Principles

You do not have to be a profound author to write good reports. You simply need to be able to remember your experience and convey that in a way that makes it easy for an audience to understand. One part of meeting that objective consists of following some basic writing principles, and the other part is understanding what to include when describing your experience. The following section discusses some general writing principles that will ensure the success of even the most reticent report writer.

12.2.1 Organization: Headings and Chronological Order

The use of headings as a tool to organize reports is helpful to the author as well as the reader. Headings automatically give you an outline of what you want to cover in your report, and they refocus the reader as they are reviewing your report. Headings are also useful to individuals like prosecutors who will be referencing your report multiple times looking for various pieces of information. If you have headings in your report, it makes it that much easier for the prosecutor to find the information they are looking for, or for you to locate it to refresh your memory on the witness stand.

Animal cruelty investigations may span weeks or months, and some animal cruelty crime scenes are vast, resulting in an overwhelming amount of information to include in a report. One of the

Animal Cruelty Investigations: A Collaborative Approach from Victim to Verdict™, First Edition.
Edited by Kris Otteman, Linda Fielder, and Emily Lewis.
© 2022 John Wiley & Sons, Inc. Published 2022 by John Wiley & Sons, Inc.
Companion website: www.wiley.com/go/otteman/victimtoverdict

best ways to meet this challenge is to write your report in chronological order. If events or findings in the future relate to something from earlier, you can draw those connections when you get to the later point in your report or in your conclusion where you tie everything together. When you break down the warrant execution, the investigation as a whole, or the medical exam procedure chronologically, and tackle each piece individually, it is much less daunting. Another option is to write an initial report after an event like a search warrant or a forensic intake exam, and then continue to write smaller supplemental reports as the investigation and veterinary treatment continue as a way of keeping yourself organized and thorough.

12.2.2 Topic Sentences

The single writing principle that can elevate your reports the most is the use of topic sentences. When you begin a paragraph, the first sentence should give the reader an idea of what to expect in the following sentences that make up the paragraph. If you are writing a witness statement about assisting with the execution of a search warrant, an example of a topic sentence might be:

> I approached the house and the first room I entered and searched was the kitchen.

Your paragraph would then go on to describe the kitchen. If there was a lot to describe about the kitchen, you could break your paragraphs into aspects of the kitchen: the sanitation, the animals, and the evidence you documented or collected from the kitchen. The topic sentences would be as follows:

- When I entered the first room, the kitchen, I was overcome by the poor sanitation. [Go on to discuss the details of the poor conditions.]
- The kitchen contained several animals housed in various crates and containers. [Go on to discuss what the animals looked like, where, and how they were housed.]
- While processing the kitchen, I marked evidence to be seized, and documented the conditions with photos. [Go on to discuss how you determined what was evidence, what you marked, and how you documented it with photos.]

Topic sentences force you to organize your writing in a way that will help the reader follow your train of thought. It can be helpful to make a topic sentence outline of your report first, so you can determine whether it flows in a way that mirrors your experience. This can also help you identify holes in your narrative and realize what you might be forgetting.

12.2.3 Passive Voice

Particularly in report writing for criminal cases, be aware of and avoid using the passive voice. By avoiding the passive voice, you are telling the reader who did the action in the sentence. If you reread a sentence and you cannot name the person who did the action, you probably have used the passive voice. Here is an example in the context of a veterinary report:

- *Passive voice:* "The tissue samples were sent to the lab for testing."
- *Active voice:* "CVT Jane Doe sent the tissue samples to the lab for testing."

The second sentence tells the reader who sent the samples. This informs the prosecutor or the defense attorney that Jane Doe is who they need to call as a witness if they have questions about the process of sending the samples or to establish the link in the chain of custody for that evidence. Sentences written in the passive voice creates unnecessary confusion around who was involved and their role.

We use the passive voice when we talk and write to each other casually, so it can be hard to identify at first. Most computer programs offer a way to automatically highlight the passive voice in your writing. Once you are aware of how you tend to use the passive voice and what it looks like, it will become easier to spot or catch yourself before you write a sentence in that way.

12.2.4   Proofread

When you have already invested a lot of time in generating a report, the last thing you want to do is spend time rereading it, but proofreading is a necessary step in the report-writing process. First, you must review your own work looking for typos, skipped words, missing information, or confusing paragraphs. Do not rely entirely on computer programs to catch all spelling and grammar errors. This is a good time to keep an eye out for words – common in these reports – that a spell check program will not catch because it does not know if you meant matts or mats, human or humane, statue or statute. The next step is to recruit someone to proofread it for you. Having a different person review your writing can bring to light areas or wording you did not realize needed clarity or typos your eyes missed in your own read-through.

Also, keep these writing tips front of mind when you are proofreading for a colleague. Make it a policy in your organization that reports undergo review for clarity, grammar, punctuation, and spelling before they are finalized. It is important to distinguish those purposes of review and refrain from editing the author's voice, opinions, perspective, or experience. If all your co-workers are also generating reports about the same case, it is best practice to finish authoring your report before you proofread another's.

12.2.5   Jargon

Every field utilizes terminology unique to its discipline and using that vernacular in a report can confuse an audience that is not experienced in the field. It is important, especially in the veterinarian's report, to use the most appropriate word for what you are describing, even if it is jargon or a technical term. If that is the case, then a parenthetical needs to follow, giving a lay explanation of the term or phrase. For example:

> The radiographs (X-rays) show a fracture of the left femur (large bone between hip and knee) and dislocation of the coxofemoral (hip) joint.

If you are accustomed to abbreviating a term, resist doing that in a report and spell out the word or phrase at least once, but ideally throughout the report. For example:

> The horse had a body condition score (BCS) of 2 out of 9.

It can be helpful to have someone proofread your report who is not an expert in your discipline and can identify words or phrases that are confusing. For example:

> I attempted to make contact with the suspect on Wednesday at 1500 hours.

A person who does not work in law enforcement or regularly read reports from law enforcement officers will wonder what "make contact with" means. It is unclear if that means a phone call, an email, or a knock on the door. The use of military time may also trip up some audiences. While this becomes second nature to law enforcement, a jury or veterinarian may get distracted from reading the report because they are doing the mental calculation of what time "1500 hours" is.

12.2.6   Quoting

Quoting witnesses and suspects in your reports can be extremely valuable to prosecutors, when done correctly. It is critical that you *do not* put a statement in quotes, unless you are certain that you are quoting the statement exactly as the person said it. If you want to modify the pronoun or tense of the quote to make it flow better with your sentence, you can identify those changes with brackets in the quote. For example:

> "I saw [John Smith] kick the dog on the left side of her body."

Try not to use quotations excessively and reserve them for highly relevant and impactful statements.

12.3   Crime Report

This section is particular to the reports that law enforcement officers generate in animal cruelty cases. Officers receive much training on report writing, but it is important to solidify good report-writing principles through repetition and point out what might be unique to animal cruelty case reports.

12.3.1   Include Sensory Details

By including details about your sensory experience at a crime scene, you are providing important evidence in the case. It is important for a prosecutor to know if you could smell, for example, an animal's infected wound from another room in the house. They need to know if you could easily feel an animal's ribcage when you ran your hand over its side. Be aware of your senses when you are on the scene and make note of what you are experiencing through each of them.

12.3.2   Include Statements from Individual Co-Suspects

When you have more than one individual who may be a suspect, make sure you are including the statements that are specific to each person, and not the group of individuals (see Chapter 5, for more information about interviewing and multiple suspects). If there are many individuals referenced in your report, it will be helpful to the reader if you can identify their relationship to one another as you discuss their statements or role. For example:

> Jane Doe, John's wife, proceeded to walk with me out to the barn to see Anna, the horse reported to be thin.

12.3.3   Explain Where You Are Physically

Law enforcement officers must set the scene for the reader by describing where they are when they are doing the investigating (i.e. on the phone, at the neighbor's apartment, in the veterinary clinic), but it becomes even more crucial to do so when they are communicating with the suspect. Even when an individual is not physically restrained, the circumstances of where and how a law enforcement officer interacts with them can create a custodial environment. Because certain laws are implicated when a person is taken into custody (duty to give the Miranda warnings, for example), a law enforcement officer needs to provide as many details as possible about the location and circumstances of their interaction with a person suspected of a crime. These details are what a prosecutor will rely on in the event the interaction is called into question.

12.3.4   Document Delivery of Warnings or Notices

Many animal neglect cases can be resolved through education and warnings, but if those warnings are not heeded, they become the foundation of meeting the required mental state for the crime. Any resources an officer recommends or arranges for a suspect must be documented in the officer's final report on that case. Even if the case has not resulted in a criminal citation, it is relevant the owner of the animal has been made aware of what is required for the care of that animal and the resources available to provide that care.

Some states include a notice requirement connected to seizing animals. For example, in many states a suspect must be personally notified that there are costs that will accrue in connection with their seized animals. If you told the suspect this on the day of the warrant or if you handed the suspect any paperwork indicating this, then it is very important to include that in your report. Similarly, if you informed the suspect of the remedies available to the animal care agency holding the seized animals – preconviction forfeiture or lien foreclosure – memorialize that notice in your report.

12.3.5   Include Behavior of the Animals

Documenting the behaviors of the animals you encounter will be helpful for the experts utilized in the case and to the ultimate fact finder in the case. Even if you are not an expert on the particular animal you have encountered, be sure to take the time to document the behavior you are witnessing. Just as the behavior of humans gives you insight into their state of mind or their comfort level around particular individuals, so does the behavior of animals. The veterinarian assisting in the case can use your report to inform their assessment of the animal(s). For example, if a dog chooses to position itself behind an officer in full uniform, rather than next to a person the dog is familiar with, that is very unusual behavior and worth noting. Other examples are if you notice an animal continuously circling or pacing, or if you find a cat curled up tightly in a corner, or behind some furniture. Take note of how the animal reacts if the suspect gets upset while talking with you or makes a large gesture. If you are accustomed to documenting the behavior of the humans you are interacting with, the same applies to the animals in your cases.

12.3.6   Investigator Notebooks

There is no expectation that you must commit to memory everything that happened on the scene or during an interview, but there is an expectation that whatever notes you take end up in your crime report. Do not create a discrepancy between your report and your notes from the field. The notes from the field form the basis of your report, where you will supplement those notes with additional details of what you observed, heard, smelled, or touched.

12.4   Veterinarian Reports

Veterinary reports are crucial to a thorough animal cruelty investigation. While the foundation of many of these reports is the standard medical notes generated while practicing veterinary medicine, the reports *must* go beyond that if you are a lead veterinarian in an animal cruelty investigation. Understand that, even though you are supplementing the standard medical notes with additional findings or opinions regarding animal cruelty, this does not mean you are speaking outside the scope of your expertise or experience. A veterinary report in an animal cruelty case may take a different form than you are accustomed to, but the information you are presenting is well within your knowledge base given your experience, and the professional training and continuing education that are required of veterinarians. The veterinarian brings the medical findings to light and explains the relevance of these findings to the health of the animal by finalizing opinions and conclusions.

Depending on the nature of the case, you may only end up generating a single report or you may author several reports. A case may warrant an initial report and findings with a follow-up of supplemental information, such as progress of the animals, laboratory results, or other information. If the volume of the report seems overwhelming, take the time to plan for how you will arrange the information you have collected, and then stick to that plan. If you just start writing without a plan, it increases the likelihood that you will leave out information and spend more time than necessary in your editing/review process. Your plan may include sections as recommended here with a general outline to start. Breaking the work down into specific areas facilitates accurate and efficient writing.

12.4.1 Initial Veterinary Report

The initial veterinary report will likely be the longest. Whether there is a single victim animal or over 100 victim animals, the nature of the information you provide is the same.

12.4.2 Crime Scene

If you were present during a search warrant execution or you were given access to the location where the violation/investigation took place, begin your report with those observations. If you took notes while you were on the scene, be sure to include the information from those notes in your report and the notes themselves in the discovery to the prosecutor on the case (see Chapter 9, for the type of observations and notes that are expected of a lead veterinarian on the scene). (See Appendix B, for examples of veterinary on scene assessments.)

12.4.3 Description of Victim Animal Population

Prosecutors need information specific to individual victim animals to issue charges in a case, but that does not negate the value of discussing the victim animal population as a whole. In cases involving several animals removed from poor living conditions, it is worthwhile to include information that demonstrates the magnitude of the neglect and to explain how the neglect or injury to the population as a whole relates to the individual animal. The following are examples of statements a veterinarian can include in their report to help the reader understand how widespread the issues were in an animal neglect case:

- Anemia (low red blood cells and hemoglobin) consistent with heavy parasitism and starvation was found in 12 of the adult dogs. High CK (creatine kinase, muscle enzyme), high eosinophil (white blood cell that may increase with heavy parasite loads) counts, and electrolyte changes were also found in many of the dogs, again, consistent with malnutrition and heavy internal parasite load. These changes indicate muscle wasting or breakdown as a result of prolonged lack of adequate nutrition.

- 37% of results have increased CK, which is an enzyme that is released by muscle when trauma or cell breakdown occurs.
- The body condition scores for this population of dogs:
  - 41% scored less than 2
  - 24% scored less than 3
  - 21% scored less than 4
  - Only 14% scored in the low range of acceptable body condition.
- All the animals had signs of chronic (long-term) exposure to feces and urine, including fecal material that was dried and stuck to their paws, tails, and ventral abdomens. The animals all had a very strong odor of ammonia, due to chronic exposure to feces and urine in a confined area. Chronic respiratory infections were present in all the animals also. Prolonged exposure to animal waste (and subsequent ammonia) not only predisposes, but also worsens the symptoms of respiratory tract disease.

12.4.4 Physical Exam Findings

The approach to reporting your physical exam findings will differ, depending on how many animals are involved in the case. If few animals examined, then you can report all your findings for each animal directly in your report document. If you have examined numerous animals, it would be beneficial to utilize other means of conveying the information. In every case you need a physical exam form for each animal you examine. Include these exam forms in your primary report as an attachment and reference them throughout your report. Summarizing physical exam findings in an Excel spreadsheet that includes all the information from the exam forms in one location is an efficient and helpful process that illustrates the overall findings in a population of animals. This also provides methodology that you can continue to update and produce in connection with your initial and supplemental reports. A word of caution: every time you enter your findings into a different format it creates an opportunity for errors and typos. Make sure whoever is charged with creating a spreadsheet of data taken from exam forms is double- and triple checking their work even before you, as the lead veterinarian, review it.

Once you have all the specific exam information in one location (i.e. attachment of individual exam forms or Excel spreadsheet), use your report to highlight particular cases that exemplify the issues found in the population or cases where you documented extreme neglect. Using exam forms and a summary is helpful whenever a case involves a variety of species or a group of over five animals. Managing the information, drawing conclusions, and communicating the findings using these methods improves clarity and reduces the possibility of errors or omissions.

(See Chapter 7 for more on the specific information veterinarians should include in their report from the forensic examinations.)

12.4.5 Photos

Whenever possible, insert photographs or diagrams directly into your report. These images will help the prosecutor specifically identify the animal for charging purposes and add clarity to the conditions you are describing. When you are reporting your findings on a victim animal, include their identifying information and a full-body picture of that animal. When describing specific conditions, a wound for example, include a photo of the wound with a caption indicating what the photo is of and where it is located on the body of the animal. Sometimes including a full-body picture with a circle or an arrow identifying the wound can be helpful. In cases involving projectile wounds or fractures displayed in radiographs, insert an image in the body of the report and then add arrows or circles to indicate what you are referring to in your findings (Figure 12.1).

Photos are particularly powerful in a veterinarian's report when they connect the conditions found on the scene with the injuries or wounds found on the animal. For example, if an animal was kept in a small area or cage that was saturated with urine, the veterinary report will include, if possible, a photo of the cage flooring next to a photo of the animal's urine-scalded feet that resulted from that living condition. All photos taken in the course of the veterinary exam must accompany the report as an attachment.

12.4.6 Terminology and Laymen's Terms

For veterinarians it is particularly important to include laymen's terms in your cruelty case reports. Of course, you can use the terminology your profession uses to describe findings in a physical exam, but because veterinarians are not the primary audience of the report, also include parentheticals that make the information accessible. One way to think about how to write your report is to do so in the same way you would explain a condition or a finding to a client at your veterinary practice. Your medical notes might use phrases and abbreviations that anyone in the profession would understand, but when you talk with your client you change your language to convey what you found on their animal. This does not mean you have to write everything twice. You can use the scientific term for the finding and then include a quick

Figure 12.1   The circles were added to this radiograph in the veterinarian's final report to identify and highlight for the reader both the recent fractures and the healed fracture referenced in the text of the report. *Source:* Oregon Humane Society.

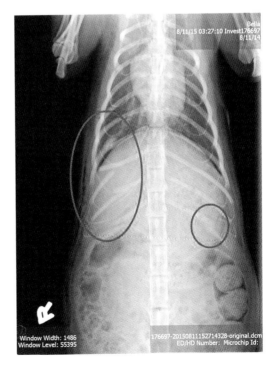

parenthetical that adapts it to the average reader's level of understanding. Here are examples of how a veterinarian can do that in their reports:

- "... injuries are acute (rapid onset, very recent). . ."
- "The rate of healing callus formation (repair of the bone) depends on several factors. . ."
- "... the cat's upper and lower jaw anterior (front of the mouth) are darkened. . ."
- "Medical notes record injected sclera (hemorrhage and inflammation of the whites of the eyes) with healing burst vessels."
- "... the right ear pinna (flap) is reddened."

12.4.7 Conclusion

The conclusion is the point you have been working toward from the beginning of your assessment of the animal(s). This part of the veterinarian's report is *so* important. The conclusion is where you distill all your findings into your expert opinion with respect to rule-outs, causation, timeline, pain and suffering, and long-term impacts to the animal(s). Trust your expertise and your experience and articulate your conclusions with confidence. For example:

> The conditions in which Bella lived, which I am aware of based on the photos I observed, do not meet the legal minimum standard of care for a pet in this state. Once she became injured her ability to protect herself from the environment or get to food or water was eliminated. She suffered from chronic infections and cancer that should have been examined and treated by a veterinarian. These conditions existed for many months. Her recent neurologic injury likely occurred as a result of the combination of arthritis in her spine, injury by the cable, and the chronic illness she suffered. These elements combined created suffering and injury from which she could not recover.
>
> Failure to meet the minimum standard of care for a dog in this way is a violation of state law. Based on my examination of the evidence, examination of Bella, and assessment of her condition, she was a victim of long-term neglect and suffering.

12.4.8 Necropsy Report

A necropsy report generally will follow the same structure as a report on a physical exam with a few nuances. First, you want to be sure to include how the animal arrived on your necropsy table. Include information about who the investigating agency is, who the lead investigator on the case is, who brought the animal to you to begin the necropsy procedure, and how the animal was packaged when presented to you for necropsy. A photograph of how the animal was packaged and how it looked when it was removed from the packaging supplements this part of the report well. Including that information will help underscore the chain of custody for that piece of evidence and further legitimize your report and necropsy procedure.

When recording necropsy findings, include all the same report-writing principles discussed in this chapter. Senses, initial findings, pending tests, summary of findings, and a conclusion are all very important. Include the names of assistants, such as photographers and scribes, who are present during the necropsy so the prosecutor will know who to call on, if required.

In some cases, the necropsy is the focal point of the veterinarian's work and may be a stand-alone report that includes information that is essential such as other medical records, radiographs, witness statements, rule-outs of causes of illness or injury, or it may be part of an overall report in the context of a large-scale animal cruelty case.

Use discretion in your decision to use photos and images in your necropsy report. Think about whether including the image will provide additional clarity and underscore your narrative, or whether you are just including it for the sake of including pictures. For example, if your report says you found the stomach and intestines to be empty of food, your readers can picture what that looks like and understand what that means without you including a photo of the open abdomen and stomach. That is not to discourage you from including photos, which are enormously powerful in any report, particularly necropsy reports, but to encourage you to be discerning in doing so. Most people who will read your report will not be able to distinguish areas of concern in the interior of an animal, so you should reserve the use of a photo for the instances where it provides additional clarity and impact to what you are describing in your report. For example, if your report focuses on fractured ribs, then clearly illustrate your findings by supplementing the written word with one good photo that explicitly shows the broken bone. Choose photos that can be labeled and clearly explained, remembering that individuals reading these reports have little to no experience in interpreting this information and it is your responsibility to deliver information in a manner that is understandable to the reader. Knowing your audience makes your report more useful to the criminal case.

12.4.9 Supplemental Veterinary Reports

As you continue to provide treatment and rehabilitation to evidence animals, you will gain more insight about their initial injuries or illnesses. Memorialize these insights in a supplemental report. If further medical work up has caused you to reconsider your initial diagnosis or conclusion, then report that, and explain why. Do *not* revise your original report and resubmit it to the prosecutor or law enforcement agency. It is substantially more helpful if you explain why you diagnosed something initially one way and then explain what changed since then that has resulted in your current diagnosis. If toxicology reports or other data come in later that are relevant, explain this and advance your conclusions in a supplemental report.

It can also be valuable to submit a supplemental report to confirm or underscore your initial conclusion. For example, if you are presented with an emaciated dog and conduct the typical rule-outs of intestinal parasites or an obstruction, you are likely to conclude in your report the dog is emaciated due to lack of nutrition (i.e. food). If after three to four weeks the dog has regained a significant amount of weight and the only intervention you have provided is proper nutrition, you can then generate a supplemental report saying as much.

If further injuries or illnesses are discovered over the course of your treatment, then reporting those can also impact the crimes being charged by the prosecutor. Identify the animal in the same way you did in your initial report so there is no confusion.

12.5 Witness Statements

12.5.1 Who Generates?

Anyone who assists with processing an animal cruelty crime scene, plays a role in evidence collection, who interacts with a suspect in an investigation, or who witnesses a crime occur must generate a witness statement. Your operational policies need to include the requirement that staff produce witness statements, whether you work in the veterinary field, the animal care field, or in law enforcement. It may seem excessive to have five animal handlers generate witness statements in responding to the same scene, but any one of those animal handlers could have noticed something the others did not and could be called to the witness stand to testify about it. Ask everyone involved to write a short statement that includes their role, duties, and processes during the operation. It is not the responsibility of nonveterinary professionals to include medical or behavioral opinions in these reports.

12.5.2 Generate Quickly

The first 24 hours after a search warrant execution in which animals are seized are filled with important tasks, including generating a witness statement. The more time goes by the fewer details you will remember. If you write the report in the first 24 hours or within a few days of the experience, you will still acutely remember how it smelled, for example, and what you encountered during your role on the scene. Make every effort to preserve the details of your experience because it is all relevant to the case.

12.5.3 Form

There is no industry standard for the form a witness statement needs to take. It is more important that you generate a statement than what it looks like. If it is easier for you to write in bullet points than to generate a narrative in paragraphs, then do that. Given there is certain information that every witness statement needs to include, it would be helpful if agencies frequently involved in animal cruelty cases had a template for their employees to use that prompts inclusion of that information (see Appendix C, for an example template for a witness statement.)

12.5.4 What to Include

Regardless of the format of the report, there are certain pieces of information that need to be included in every witness statement:

- *Contact information:* You are generating the report because you are a witness; this means the prosecution needs to know how to contact you. Be sure to include addresses where you can receive subpoenas for trial and understand that your report will be included in discovery to the defense.
- *Role:* Make very clear what your role was in relation to the case or the scene processing. Listing the role(s) you had will help the prosecutor know what you will be able to testify about, and it helps the broader audience understand the scene-processing plan and why each role was necessary.

  Details: Include as many details as you can remember with certainty. Begin with basic but important details like the location you are writing about and the date you witnessed the information you are writing about. It is also helpful to include the names of other agencies and individuals who were present.

  Animal cruelty cases often take over a year to go to trial and your report is what you will need to rely on to refresh your memory to give testimony. Think about what your future self would want to remember from that experience. A detailed report paints the picture of the scene for individuals reviewing the case who were not there. Simply saying you "entered a dirty barn that was crowded with stuff" is not going to be enough information for someone to understand what you witnessed. Like the crime reports, use all your senses to help describe your experience.

If you talk about a particular animal on the scene, specifically identify it with its evidence label, if possible. If the animal is referenced with the same unique identifier across multiple reports, then all that information can be used in relation to that specific charge. If you are making broad statements about groups of animals on the scene or a single animal without identifying it, then that information is used differently in the case.

Temper emotions: How the experience or the scene made you feel emotionally is not one of the five senses you should be using to describe accurately what you witnessed. Providing a high level of detail does not equate to a highly emotional report. That is not to say these are not high-stress, highly emotional situations, but the witness statement is not the appropriate venue for details of that nature. In addition to tempering your emotions for report-writing purposes, try not to surmise what emotions the victim animals might have been feeling at the time. Do not let this prevent you from including your reactions and experience in your role though. For example, saying "The sheer number and advanced state of emaciation of the animals housed in the barn was shocking to me" is different than saying "As I walked by one emaciated animal after another, their sorrowful eyes expressed relief that we were there to help them" or "The sheer number of emaciated animals housed in the barn made my heart sink, thinking of how long they had suffered in those conditions." Stick with detailed statements about what you experienced (saw, smelled, heard, touched) and your role.

You can also include quotes in your witness statement. Only include a quote in your report, if you can quote it exactly as it was said. If you are confident those were the exact words the person used, then include the statement. If you would not be able to testify under oath that is what the person said, then paraphrase what you heard rather than putting it in quotes.

- *Who can corroborate?* Include the names of others who would have witnessed what you did. It is not necessary to have multiple witnesses to every part of processing a scene, and it would not be a good use of resources to assign two people to every task. However, if you are processing a building or an area at the same time as another person, it is worth mentioning that in your report so the prosecutor knows who could corroborate the details you are including.
- *Relevant experience or expertise:* Do not shy away from making the reader aware of any experience or expertise that adds credibility to statements you are making. If you have worked in a dog shelter for over a decade and you notice a dog on the scene displaying behavior you know to be an indicator of stress, then feel confident including that in your report. If you were raised on a farm such that you are familiar with the noises made by certain livestock, this could be relevant to mention if you note something unusual on the scene about the sounds emitted from a victim animal. You need to pair the statement of what you saw with the reason you have confidence in making that statement, i.e. your experience or training. It is not necessary to write an exhaustive list of all your credentials, but if you have significant experience in animal welfare, husbandry, evidence collection, or veterinary science, then consider highlighting that in your report or attaching your curriculum vitae (CV).
- *Can include pictures:* Much like the crime report and the veterinary reports, including photos in the body of a witness statement can be helpful to the reader. As a witness, avoid including any photos in your report that depict scenes you did not personally witness. You do not have to be the person who took the picture, but you must be able to say that is exactly what you saw and the way you saw it, on the day in question. Do not rely on pictures to relay your experience – your report needs to be your words about what you noticed and experienced.

12.6 The Case Packet

12.6.1 Importance

It is incumbent upon the agencies and individuals presenting the culmination of an animal cruelty investigation to a prosecutor to do so in an organized fashion that represents the effort that went into building the case, and in a way that is easily navigated by the attorneys evaluating the case for charges and prosecution. These investigations involve multiple witnesses, a significant volume of veterinary records and diagnostics, even more paperwork related to the daily caretaking of the evidence animals, in addition to any number of witness statements that are generated over the course of the investigation and holding and evaluation of evidence. Prosecutors are inordinately busy and are not confronted with animal cruelty cases on a regular basis, making them unfamiliar with case assessment and the evidentiary hallmarks. It is in the best interests of everyone involved to provide the case materials to them in a format that facilitates quick understanding of the applicable laws, the facts, and the supporting evidence. Animal cruelty cases are challenging to prosecute to begin with, so adding the additional burden of sifting through a stack of documents or confusing flash drives could result in strong evidence being overlooked or simply a decision not to pursue charges.

12.6.2 Process

Communication and organization are the key to making a useful case packet a successful endeavor. The assisting animal care agency and/or veterinary clinic need to communicate with the lead law enforcement agency on the case to determine the proper channels to deliver the evidence to the prosecutor's office. In most cases, the assisting agencies could work together to compile the evidence and submit the packet to the lead law enforcement officer to provide to the prosecutor along with the crime reports. If the prosecutor has been working collaboratively with the assisting agencies and the law enforcement agency, then it might be acceptable to deliver the case packet directly to the prosecutor, while providing a duplicate copy to the law enforcement agent on the case.

Designate a point person for the collection and compilation of the documentation. The first duty of this person is to create a feasible timeline for submission of the materials and notify witnesses and veterinarians of a deadline for their reports. State law might dictate the timeline for charges to be filed after a criminal citation has been issued. Be aware of those timelines and intentionally provide ample time for the prosecutor to review the materials before the deadline for arraignment is imminent. The point person then needs to determine a method of receiving, saving, and organizing the information as it is submitted. It is the responsibility of the point person to review the documentation and follow up on missing items that are referenced in the documentation. For example, if a veterinary record is submitted and indicates that radiographs were taken on a particular day, the point person needs to confirm the materials submitted also include those radiographs. Be thorough so the prosecutor does not have to spend time tracking down missing information.

There are tasks the point person can be doing in furtherance of the case packet submission while waiting for the documentation from the other parties involved. Having a general idea of what the evidence consists of in the case, this person can start planning how it can most clearly be organized and presented in the packet and procure the materials (electronic or hard copy) to support their vision for the packet. There are numerous documents (discussed in detail in the section that follows) that a point person can start drafting for inclusion in the packet during this time as well.

Once all the materials have been submitted, they are organized in a meaningful, user-friendly way, and sent to the appropriate entities. The point person will include their contact information for any questions regarding the material. This will help expedite any inquiries from the prosecutor and prevent delays in assessment of the case and filing of charges. Finally, the point person needs to set an ongoing calendar reminder to continue to provide discovery for the case, when additional veterinary treatments and exams take place and daily care is provided.

12.6.3 What to Include and Why

The overarching purpose behind investing the time and effort into producing these extensive case packets is to promote serious review by the prosecutor and to make that review as easy as possible. Many of the components discussed in the text that follows are included with that end in mind.
(See Appendices B and C, for a case packet checklist and related templates.)

- *Letter to prosecutor:* Depending on the size of your jurisdiction, the prosecutor's office may only receive three or four animal cruelty cases a year, if that, making them not readily familiar with the applicable laws. One helpful thing you can do is to include a cover letter with your case packet that thanks them for their consideration of the case and proceeds to list the language of the state or jurisdiction's animal cruelty code. Even if you forget a statute or are not a lawyer and misidentify one as relevant, you are still pointing them in the direction of where to look in the code to orient themselves properly before reviewing the case specifics.
- *Case packet inventory:* Any resource you can provide a prosecutor that provides a lot of information in a quick reference format will be appreciated. By listing the inventory of the case packet in the very beginning of your submission, the prosecutor knows what to expect and will already have a bird's eye view of the case just by knowing what the available evidence includes.
- *Timeline:* The timeline zooms in the view of the case a little bit closer but still provides a general idea of the trajectory a case took and can give the prosecutor good context for the rest of the information they will review. The timeline is likely to continue to be a resource the prosecutor will refer back to when filing charges or arguing the case. It does not need to include every detail of the investigation but should include dates of events that are relevant to the investigation and the crime being alleged. For example, every date the animal was seen by a veterinarian should be included, but the timeline is not the place to list the full extent of the veterinary findings on each of those visits.
- *Witness list:* The number of people involved in an animal cruelty investigation or care of the evidence animals can be significant. By providing the prosecutor with an all-encompassing witness list, including associated roles in the case and contact information, you are easing their workload and facilitating quicker review of the case. It provides great assistance to the prosecutor if they can read the reports while simultaneously cross-referencing who each named person is with the witness list. Including the contact information makes it easier when the time comes to issue subpoenas as well.
- *Reports and witness statements:* Obviously, the reports and witness statements are crucial evidence to include in the case packet. If you have an officer's crime report, this should be included first; otherwise the reports can be organized chronologically or alphabetically by witness. Make sure you provide clear separation between each report or statement.
- *Veterinary records:* If you have a forensic veterinary report in a case, that is most important to highlight and all supporting medical records should follow. If you have different records from different clinics, make sure to clearly distinguish those from one another. This is the area of the packet to include diagnostics and radiographs as well.

- *Pictures:* All pictures taken during an investigation must be provided to the prosecutor. If you are providing a hard copy case packet, you can select a few pictures that are representative of the whole and print those out in color on full pages. You can also print contact sheets of all the photos in smaller sizes, or you can just reference a flash drive or a folder that contains the extent of the photos. Given the workload of a prosecutor and the window of time to review an incoming case, it can be helpful and impactful to include at least a few hard copy photos, in an effort to provide a lot of details in a short amount of time.
- *Body condition scoring charts:* If the veterinary records reference a particular body condition scoring chart, include copies of that chart in the case packet. Just this simple step taken off the prosecutor's plate can improve understanding of the case and receptivity to consideration of charges.
- *Restitution request or waiver:* Make sure the prosecutor knows how much it is costing the animal agency or the law enforcement agency to care for the animals associated with the case. This is important for restitution purposes and to underscore the urgency of quick decision making and action in the case overall. Provide a restitution cover letter that includes the total cost and the date that cost was determined, but also include the cost for each victim animal individually. Be *very* clear in the restitution cover letter if the costs will continue to accrue. This lets the prosecutor know to check back with you to get an updated total when the time comes for restitution or pre-conviction forfeiture (see Chapter 15). This cost can reflect veterinary exam and treatment costs as well as daily care and boarding costs.
- *Chain of custody documentation:* All the documentation around evidence preservation and chain of custody must be sent to the prosecutor. This includes chain of custody documentation for live animals.
- *CVs of experts:* Another component to include that will reduce a prosecutor's workload later is the CV of any experts utilized in the investigation. Usually this will include the lead veterinarian on the case, but if a behaviorist was consulted or another specialist was used, try to include their CVs as well. If you continually work with the same veterinarians on these cases, encourage them to update their CVs now and give you a copy to have on hand to include in these case packets.
- *Notice regarding continuing discovery:* In many animal cruelty cases the prosecutor will need the bulk of the information before the animals have fully recovered or while they are still receiving ongoing care and treatment. This is something that is generally unique to animal cruelty cases, so it is helpful to put the prosecutor (and the defense by extension) on notice there will likely be continuing medical discovery related to the case. Even though you will set a reminder for yourself to continue to provide the information at regular intervals, this shares the responsibility with the prosecutor to request that information if they continue to pursue the case.
- *Reference to included but not printed components:* If you are providing a hard copy case packet with a supplemental flash drive of materials, make sure to include a notice somewhere in the hard copy packet that there are additional materials contained on the flash drive and what those consist of.

12.6.4 Miscellaneous Suggestions

There are few steps you can take to underscore the importance and usefulness of this process and end product. First, make duplicate copies. Always retain a copy for yourself if you are the point person, so you know for certain the extent of the material you produced and you can have it as a reference if the prosecutor is having trouble locating a particular document or record. Even if you provide a copy to the prosecutor's office and the law enforcement agency, still make a third copy for yourself.

Second, send an email to the prosecutor, and/or the law enforcement agency, and yourself to document that you have sent the case packet to them, when you did so, and a synopsis of what it includes. This provides a clear reference if this step is questioned at a later date.

Create a method by which you can distinguish what material you have already submitted and what material you have not. As lab results and animal care documentation continue to accrue, you want to make sure you are not duplicating submissions to the prosecutor and creating unnecessary confusion.

Finally, encourage feedback from prosecutors on the format of your case presentation and pay heed at the trials you attend in an effort to understand ways you might improve your submission. Be open to new ways of presenting the information or suggestions of what might be helpful to include. Strive to continue to improve your submission so your cases are not only taken seriously at the prosecutorial level but appreciated.

12.7 Conclusion

The effort of everyone involved in a case is valuable, relevant, and necessary, but if there is no documentation to memorialize it, then it is almost as if it never occurred. Report writing and file organization may not be the most rewarding or captivating part of an animal cruelty investigation, but can be the difference between an acquittal and holding a person accountable for their cruelty to an animal.

13

Protective Custody (Live Animals)
Linda Fielder

When a case requires the seizure of evidence, it must be held in absolute safekeeping. This is so nothing or no one can alter the evidence from the condition it was found at the time of the seizure. When the evidence is money, a pistol, a bicycle, or a knife it is locked up in a police agency's property and evidence facility, which is a highly secure room or building where evidence is logged, tagged, and stored. It is handled only by evidence technicians, so the chain of custody is unequivocally preserved.

When seized evidence comes in the form of a living, breathing animal, be it a tropical fish, a litter of puppies, or a herd of cattle, that evidence must be held in a way that preserves the chain of custody. It must also be fed, exercised, treated for injuries and illnesses, and provided all the aspects of minimum care the species requires.

Living evidence is guaranteed to change over time. Wounds will heal, puppies will grow into adulthood, and emaciated cattle will regain their proper body condition, all while being held in Protective Custody, often for months. This chapter will outline the careful documentation, identification, and record keeping used to memorialize the condition in which animals are received, as well as the methods used for tracking each animal's movement and handling; in other words, how we apply the role of the evidence technician to the movement of animals in custody, as they are walked, treated, fed, and exercised.

13.1 The Challenge of Live Animal Evidence

The thought of holding animals as evidence can make seasoned law enforcement officers and prosecutors scratch their heads. In order to apply even the most basic rules of evidence safekeeping and Protective Custody, a seized animal would be stored in a tamperproof container in a secure room or building awaiting release or trial. While it is impossible to seal a live animal in a container to prevent a breach in the chain of custody, there are processes animal care facilities can implement to ensure no detail regarding an animal's daily care, feeding, exercise, or medical treatment creates an issue that cannot be overcome in the courtroom.

One of the most challenging aspects of holding seized animals pending trial is the fact the animal's evidentiary value is most relevant on the day it is taken into Protective Custody. This is why such care and time is invested in the first 24 hours after a seizure to discover and document the condition of every animal. Because animals are tested, treated, recovered, and rehabilitated during

Animal Cruelty Investigations: A Collaborative Approach from Victim to Verdict™, First Edition.
Edited by Kris Otteman, Linda Fielder, and Emily Lewis.
© 2022 John Wiley & Sons, Inc. Published 2022 by John Wiley & Sons, Inc.
Companion website: www.wiley.com/go/otteman/victimtoverdict

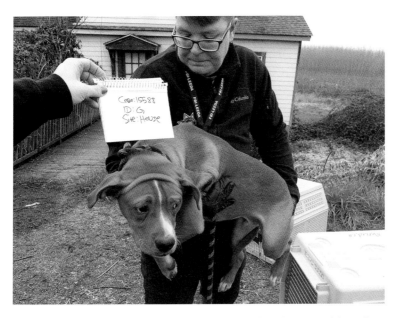

Figure 13.1   Protective Custody begins when the animal is removed from the scene.
Source: Oregon Humane Society.

their time in care, the condition on the day the animal was seized is the condition that will provide the bulk of the evidence on which judgment will be decided, not the way the animal looks or how much it weighs six months later when the case is tried [1].

So why can't these animals be rehomed or otherwise dispositioned once their evidentiary value has run its course? A starving horse will regain weight and health with proper nutrition and care, and a cat's broken leg will mend with veterinary intervention, so at the point an animal has recovered sufficiently to find a new home, why not let that chapter begin (Figure 13.1)?

The answer lies in the animal's status as property. Each animal, unless and until it is surrendered by the owner, released through forfeiture, or transferred by foreclosure of a lien for its care, remains the property of the individual or entity from which it was seized. While forfeiture and foreclosure proceedings shorten the length of time an animal must be held as evidence, too often animals are kept for months or even years beyond the time they are useful to the courts as evidence.

The burden this extended time in care places on the agencies and organizations housing the animals can be immense, and all too often prevents them from helping the animals in the first place; or it becomes a barrier to helping others that would further strain resources and require physical space.

Prosecutors and agencies must pursue all remedies available to shorten the time animals spend in Protective Custody. The veterinarian and animal care agency must perform their duties of intake, treatment, and record keeping meticulously from the moment the animal enters their care and custody until the time it is released from care.

13.2   The First 24 Hours

While the animals will receive identifying names, numbers, and photos at intake, the bulk of a case's criminal evidence is collected during the initial veterinary examination. It is important that this

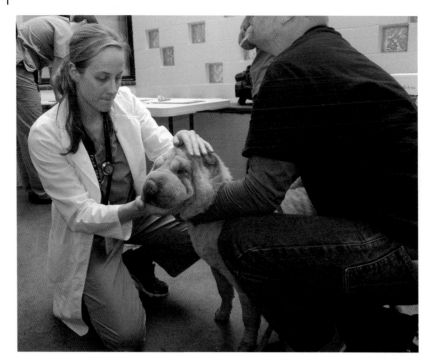

Figure 13.2   Critical evidence is discovered during the initial veterinary examination. *Source:* Oregon Humane Society.

examination takes place within 24 hours of intake so that the findings of this exam can be directly attributed to the suspect's care and treatment of the animal while it was in their custody.

The veterinarian's findings will determine the course of treatment for each animal. Under the veterinarian's direction, the process of rehabilitating and healing begins. When providing housing and care for seized animals, the veterinarian's treatment plan will influence the type of shelter, feeding, grooming, and exercise an animal requires. Ill, injured, or debilitated animals will need to be hospitalized until their conditions become stable (Figure 13.2).

13.3   Know Your Agency's Capacity

Animal care agencies must be able to provide adequate care to animals in Protective Custody and must not take on more than they can care for, or species they are unable to house properly. For example, while a seizure of 50 reptiles and amphibians may not take up considerable space in a shelter, they require specialized diets, lighting, heat support, and enclosures that a facility designed for dogs and cats is unable to provide without planning and resources. When faced with the intake of animals outside the norm for your agency, look for creative ways to meet the animals' needs without compromising the quality of their care. In the above example, an agency might be able to acquire all the needed lighting, enclosures, and heat elements for a reptile seizure by asking the community to donate supplies, soliciting help from pet shops, or reptile specialty groups, or even partnering with a zoo or university with reptile holding capacity.

While it is impossible to prepare for every scenario or have adequate housing at the ready for every species law enforcement will encounter, animal care agencies can prepare by familiarizing themselves with the experts in their area: the avian and exotics veterinarians, the equine rescue groups, those whose specialize in cattle, rabbits, goats, etc. Once you have found the experts, ask for references and check for any possible conflicts of interest between them and the suspect in the case. No one wants to find out during the trial that the avian veterinarian who examined and treated all the birds in your case is in a divorce dispute with the defendant.

13.4 Facility Set-Up and Security

The facility and enclosures your agency provide for seized animals must be appropriate for the species, age, and number of animals, and must also be secure. Security in this context refers to both the integrity of the pens or enclosures, such that animals are not able to escape or injure themselves in the attempt, and the ability to prevent access by unauthorized individuals (Figure 13.3).

All animals need shelter and containment that allows them to move about, rest comfortably, and easily access food and water. Animals removed from neglectful environments may need more than the minimum shelter and housing. They may need extra bedding if they have suffered from pressure sores or ulcerated paw pads or hooves. Newborn, old, or debilitated animals may require extra heat support, or amenities that assist mobility, such as stall pads or lowered perches. The veterinarian's initial findings, along with daily observations by care staff, will provide important information, which will be used to ensure housing is not only sufficient but supportive of rehabilitation and comfort.

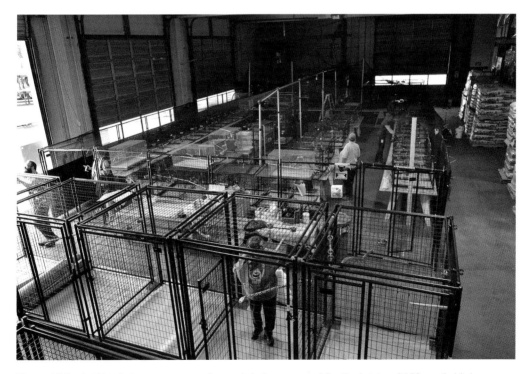

Figure 13.3 In this photo, a secure warehouse is being prepared for the intake of 150 exotic birds. *Source:* Oregon Humane Society.

Facility security is achieved when animals are held in an area away from public view and which restricts access by unauthorized personnel and the public. Security requirements can be met in several ways, from housing animals in a location separate from the main shelter, to utilizing foster homes or rescue organizations, or creating an area of your shelter that can be locked and designated for holding of Protective Custody animals exclusively. If a room or wing of the shelter is designated for Protective Custody housing but is also where the janitorial supply closet is located, the area will be accessed by unauthorized staff unless arrangements are made to relocate supplies while Protective Custody animals are held in that area. When considering security for livestock and equines that live primarily outdoors, steps must be taken to lock and fortify gates and access points to prevent entry or removal of animals by unauthorized individuals.

While the collection of evidence and adherence to chain of custody is important, it must never stand in the way of administering lifesaving care and treatment to an animal. In other words, the agency caring for an animal must never withhold emergency or necessary care in order to preserve the evidence chain of custody.

13.5   Training Staff and Confidentiality

Caring for neglected or abused animals is both stressful and rewarding. Those who provide this care, whether staff or volunteers, often feel compelled to show and tell others about the good work they are doing. Talking about cases can help offset the emotional toll that animal welfare work inflicts. In normal circumstances, animal shelters encourage their staff and supporters to spread the word about the organization's activities, but the opposite is true in the case of animal cruelty investigations and victim animals.

Information about cruelty cases must be kept confidential. The animals and all information about them are evidence and therefore must be protected. Staff, volunteers, and anyone who has occasion to know about a cruelty case within your organization or shelter must be trained regarding confidentiality. A casual conversation in a restaurant booth about a stressed Protective Custody dog may be overheard by a family member of the suspect and skewed by the defense. Even more concerning are opinions, photographs, and videos posted to social media platforms. While it is tempting to weigh in on cases of public interest when the social media conversation heats up, shelter staff, volunteers, foster parents, and veterinarians must resist this urge. Take the time annually, and before any high-profile or large-scale seizure, to train staff about the importance of confidentiality in all aspects of investigations. Agencies must develop confidentiality agreements and be meticulous about using them with all parties who interact with and care for Protective Custody animals (there is an example confidentiality agreement in Appendix C; Figure 13.4).

Staff and volunteer training does not end with matters of confidentiality. In the daily care of seized animals, consistency and uniformity of processes is even more crucial than in general shelter operations. Shelter representatives must be able to testify to the frequency and manner with which enclosures were cleaned and disinfected, the type and quantity of food provided, and any number of other details about the animals' Protective Custody experience. Consistency translates to confidence and assuredness on the stand, which underscores and bolsters the chain of custody.

The best way to be sure care is delivered according to the specific needs of the population is to create written procedures and train staff and volunteers to carry them out. It is then the responsibility of supervisory staff to check for compliance, address any concerns, and make changes to the procedures as appropriate.

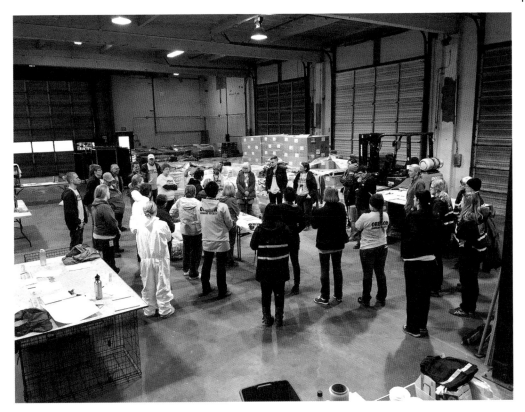

Figure 13.4 Shelter staff and volunteers must be trained on important aspects of chain of custody and confidentiality. *Source:* Oregon Humane Society.

13.6 Paperwork and Record Keeping

Records associated with seized animals are the backbone of the chain of custody. The veterinary medical record memorializes every animal's treatment and rehabilitation plan. Chain of custody logs create a record of the movement of each evidence animal for the purpose of exercise, treatment, care, and cleaning. Forms, logs, and records must be developed, utilized, maintained, and preserved. They should be comprehensive yet user-friendly, so every staff person, volunteer, or agent who interacts with the animal can easily record their activity. Most of the forms referenced in this chapter are available in Appendices B and C, for customization and use by your agency.

13.6.1 Veterinary Exam Forms

Forensic examinations differ from routine physical exams in enough ways that veterinarians should consider using an exam form or electronic template specific to criminal investigation cases. Required fields should include the patient number, animal's evidence identifier, names of all staff who assisted with the exam, date, and time performed, and the basic elements of a forensic exam such as body condition and hair coat score/assessment. Checkboxes for required exam elements such as weight, vaccines, and diagnostics ordered aid the veterinarian and staff in remembering to perform and record each element of the exam. The exam form and process are further explained in Chapter 7.

13.6.2 Protective Custody Sign In/Out Form

A record must exist in which every interaction with the animal by staff or volunteers is memorialized. Think of this as the evidence log for the animal. Forms are typically hung on a clipboard and attached to the animal's enclosure or kept in a binder in the barn or room where the animals are housed. The minimum information contained in the log includes the individual/handler's name, the animal's name unique identifier, date and time of removal and return, and the purpose of the interaction (i.e. provide food, transport to hospital, provide exercise). Completed logs become a part of the criminal case file, therefore it is important that they are not inadvertently destroyed or misplaced.

13.6.3 Other Logs and Records

Agencies utilizing third parties such as foster homes or rescue organizations for the care and shelter of seized animals must provide those parties with methods to track activities and expenses associated with the case. Feed purchase and distribution logs, daily observation logs, property access logs, and feeding charts can all be useful in multiple ways, from illustrating and supporting chain of custody, to tracking expenses associated with the animal's care.

13.7 Providing Security Without Isolation

We have stressed the importance of housing evidence animals in secure areas and maintaining thorough records of their movement and progress. It is common for Protective Custody animals to remain in care for months, and in some cases, years. Even though the animals are housed in restricted areas, their care and enrichment must not be restricted. On the contrary, agencies are responsible for ensuring that evidence animals receive an abundance of enrichment and human interaction, so their temperaments are not negatively impacted during their mandated impound. All species of animals suffer when held in isolation without opportunities to express their natural behaviors, encounter and explore items and areas that interest them, and if the species is domesticated, to receive and respond to human attention and interaction. Animals confined without enrichment become depressed, may stop eating, and often adopt destructive behaviors such as self-mutilation, repetitive behaviors such as cribbing or circling, and become fearful or aggressive toward humans and other animals. Many seized evidence animals enter an agency's care with some or all the negative hallmarks of extended periods of confinement, particularly animals used in commercial operations or subject to conditions found in animal hoarding cases. It must be the goal of the agency overseeing their Protective Custody to provide appropriate housing and as much behavioral modification training and supportive enrichment as possible, to help overcome these behaviors and prevent more damage from occurring.

Soft, comfortable, and clean bedding, a variety of toys, natural light, and regular time for exercise outside their enclosure are minimum daily requirements for most species of animals. Some livestock species respond positively when they can see or hear other animals in stalls or pens close by, while in other species this type of arrangement elicits stress and anxiety. Much research exists that outlines the ideal cage set-up for cats in a shelter with specific instructions for litter box and food bowl placement in relation to hiding boxes and bedding. Rodents and reptiles prefer enclosures outfitted with appropriate bedding or substrate for tunneling and which offer areas for hiding and sleeping such as tubes or nest boxes. If you are unfamiliar with the needs of the species in your care, do not hesitate to reach out to zoos, universities, or other reputable groups to help you create an environment and schedule that support the animals' well-being.

Environmental enrichment is an important stress reducer in all species of animals. Enrichment methods do not have to be expensive or even excessively time consuming. A paper cup filled with wet food and then frozen can provide hours of activity for a dog. Cats respond to small toys hung from their cage door, and birds enjoy foods and toys they can break open and forage through. Both staff and volunteers can be trained and utilized to provide these services. Because many times the animals are held for long periods of time in Protective Custody, they respond best to consistent schedules and familiar people providing for them. This allows the animals to feel somewhat at home in the shelter and reduces stress that follows inconsistent or sudden changes to their routine or constant introduction of new people into their environment [2].

13.8 Foster Care and Offsite Boarding

In some cases, the number and/or type of animal seized will prohibit them from being housed inside your shelter or clinic. In these cases, it is necessary to look outside the agency for appropriate placement in foster homes or offsite facilities. All the aspects we have discussed in this chapter: confidentiality, record keeping, and enrichment, also apply to animals housed outside of your facility, therefore foster or contracted caregivers must be trained and agree to follow your protocols for Protective Custody care.

Foster placements are often the most ideal way to house evidence animals because they mirror a home environment and provide the most enrichment and least stress for the animal. Placements must be thoughtful, however, so that both the caregiver and the animals are set up to succeed.

It is the agency's responsibility to ensure that foster homes or offsite facilities are safe and secure options for housing evidence animals. A representative from your shelter or agency may need to inspect barns, homes, or pastures to make sure fencing and gates are in good working order, areas are free from environmental and structural hazards, and that all environmental needs of the species will be met. Your agency must then select animals that are good candidates for foster placement. They should not be escape prone, aggressive, overly fearful, or medically fragile. Animals with more complex needs should be placed with experienced caregivers.

Foster caregivers and offsite boarding facilities must be provided with all the resources and information they will need to care for the evidence animal successfully. This will include detailed feeding and medication instructions, emergency contacts and protocols, training, and behavior tips and strategies, and processes for contacting shelter or agency representatives with any questions or concerns.

Foster caregivers must understand that the holding agency is ultimately responsible for all decisions related to the animals and they are required to strictly follow veterinarian's instructions for care, treatment, and feeding. When animals from a large-scale starvation case are sent into individual foster homes, caregivers often feel compelled to research and provide supplements, special diets, and treats with the intent to help their foster animal gain weight and condition more rapidly. While the intent is admirable, it complicates the investigation when animals are not rehabilitated in the precise way the attending veterinarian has prescribed.

Foster caregivers and offsite boarding facilities must be trained to utilize chain of custody forms as well as other procedures your agency requires for supply acquisition or reimbursement, progress notes, medication logs, etc. All caregivers who will interact with or be responsible for daily care should receive training on processes as well as agree to confidentiality and communication requirements. Foster families should refrain from posting photos or information about their Protective Custody animal on social media platforms, for example. Your agency must not be prone to an "out of sight, out of mind" attitude regarding foster animals; on the contrary, staff should conduct routine periodic check-ins with caregivers to monitor progress and address any questions or concerns as they arise. In some cases, and often to the dismay of shelter staff and foster caregivers, the court may rule that an animal be returned to a suspect. Include this possibility in your foster caregiver trainings so volunteers understand this possibility.

13.9 Routine and Emergency Veterinary Care

Protective Custody animals require preventative veterinary care such as vaccinations and deworming while they are in your shelter. By vaccinating animals immediately on intake, your agency is offering a degree of protection against diseases such as parvovirus, equine strangles, internal and external parasites, etc., which can be a risk in shelters and group housing arrangements. These procedures are considered baseline veterinary wellness care, are noninvasive, potentially lifesaving, and easily justified at trial as necessary to the maintenance and health of animals held as evidence.

Other medical care to address illness and injury will be administered as needed throughout the animals' stay. Staff and volunteers providing daily care must be observant to changes in health or behavior and bring concerns to a veterinarian's attention immediately. While evidence animals may not be sterilized or receive elective medical procedures, they must receive veterinary care and treatment for any illness or injury that causes discomfort, pain, or distress. For example, while one may argue that grooming a dog is not an essential procedure, if the dog is matted and uncomfortable as a result, or if the coat condition was deemed unacceptable during the veterinarian's examination, it is within the agency's scope of duty to provide grooming and bathing to relieve the dog's discomfort. As a baseline, remember that animals must not suffer neglect while in your care, and so your agency must be vigilant to any medical changes or decline in condition throughout an animal's Protective Custody stay and provide swift and adequate treatment as needed.

Emergency care procedures and contact information must be distributed to staff, volunteers, and foster caregivers, with emergency contact information posted prominently and available for use.

13.10 Death in Care and Euthanasia Considerations

Sometimes, expectedly or unexpectedly, a Protective Custody animal will die while in your agency's care. By proactively creating policies and procedures to address an animal's death in custody, some of the stress associated with such an event will be alleviated.

Any time an evidence animal dies in care, the process of careful documentation and investigation into the cause of death is immediately set into motion. As with any aspect of a criminal investigation, documentation is key. The individual who discovers the deceased animal is responsible for recording the time of discovery and generating a report detailing the incident. When possible, the animal and its immediate environment should be photographed. A veterinarian must be contacted without delay, and efforts undertaken to determine the cause of death. Diagnostics and necropsy are routinely utilized in such cases. Likewise, the prosecutor assigned to the case must be immediately notified, as they are the ultimate party responsible for the safekeeping and disposition of the evidence in their case. If the cause of death is not immediately known, the law enforcement agent or investigator assigned to the case will also want to know about the incident and determine whether additional investigation is warranted.

It is important to have a plan in place for the rare but critical incidents in which a Protective Custody animal requires emergency euthanasia. Tragedies or emergencies can happen any time of the day or night and, while they are never easy to navigate, by having procedures in place and emergency contact information readily available, your agency can facilitate a rapid and humane response to end an animal's suffering.

Euthanasia may be appropriate in cases of critical untreatable illness or injury from which the animal is not likely to recover and that is causing pain and suffering that cannot be relieved by treatment and medication. These cases may come on quickly, such as a livestock animal attacked by a predator, or may progress over time, such as a cat with leukemia that has affected the animal over a period of months or years.

Euthanasia of animals not owned by your agency requires a strict adherence to policy and procedure as well as the direct involvement of a licensed veterinarian, preferably knowledgeable about the case and the animal victims. The veterinarian will guide treatment or euthanasia decisions, with the consideration that the animals are in Protective Custody status. It is always advisable to alert the case prosecutor as soon as possible in the euthanasia decision process. While the veterinarian is the ultimate expert on the matter from a medical perspective, the prosecutor is responsible to the court to account for the evidence. Some circumstances will allow for thorough communication with the prosecutor prior to an animal being euthanized, but in emergency situations, humane principles of veterinary medicine and the animal cruelty code in the state will mandate euthanasia more expediently than you may be able to notify the prosecutor. Documentation is also paramount in all euthanasia decisions. Photos and video are helpful to record the condition of the animal, as are detailed medical records and reports from the treating veterinarian, which will be submitted to the prosecutor in a timely manner and become part of the case file. The veterinarian or prosecutor may decide that a necropsy of the animal post euthanasia will contribute important information to the case. In these instances, the agency or the veterinary staff will be responsible for properly packaging and transporting the body for necropsy.

The agency will hold the bodies of deceased animals as evidence until released by the proper authority. If there is no means to do this, then the prosecutor should coordinate with the defense prior to disposal of the remains.

13.11   Offspring Born in Care

Ideally, if evidence animals were seized pursuant to a search warrant, unborn animals were included in the affidavit as evidence to be searched for and seized. By including unborn offspring in the search warrant, any animals born in Protective Custody immediately become evidence in Protective Custody themselves and are also subject to forfeiture or foreclosure proceedings. Agency staff will be responsible for recording the birth and assigning an evidence identifier to the animal, and immediately beginning chain of custody records for the newborn animals. It is considered best practice to arrange for a veterinarian to examine newborns as soon as it is practical and safe to do so. Newborn animals may suffer from abnormalities or conditions attributed to the neglect or abuse of the mother. The veterinarian must generate a supplemental report regarding their findings and observations.

Newborns receive the same monitoring and care such as preventative vaccination and deworming on the same schedule as any owned or sheltered animal would receive. As with any evidence animal, newborns may not be subjected to nonessential procedures, such as tail docking or dewclaw removal, as these are not necessary to the health or comfort of the animals.

Prosecutors and law enforcement agencies should also be notified immediately when animals are born in care. Be prepared to report their identification numbers so they can be entered into the databases of these entities as additional animals attached to the case.

If the shelter or facility where the mother and newborns are housed exposes them to substantial risk of infectious disease or undue stress, the agency should prioritize placing the animals into the least populous or stressful area of the shelter to preserve their health and well-being. Foster placement can be ideal for newborns as they are less likely to be exposed to infectious disease and can enjoy a quieter and less stressful environment.

13.12 Conclusion

Finding the space and resources to hold animals in Protective Custody can be a hurdle for some agencies and jurisdictions. Grants are available to assist with the cost of holding animals in cruelty cases. A list of organizations offering cost of care grants can be found in Appendix D. It is disheartening to hear of agencies that are reluctant to take on large scale cruelty investigations because of the cost of lengthy Protective Custody periods. By pursuing all remedies for forfeiture or foreclosure that are available in your state, utilizing volunteers and foster homes for care, and seeking grants to offset the financial impact, agencies are better equipped to respond when the need arises.

References

1 Bernstein, M. and Wolf, B. (2005). Time to feed the evidence: what to do with seized animals. https://elr.info/sites/default/files/articles/35.10679.pdf (accessed 17 August 2021).
2 The Association of Shelter Veterinarians (2010). Guidelines for standards of care in animal shelters. https://www.sheltervet.org/assets/docs/shelter-standards-oct2011-wforward.pdf. (accessed 30 May 2021).

14

Media and Fundraising

Emily Lewis

Animal cruelty cases often gain traction with local and even national news, and every organization or agency involved in a case must prepare ahead of time for how to respond to media inquiries and coverage. Also, due to the frequency with which animal cruelty cases utilize a nonprofit animal rescue entity for animal handling, processing, or holding, the issue of fundraising becomes relevant.

In keeping the public informed about an animal cruelty case or investigation, agencies and individuals must do so in a way that does not jeopardize the integrity of the investigation and balances the accused's right to a fair trial. In their mission to report the news to the public, representatives from the media are likely to contact any person with a connection to the case. It is important to have clarity around how to navigate these interactions, whether you were the examining veterinarian or are the lead officer working the case.

One of the advantages of widespread media coverage of a case can be the support it generates for the animal care agencies providing for the victim animals. Even if the media is not driving a fundraising effort, these cases are inordinately expensive, and the nonprofit animal care agency will need to acquire funding to support their work. However, there are several ways a fundraising or marketing campaign can undermine a criminal animal cruelty case. This chapter will discuss the potential pitfalls of fundraising in these cases and make suggestions on how to respond or avoid those pitfalls.

14.1 Media Coverage

With the 24-hour news feed exploding across multiple platforms and literally at the fingertips of the public, it is important to understand and plan for the media's role and impact in your animal cruelty investigations.

14.1.1 Types of Media Coverage

News stories take may forms and utilize multiple platforms. Be aware of each of these venues as you might need to generate a policy that addresses the nuances of each.

Animal Cruelty Investigations: A Collaborative Approach from Victim to Verdict™, First Edition.
Edited by Kris Otteman, Linda Fielder, and Emily Lewis.
© 2022 John Wiley & Sons, Inc. Published 2022 by John Wiley & Sons, Inc.
Companion website: www.wiley.com/go/otteman/victimtoverdict

14.1.1.1 Print News

Reading the morning paper is less common than it once was, but local newspapers continue to have an interest in stories involving animals, particularly if cruelty is involved. These can range from large media outlets, like a nationally distributed newspaper, to small newsletters distributed to a limited number of local residents. Regardless of the size of the publication, it is almost certain to be published online as well as in print. Print news engages in investigative and in-depth reporting more frequently than other types of media.

14.1.1.2 Television News

Local news networks commonly pick up and report on stories about animal cruelty cases. Often this type of reporting takes place close in time to a milestone in the investigation or case, such as a search warrant execution or an arrest. These networks value timely, impactful stories that will catch the interest of their audience in the small timeframe they have to do so.

14.1.1.3 Radio

Though the news stories reported over local radio stations tend to shadow the stories that were picked up by the television networks, it is likely there is less reporting via the radio than all other media platforms. That being said, some public broadcasting stations may engage in similar investigative and in-depth reporting to their print media counterparts.

14.1.1.4 Social Media/Internet

Though newest on the scene of media and reporting, social media is far and away the biggest venue for reporting the news to the masses. Social media is essentially an online community where people congregate. It is the most interactive platform, meaning the consumer often engages in commenting on stories and posts. All print, television, and radio entities will also use social media to disseminate their information. Some media outlets exclusively rely on the Internet to broadcast their stories, either via podcasts or by using common social media platforms. Not only does social media act as an outlet for any journalistic endeavor, it also functions as an extremely efficient method of propagating existing news stories.

14.1.2 Objectives in Media Coverage

Interacting with the media can be anxiety inducing and/or time consuming, but the objectives of the media and the individuals involved in animal cruelty investigations do not run counter to one another in every circumstance. In many ways the media gets the word out to the public regarding animal cruelty laws, prevention, and efforts made against animal maltreatment. It is worthwhile to foster a good relationship with the primary media outlets in your jurisdiction. Take time to meet the reporters and discuss how you can work together to inform the public without jeopardizing the important work.

14.1.2.1 For Law Enforcement or Investigating Agencies

Most law enforcement entities have experience interacting with the media. In fact, many agencies designate someone as the primary point of contact for all media inquiries, referred to as the "Public Information Officer" (PIO). The purpose of the PIO is not simply to act as a buffer between the agency and the media, but to pursue certain objectives through that interaction. One objective may be to seek the public's assistance with an investigation. For example, the media can help get the word out that an agency needs assistance locating a particular vehicle or a person who is suspected of a crime like animal abandonment. Law enforcement also engages with the media to inform the public that they investigate cases of animal cruelty for public safety purposes. Given the substantiated link between animal crime and human violence, there is an objective to inform the public and promote the understanding of the seriousness of animal crimes. In some cases, it might become an objective of law enforcement to make a statement to the media that curtails rumors or misinformation about a case that would or has led to a safety issue for someone involved, be it a witness or a suspect.

14.1.2.2 For Animal Care Agencies

Animal care agencies assisting with animal cruelty investigations also have varied objectives when interacting with the media. Primarily, the organization wants to inform the public about the valuable role they are playing in the community. Also, many of the animal agencies assisting in these cases rely on donations to sustain their work and they need the public to be aware of the increased demand on resources when they take in animals from an animal cruelty case. It also creates an opportunity to manage the influx of public correspondence with respect to inquiries about volunteering and adoption opportunities connected with the victim animals.

14.1.2.3 For Veterinarians

Veterinarians may be less likely to respond to media requests related to cases they have participated in, but when they do engage, it can be in furtherance of their own objectives as well. Through the media, veterinarians have a platform to galvanize the profession to report animal cruelty (as is their duty in many states) and participate as an expert in these investigations. They can also combat any ill will circulating about their decision to report or participate in a particular case. Notably, the veterinarian is the person who can speak on behalf of the victim, as appropriate, to relay the seriousness of the incident and the importance of the investigation.

14.1.2.4 For Media

The media's primary objective is to inform the public. Reporters seek transparency in government and matters of public safety; both of which are relevant to animal cruelty cases. Of course, the various media outlets vie for consumers of their information, and therefore also have the objective of presenting interesting stories and doing so first. Animal cruelty investigations or arrests almost always resonate with the public. The media's goal when it comes to reporting on those cases is to provide the public with as much information as they can garner on the topic, with a preference for details about the crime committed, the evidence uncovered, the person accused, and location of the incident.

14.1.3 Defendant's Rights

When it comes to coverage of a case in the media, a defendant is afforded rights under the law. Constitutionally, the defendant has a right to a fair trial by an impartial jury [1]. Media coverage can create enough backlash and/or rumors that it taints the defendant's jury pool [2]. The defendant also has a constitutional right to privacy [3], preventing the media from accessing their property during a search warrant execution and from publishing information that is not a matter of public record. Laws regarding who is subject to public records laws and what constitutes a public record will differ by state and are important to review when engaging in criminal investigation work. If the accused is a juvenile, they are extended even more protections under the law with respect to disclosure of identity and details of location. Finally, it is important to remember that the defendant also has a right to communicate with the media.

14.1.4 Risks in Media Coverage

Even though there are benefits to media coverage of an investigation or prosecution, there are significant risks posed by that coverage as well. It is generally understood now that any news story will live forever online. This means that any quote made by an expert witness veterinarian, supervisor of seized animal care operations, or investigator on a case can be found and used at trial in attempts to, for example, discredit a witness or demonstrate bias. It also means that any photographs taken by or given to the media can be called into question during the criminal trial and any related civil suits. If television media is invited to record footage, anything they have captured and aired can be presented at trial if it is relevant in some way; for example, if there is video of how the evidence animals are being processed.

Depending what information is included in a media story, it can interfere with the jury pool. The media commonly reports on a defendant's criminal record or admissions they have made with respect to the current case [4]. These are examples of information that may not be permissible evidence introduced in the trial setting, but jurors will have already heard it. Increased media coverage of a case can cause future jury members to form a conclusion about guilt prior to the trial even commencing. There are tools available to attempt to remedy those issues – targeted voir dire questions, judicial orders, delay of trial, change of venue – but these are seldom employed and not likely to resolve the issue when they are [5]. Regardless of whether a court finds that a jury has been prejudiced against the defendant by public media on a case, the goal is for a guilty verdict to result from evidence that proves the elements of the crime, not that the media will control the scales of justice.

The way news is currently disseminated exacerbates the risks that are inherent to media coverage of an animal cruelty investigation. With the ability of social media to act as a springboard for any story, the reporting of your case could travel outside of your jurisdiction and be picked up by national media conglomerates in a matter of minutes. This can create a flood of public response, be it positive or negative, that can quickly spiral out of control resulting in diverted resources and increased likelihood of misinformation.

14.1.5 Existing Guidelines

14.1.5.1 For Media

The First Amendment right to "freedom of the press" [6] does not afford the media unchecked authority to seek and disclose any details of a case in any manner they choose. There are several national and international professional journalism associations that publish ethical codes of conduct, with common themes of truth and accuracy, minimizing harm, and impartiality.[1] Additionally, many state bar associations and court systems issue rules and guidelines for journalists engaging in courtroom reporting.[2]

---

1 Society of Professional Journalists (n.d.). SPJ code of ethics. https://www.spj.org/ethicscode.asp (accessed 30 May 2021); New Leaders Association (n.d.). ASNE statement of principles. https://members.newsleaders.org/content.asp?pl=24&sl=171&contentid=171 (accessed 30 May 2021); International Federation of Journalists (2019). IFJ global charter of ethics for journalists. https://www.ifj.org/who/rules-and-policy/global-charter-of-ethics-for-journalists.html (accessed 30 May 2021); The Associated Press Managing Editors. (1994). Statement of ethical principles. https://web.archive.org/web/20080622123407/http://www.apme.com/ethics (accessed 30 May 2021).
2 United States Courts (n.d.). A journalist's guide to the federal courts. https://www.uscourts.gov/statistics-reports/publications/journalists-guide-federal-courts (accessed 30 May 2021); Oregon Newspaper Publishers Association (n.d.). News media and the court. http://orenews.com/news-media-court (accessed 30 May 2021).

14.1.5.2   For Law Enforcement

The overarching guideline for law enforcement in their interactions with the media is not to pro-vide information that would jeopardize an active case or violate confidentiality constraints. The state law must inform the communications policies that law enforcement agencies draft and imple-ment, so it is clear what information is protected and what information is permissible to release. Generating a policy is of utmost importance and will create consistency and uniformity in how officers interact with the media and what information they convey.[3]

14.1.5.3   For Veterinarians

The guidelines relevant to a veterinarian's interaction with the media will depend in part on their role in the investigation. Generally speaking, state licensing boards and the American Veterinary Medical Association (AVMA) issue rules and guidelines veterinarians are expected to follow [7]. These rules might require confidentiality when it comes to information about a patient and/or client [8]. If a veterinarian works as the lead doctor on an animal cruelty case, that veterinarian can be deemed an agent of the investigating agency. As an agent of the agency, the veterinarian would have to keep the same confidentiality on open cases as their law enforcement partner. Similarly, if a veterinarian is a primary witness for an ongoing animal cruelty case, it is outside the scope of their authority to disclose information that would have the potential to jeopardize the investigation.

14.1.5.4   For Prosecutors

Prosecutors have very clear guidelines with respect to interactions with the media about their criminal cases. These guidelines even extend to the agencies and individuals assisting with the investigation of those cases. In their Model Rules of Professional Conduct for lawyers, the American Bar Association (ABA) includes the following under the "Special Responsibilities of a Prosecutor":

> [E]xcept for statements that are necessary to inform the public of the nature and extent of the prosecutor's action and that serve a legitimate law enforcement purpose, refrain from making extrajudicial comments that have a substantial likelihood of heightening public condemnation of the accused and *exercise reasonable care to prevent investigators, law enforcement personnel, employees or other persons assisting or associated with the prosecutor in a criminal case from making an extrajudicial statement that the prosecutor would be pro-hibited from making. . .* [9]
>
> (Emphasis added.)

All 50 states use this model rule as an outline to their respective state rules [10]. More than likely the prosecutor's office will have written policies directly related to their interactions with the press [11].

14.1.5.5   For Animal Shelters/Rescues/Sanctuaries

There are no laws or professional rules of conduct specific to animal shelters, rescues, and sanctu-aries when it comes to interactions with the media. When these organizations are holding or car-ing for animals involved in a criminal animal cruelty case, they are doing so as agents of the

---

3 International Association of Chiefs of Police (2019a). Considerations document: Media relations. https://www. theiacp.org/sites/default/files/2019-08/Media%20Considerations%20-%202019.pdf (accessed 30 May 2021); International Association of Chiefs of Police (2019b). Concepts and issues paper: Media relations. https://www. theiacp.org/sites/default/files/2019-08/Media%20Paper%20-%202019%202.pdf. (accessed 30 May 2021).

enforcing entity. That means the guidelines that apply to that enforcement entity extend to the animal care organization with respect to those specific animals.

14.1.6 Different Phases of the Case

The phase an investigation or case is in – beginning, middle, or end – will influence how you can or should respond to media inquiries. At certain points in an investigation some information becomes public record and you may decide to share more information. In other cases, you may want to take extreme precautions at every phase of the investigation despite what information becomes public record, in order to protect witnesses, other victims, or the suspect(s) involved in a case.

14.1.6.1 Report Made, Beginning of Investigation

Occasionally, news outlets will learn that a situation has been reported and that your agency may be involved. This is one of the simpler inquiries to navigate. At the beginning of an investigation there is not much information you can relay to the public because it has a higher potential of impacting the ongoing investigation. Typically, at this phase, an agency could confirm they are investigating but politely decline to comment further on an open investigation. Your agency policies may prohibit you from either affirming or denying that an investigation is taking place. There is too much left to learn at this phase of an investigation to be sharing any findings or theories with the media.

14.1.6.2 Ongoing Investigation into Chronic Issue

Animal cruelty investigations can take weeks or months to complete, and the media may request an update about an investigation that has been on their radar. Again, it is likely that disclosure of details to the media would hinder the ongoing investigation and potentially put involved parties at risk in this phase of an investigation. In this situation you may want to take the opportunity to educate the media (and thus the public) about why these cases can go on for weeks or months and simply decline to comment on the specifics of that ongoing investigation.

14.1.6.3 Search Warrants

The execution of a search warrant in an animal cruelty case is an event that will pique the interest of the media. It may also be the first point in the investigation that information will be accessible to the media through public record avenues.

During Execution of the Warrant Some journalists listen to police scanners and learn about search warrant executions as they are actively occurring. In animal cases, the number of vehicles and personnel needed to execute a warrant service can be significant, making any staging area conspicuous as well. As mentioned in Chapter 9, it is important to plan for media presence at the search warrant location and designate a person to interface with them. Members of the media should never be permitted to enter the scene of a search warrant without express permission of the judge or the lead investigator on the case. Note that this includes media personnel who may be employed by the assisting animal care agency or veterinarian. Without specific authorization otherwise, media personnel must stay relegated to areas open to the public.

Immediately After the Search Warrant Execution Immediately after the search warrant execution the media may have an interest in documenting the seized animals arriving at the animal care facility. Again, the media should be restricted to areas open to the public.

The PIO for the investigating agency or the animal care agency may be documenting the animals' arrival in a preapproved manner that may later be disseminated to the media (and included in the case file), but members of outside media outlets should not be permitted to document any part of the process involving the animals' arrival, unloading, or veterinary examinations.

Creating a plan for footage collected by internal PIOs allows an agency to meet their objectives of informing the public without jeopardizing their case. When outside media are permitted to take photos and video it is difficult to get duplicates of that footage to include in discovery.

Once the search warrant return has been made, in most cases the media is able to access the documents via public record channels. In some ways this alleviates the decision of what information an agency should release to the media because the search warrant documents will provide a significant amount of detail. In other ways it can make the rest of the investigation more difficult if there is a large public response to the information released by the media. It can be helpful to draft and issue a press release close in time to your search warrant return in order to anticipate interest and have a vetted statement to rely on in your responses. See Appendix C for sample press releases issued in animal cruelty cases.

14.1.6.4 After Citation or Arrest

Citation and/or arrest in a case is another newsworthy development. Use caution at this point in your conversations with the media because, if arraignment has not occurred, then the suspect has not been officially charged with the crimes for which they were cited or arrested. Additionally, due to the public's historically emotional and vehement reaction to animal maltreatment, releasing their name and exact address can put a suspect and their family at risk. Of course, a custodial arrest will result in some documentation that is available to the public, but it does not mean that you are required to or should provide it in your press releases or interviews with the media.

With strict adherence to the internal policy on media interactions, the lead veterinarian on a case may issue a statement to the press. Keep in mind that this statement can be used during trial for any relevant purpose, including discrediting and bias. For that reason, the veterinarian's statement needs to be consistent with the report they submitted in the case and be limited to factual findings. For example, "Many of the cats were anemic and suffered from severe dental disease," or "The dog in this case sustained multiple bone fractures and is currently receiving ongoing treatment for these serious injuries." Instead of statements infused with legal conclusions or opinions about the defendant, for example, "The animals were severely neglected based on their skeletal conditions. It is clear the owner was too lazy to purchase adequate food for them."

14.1.6.5 Pending Trial

The period between when a suspect is arraigned and when the trial or plea agreement occurs can be quite lengthy unless the suspect is in police custody. When a person is being held in custody (i.e. jail), there are strict timeframes that expedite the charging process to ensure that an individual is not kept against their will for a prolonged period of time. During this time, the media may follow up with involved agencies or individuals to inquire about the status of the case, condition of the animals, or the availability of the animals for adoption. Any information released to the media should already have been produced in discovery for the case. Said a different way, the media should not have information before the prosecutor and defense have it in their possession. Again, always refer the media to the lead investigating agency before providing any updates about an active case.

14.1.6.6 During Trial

There are journalists who monitor the court dockets and will know when a case is set for trial. The media will be subject to the court rules for cameras and media presence in the courtroom during trial, but that does not always explicitly prevent contact with agencies or witnesses outside the courtroom. First and foremost, adhere to the policies your agency has generated with respect to communications with the media. While trial is ongoing, do not provide any information to the media aside from using the appropriate spokesperson to confirm that the trial is underway. Witnesses are not permitted to discuss the case outside of the courtroom and that extends to representatives of the media.

14.1.6.7 After Trial

Once the trial has concluded, additional information can be released to the media. Typical posttrial press releases will include: the charges the defendant was convicted of, which judge oversaw the trial, and, if available, the terms of the sentencing. If you are displeased with the sentence or how the trial was prosecuted, airing those grievances through the media is not an appropriate way to address them. In most cases trials are open to the public and the public can request trial transcripts. This makes the information provided in testimony a matter of public record, allowing you to reference it without jeopardizing discovery rules or the viability of that evidence in the case. As an assisting agent of the lead law enforcement agency on the case, you have a duty to be very factual in the information you are providing to the public and to avoid statements that would inflame the public or exaggerate the facts of the case.

While maintaining a good relationship with the media is important, be careful not to stray from your agency's policies in your interactions with them. If resources allow, it is a good idea to designate a person to be responsible for coordinating and interacting with the media. Ideally this person would have some experience working with the media or a background in public relations/communications. If you are assisting law enforcement with a case, remember to refer media to the lead investigating agency or confirm with the agency how they want you to respond to inquiries.

14.2 Handling Negative Press

Working in animal cruelty investigations does not exempt you from negative press. Even though animal cruelty cases are generally viewed as rescue stories and the media reports on them in a positive light, these stories still often garner negative comments or response. The media typically does not have the full complement of information on a case and, as such, what they report has the potential to create discourse in the community. Veterinarians can be criticized for reporting clients. Animal care agencies can be challenged for charging high adoption fees for rescued animals. Law enforcement agencies are susceptible to critiques of their investigation and lack of empathy in removing animals from an individual's home. All entities can be admonished if any of the animals from a case are euthanized, regardless of the reason. These are all common laments surrounding animal cruelty investigation work and, with the help of social media, can spiral quickly into a public relations nightmare.

As an agency or a participant in the case, you must be thoughtful, well-prepared, and cautious in how you respond. After investing significant time and resources into investigating and rescuing animals, you may feel compelled to give clarity if a different narrative is emerging in response to the media's release. Making a plan for negative press is a worthwhile endeavor and has the likelihood of mitigating the damage quickly. In some cases, not responding will be the best response; this is known as "starving the story." Attempting to refute every allegation in the comments section of a news story or in the feed of a social media account is likely to perpetuate the firestorm rather than temper it. It may also be damaging to the case. The news cycle grows increasingly more fleeting and requiring that your staff and volunteers refrain from commenting facilitates a quick fading of interest. This is the time when positive relationship-building with the media pays off. In cases where a suspect or other member of the public is attempting to paint you in a bad light, the media controls whether a story gets released and how the information is conveyed. Take the time to understand how law enforcement and public relations professionals handle situations involving negative press, so you can be prepared to act quickly and decisively.

14.3   Internal Communications Policy

Any agency that engages in animal cruelty investigations should have a communications policy specific to those investigations. This affords your agency consistency in interactions and a reference, when necessary, on the witness stand. See Appendix C for an example communication policy document. As with every policy you generate, once you have put the effort into its creation, make sure you pair that with adequate training for staff and volunteers to ensure adherence.

14.4   Fundraising

Animal cruelty investigations can fall short of action taken to remedy a situation solely due to lack of funds. This can come in the form of lack of resources to investigate, the cost of adequate veterinary forensics, or the financial burden of caring for animals as the criminal justice process is carried out. Animal cruelty investigations are expensive, and it is necessary for assisting agencies to support this work through fundraising. Generally, in this section we refer to "fundraising" in the context of seeking money to help pay for the care and treatment of animals in an active criminal case. This is distinguished from the fundraising that is done to facilitate the ability of the organization to do similar work in the future.

14.4.1   Why Is Fundraising Necessary?

Animal cruelty cases involve living evidence that, under state laws, require a minimum level of ongoing care. The cost of providing that care is often a prohibitive factor in addressing these crimes. First, an assisting animal care organization must create space to house the Protective Custody animals. This displaces the space used for non-case-related animals that are presumably available for adoption. Depending on how long the Protective Custody animals are held, the animal care organization could have housed and adopted out three to five to ten times that population of animals in the space being occupied by the Protective Custody animals. So as not to displace adoptable animals, the animal care agency would need to procure alternative temporary housing facilities for the Protective Custody animals and then, in most circumstances, retrofit that space to accommodate that particular species of animal. All this has a significant financial impact on the assisting animal organization that they would not otherwise have experienced but for the crime of animal cruelty being committed by the defendant.

Not only do the assisting agencies have to expend money on the space to house the animals, but also on the workforce necessary to care for them. This includes, but is not limited to, providing food, water, sanitation, enrichment, and medication multiple times a day. Even if an agency already has a workforce employed to care for a certain number of animals that now happen to include Protective Custody animals, this population of animals almost always requires a higher level of care, at least initially, and more time providing that care.

None of these costs are eliminated by the use of foster homes for Protective Custody animals. Again, using foster homes for the purpose of Protective Custody animals means those homes are not available to other animals, which then remain, at a cost, in the animal rescue facility. Additionally, a foster care program does not run without oversight and the organization will be using staff to coordinate the logistics of processing foster applications, training foster homes about the policies related to the Protective Custody animals, sending the animals into foster, responding to inquiries and concerns of the foster while they have the animal(s), and ensuring that foster animals get medical checkups when they are due. Many agencies will provide the food and equipment necessary to foster the animal and, if they do not provide that, they are paying for the animals that remain in the shelter who would otherwise be in foster care. Again, if this impacts the number of animals a rescue organization can move through to adoption, it results in a decrease of a significant revenue stream used to fund its operation.

The conditions that result from animal cruelty require veterinary care that is costly as well. To conduct a forensic examination, a veterinarian must have the resources to engage in any diagnostics necessary. This can include blood tests, tissue sample testing, radiographs, ultrasounds, and even full necropsy or toxicology testing, not to mention the cost of the veterinarian and their staff's time in conducting the exam. Once the exam is complete, it is likely the animal will need ongoing care for any number of issues. It is the investigating agency's responsibility to get assurances that this level of minimum care is being met and they or another entity must incur the cost.

It is a disservice to the community and to the victim animals if financial concerns are a barrier to conducting thorough animal cruelty investigations. The agencies providing resources to ensure those cases do not fall victim to a shoestring budget must be permitted to seek financial assistance through fundraising, and not be disparaged for doing so. As we will explore in the remainder of this chapter, the caveat to fundraising during an active criminal case is that it cannot impinge on a defendant's rights, and it cannot jeopardize the case in a material way.

14.4.2   Vulnerabilities Created by Fundraising

The need to seek additional outside funding while caring for Protective Custody animals must be balanced with the risk of jeopardizing the case. If your organization played a role in the collection of animal evidence or treatment of evidence animals, you are essentially an agent of the law enforcement entity investigating the case. Under no circumstances should requests for donations or fundraising campaigns use any rhetoric that passes judgment on the accused prior to adjudication. Only facts can be used in the fundraising materials about criminal cases; this requires restraint from pontificating about the conditions at the scene or the health and emotions of the animals. Realize that by choosing to fundraise during an active criminal case, you are providing the defense with grounds to question witnesses on bias and to challenge restitution sought; essentially you are making the prosecutor's job more difficult. You may also be exposing the organization to civil liability should the fundraising materials stray from or exaggerate any facts of the case. Another concern is the impact of fundraising on the judge or jury in a case. If, based on evidence presented, the decision maker feels that the victim animals have sufficiently recovered and the animal care organization has been made whole through donations, it has the potential to sway their assessment of the seriousness of the violation.

There is less risk associated with seeking donations from a narrow, targeted audience. Using information from press releases to draft a request to a specific major donor for financial assistance in a case exposes that case to fewer vulnerabilities than a public campaign. In these situations, you can employ confidentiality agreements and get other assurances that the information will remain private and not publicized. Regardless of the size of the audience, you may be required to disclose your fundraising activity if it is connected directly to a particular case.

14.4.3 Traditional Methods of Fundraising

While governmental agencies or for-profit veterinary clinics may be restricted in how they can fundraise, nonprofit animal care organizations have a variety of ways to sustain their missions financially. The most traditional avenues are individual donors, grants (foundations, corporate, and government), fundraising events, estate bequests, and earned income (i.e. adoptions). Appealing to the donor through most of these methods requires focusing on a specific donor or a particular group of donors, but some fundraising strategies are geared toward an appeal to the general public.

Regardless of the method, sharing a story about a victim of animal cruelty tends to inspire more and bigger donations than other anecdotes. Because the nonprofit wants to motivate the individual or the foundation to contribute to their organization, the staff pursuing the donations may be prone to use emotional language and vivid adjectives when telling the stories of the nonprofit's work. In the context of fundraising in connection with a criminal case, that can become problematic.

14.4.4 Timing

A criminal investigation goes through many phases and not every phase is an appropriate time to consider fundraising. In fact, fundraising should be off the table completely between when a situation is reported and the decision to remove animal(s), and even long after that in many cases. If an animal care agency is called to assist in the removal and housing of a large number of animals, representatives from that organization might start to make a plan about how they are going to offset the financial impact of that event. The unpredictable nature of animal cruelty cases is such that actually securing donations or grants in advance would be irresponsible from a fiduciary standpoint.

Once the organization is actively incurring costs associated with the case and the animals, there may be appropriate ways to fundraise. If a press release is to be issued, it can include information about how to donate if the lead law enforcement agency approves. Staff of the animal care organization can approach specific donors or foundations to seek financial assistance for the case if sensitive information related to the case is kept confidential. Fundraising after a case has been adjudicated to secure funding for future case assists allows for a more detailed pitch and less risk as it relates to the case work.

14.4.5 Fundraising and Restitution

Some judges and attorneys may find restitution and fundraising for the costs associated with a case to be mutually exclusive. This is a risk worth considering in your decision on whether to fundraise in connection with a particular case.

There are arguments available to a prosecutor to refute the idea that restitution should be offset by donations an animal care agency received. Members of the public would cease to donate if that donation turned into a windfall for an individual convicted of animal cruelty. It is not the public's responsibility to pay for the harm caused by the defendant. Restitution is part of the sentencing process, and it is part of holding that person accountable for the outcome of their criminal conduct. Permitting a reduction in restitution is not in keeping with the intent of restitution in these cases.[4] The vast majority of animal care organizations are not going to be seeking donations specifically earmarked for a particular case. The money will go into their operating budget and will likely be used to replace the funds taken away from the animals they routinely assist in their community. Finally, across the board, animal care agencies lose money when assisting with these cases. If they receive donations, they rarely come close to covering the added costs, and adoption fees fall woefully short of actual costs of care as well. If restitution is awarded, it is often reduced and, if paid at all, paid over the course of many years.

Despite the arguments available in favor of the defendant paying the full restitution amount, prosecutors and animal care agencies should be prepared to produce documentation of donations related directly to a case. If ordered to submit donation information, it is within the organization's right to contest any requirement to produce donor names and personal information. The sum of money and what it was spent on is what is relevant, not who made the donation. Include The staff time spent procuring and processing the donation is also relevant and should be included. A defendant should not have the full value of a donation credited to the costs they owe for the care of the animals they victimized if some of the donation was utilized for other purposes related to the case.

There are ways to resolve any ambiguity between restitution and fundraising. Agencies involved in animal cruelty investigations need to meet with the local prosecutor ahead of time to understand their state's laws on restitution in criminal cases and how the case law has interpreted those statutes (Box 14.1). Using that insight, plan to receive donations during a time when you are assisting with a case. Another option is to finesse the language you are including on your fundraising and marketing materials about the case. Instead of seeking funds specifically for or because of that current case, ask the public to support your continued work "on cases like these." Removing the direct correlation between a supporter's donation to your organization and the immediate case at hand can help remove ambiguity when discussions regarding restitution take place.

14.4.6 Guidelines for Necessary Fundraising

If the risk to the case is too great, there are alternatives to fundraising in direct connection with an active case.

14.4.6.1 Do Not Use Active Cases

Once a case has been adjudicated there is more information to share with interested donors. If you stagger your fundraising campaigns and use past, closed cases there is significantly less risk to the case and the organization. Additionally, you can use more compelling images and concrete language about the scene, the charges, and the outcome. Using this strategy of fundraising also facilitates the use of follow-up stories on recovered and rehabilitated animal victims. Waiting to fundraise on a case until it has resolved gives you the benefit of being able to tell the whole story and connect the outcome with the work you continue to engage in.

---

4 *Mahan vs. State* (2002) 51 P.3d 962; *State vs. Burr* (2001) 147 N.H. 102, 782.

Box 14.1 Example

The state of Oregon went so far as to address the uncertainty by amending their legislative findings and their sentencing laws:

Oregon Revised Statutes §167.305(6):

(6) A government agency, a humane investigation agency or its agent or a person that provides care and treatment for impounded or seized animals:

  a) Has an interest in mitigating the costs of the care and treatment in order to ensure the swift and thorough rehabilitation of the animals; and

  b) May mitigate the costs of the care and treatment through funding that is separate from, and in addition to, any recovery of reasonable costs that a court orders a defendant to pay while a forfeiture proceeding is pending or subsequent to a conviction;

Oregon Revised Statutes §167.350(1) (b):

If a government agency or a humane investigation agency or its agent provides care and treatment for impounded or seized animals, a court that orders a defendant to repay reasonable costs of care under paragraph (a) of this subsection may not reduce the incurred cost amount based on the agency having received donations or other funding for the care.

14.4.6.2 Wishlists

Wishlists are a creative alternative to fundraising that pose less risk to an active case. Particularly in cases where your organization must collect supplies, such as bird cages or reptile enclosures, a wishlist can often be a way that donors can contribute to the cause while you get the equipment you need. On many platforms you can preload your wishlist and then make it live when the case is made public. At that point you can direct the public and other donors to the wishlist if they want to help.

14.4.6.3 National Organizations

There are national organizations, foundations, and charities in place that will provide grants to assist with criminal cases without requiring disclosure of important details about the case. For example, the Animal Legal Defense Fund can provide expedited grants for veterinary forensics and daily costs of care for animals connected to a criminal investigation or prosecution. The Association of Prosecuting Attorneys offers grants in cases of cruelty involving dogs [12]. PetSmart Charities and Banfield Charitable Trust and the American Society for the Prevention of Cruelty to Animals (ASPCA) are examples of other national entities who can assist financially without jeopardizing a case.

14.4.6.4 Funding from Law Enforcement

On occasion the budget of a law enforcement agency will include money for animal cruelty casework. Leadership at the animal care agency called upon to assist must discuss who will bear the financial cost of the care and treatment of the victim animals in advance of the intake. Sometimes these discussions can result in interagency collaborations that prove sustainable across future cases as well.

14.4.6.5 Specific Donor Asks

Nonprofit animal care agencies have the option of approaching a targeted donor with a request for financial assistance in a case. If the supporter requires certain specifics about the case, make sure law enforcement is aware and involved if they choose and have the donor sign a confidentiality agreement before disclosing any information about the case to them.

14.4.6.6 Designated Fund for Future Cases

Agencies can initiate a fund that supporters can contribute to throughout the year that will be used for casework when it occurs.[5] This money will not be tied to a specific case and gives an agency the flexibility to be able to respond in the moment to an urgent animal cruelty case.

References

1 Constitution of the United States, Amendment 6, (1791) (USA).

2 Simpler, M.F. (2012). The unjust "web" we weave: the evolution of social media and its psychological impact on juror impartiality ad fair trials. *Law Psychol. Rev.* 36: 275.

3 Constitution of the United States, Amendment 4, (1791) (USA).

4 Dee, J. and Hans, V.P. (1991). Media coverage of law: its impact on juries and the public. *Am. Behav. Sci.* 35: 136.

5 Dee, J. Hans VP. Media coverage of law: its impact on juries and the public. *The American Behavioral Scientist. 1991 Nov/Dec* 35: 136.

6 Constitution of the United States, Amendment 1, (1791) (USA).

7 American Veterinary Medical Association (n.d.). AVMA policies. https://www.avma.org/resources-tools/avma-policies?f%5B0%5D=policy_topic%3A1816 (accessed 30 May 2021).

8 American Veterinary Medical Association (2019, updated 2021). 2019 Model veterinary practice act. https://www.avma.org/sites/default/files/2019-11/Model-Veterinary-Practice-Act.pdf (accessed 30 May 2021).

9 American Bar Association (n.d.). Rule 3.8 Special responsibilities of a prosecutor. https://www.americanbar.org/groups/professional_responsibility/publications/model_rules_of_professional_conduct/rule_3_8_special_responsibilities_of_a_prosecutor (accessed 30 May 2021).

10 American Bar Association CPR Policy Implementation Committee. (2020). Variation of the ABA model rules of professional conduct rule 3.8: Special responsibilities of a prosecutor. https://www.americanbar.org/content/dam/aba/administrative/professional_responsibility/mrpc_3_8.pdf (accessed 30 May 2021).

11 The United States Department of Justice (2018). 1-7.000 – Confidentiality and media contacts policy. https://www.justice.gov/jm/jm-1-7000-media-relations (accessed 30 May 2021).

12 Association of Prosecuting Attorneys (n.d.). National dog abuse investigation and prosecutor assistance application. https://www.apainc.org/programs-2/animal-abuse-prosecution-project/national-dog-abuse-assistance (accessed 30 May 2021).

---

5 An example of this type of fund is the Velvet Assistance Fund used for emergency care for animals: DoveLewis (n.d.). Velvet Assistance Fund. https://www.dovelewis.org/community/financial-medical-aid/velvet-assistance-fund (accessed 30 May 2021).

15

Forfeiture, Surrender, and Related Legal Remedies
David Rosengard

When it comes to animal cruelty, that the *animalness* of those creatures victimized by criminal cruelty is relevant may seem so obvious as to be dismissible. If the victims of animal cruelty were not animals, we would, after all, not be discussing the issue as animal cruelty.[1] However, this seeming tautological simplicity of it mattering that dealing with animal cruelty involves dealing with animals belies the complexity of what the involvement of animals means for both responders on the ground and legal practitioners involved in animal cases.

One of the places where animal cases have given rise to complex practical and legal scenarios grows out of one seemingly simple question: after you have seized the animal in a cruelty case, what do you *do* with that animal?[2] Law enforcement and the legal system are no strangers to evidence seized during the investigation of criminal cases – there is no shortage of best-practice procedures and case law illustrating who owns such evidence, whether (and when) it shall be returned to its owner, in what condition the evidence should be kept, and so forth. Nor is there a lack of material discussing the position of victims within the criminal justice system. Animals seized pursuant to cruelty cases, however, occupy a position that does not neatly fit in either the traditional categories of victim or inanimate evidence. Statutory law, rescue organizations, law enforcement agencies, prosecutors, and animal legal advocates have all had to grapple with the unique position animals occupy, as they resolve postseizure animal issues.

---

1 In the interests of clarity, throughout this chapter I will use "victim of crime" to refer to someone who has been harmed by a criminal act in a fairly direct fashion, whether or not they qualify as a crime victim under a given jurisdiction's law. Conversely, I will use "crime victim" to refer to someone who meets a given jurisdiction's requirements to have legal status as a crime victim. In contexts where the distinction between the two is inconsequential, I will simply use "victim." So, for example, an animal who has been criminally neglected or abused is a victim of animal cruelty – but may nor may not be a crime victim, depending on the jurisdiction where the case is being heard, and what issues are being litigated. Cf. *State vs. Nix*, 355 Or. 777, (2014)*; People vs. Harris*, 405 P.3d 361, (2016).

2 Throughout this chapter I assume that the animals in question have been seized pursuant to a search warrant or other reasonable circumstances – that the seizure is, in other words, valid. For factors underlying validity of seizure, warrant drafting tips, or issues implicated by a warrantless seizure, please see Chapter 9.

Animal Cruelty Investigations: A Collaborative Approach from Victim to Verdict[TM], First Edition.
Edited by Kris Otteman, Linda Fielder, and Emily Lewis.
© 2022 John Wiley & Sons, Inc. Published 2022 by John Wiley & Sons, Inc.
Companion website: www.wiley.com/go/otteman/victimtoverdict

15.1   Seized Animals and Reasonable Minimum Care

Though animal cruelty victims are property, just as is traditional evidence, they cannot be dealt with in the same way. While the goal for seized property is typically to preserve the item taken as statically as possible, this is not an option in animal cases, for the simple reason that animals are not things. Unlike objects, animals – as living creatures – need sustenance, shelter, and care: a statically preserved animal is a dead animal. At a minimum, seized animals require maintenance care: the reasonable necessities for them remaining healthy. Moreover, given that animals seized pursuant to cruelty cases are often seized precisely because they have been neglected, abused, or otherwise subject to unlawful harm, those animals often additionally need ameliorative care, more than what they would need had they not been criminally harmed.

It is worth noting that declining to provide this sort of maintenance and ameliorative care is not an option available to the agency who has custody of seized animals. Failure to provide seized animals with reasonably necessary care conflicts with the statutory duty to refrain from conduct constituting animal neglect. Treating a seized animal like other forms of seized evidence – logging the animal into evidence storage and leaving them there until needed for litigation – would actually implicate the responsible agency in committing animal cruelty by failing to provide an animal in their custody with necessary food, water, shelter, and care. Similarly, for a custodial agency to forgo providing for the reasonable care of an animal who was seized because of their exposure to neglect, abuse, or other cruel conduct would result in an absurd outcome vis-à-vis cruelty law. One of the reasons modern animal cruelty laws exist is to protect animals from suffering[3] – seizing such an animal, only to then inflict further suffering upon them cannot be the appropriate outcome. Finally, the seized animal remains the property of their owner (often the defendant in the associated animal cruelty case) – despite being under the care of the custodial agency. Should the owner successfully retain ownership of the animal in question – whether through charges not being filed, a civil hearing prior to conclusion of trial, through a not guilty verdict, or otherwise – they are unlikely to be pleased to discover that their animal has degraded or died because the custodial agency declined to provide reasonably necessary care. Such a scenario, in turn, may well give rise to successive additional rounds of litigation.

Choosing to kill seized animals rather than providing them with reasonably necessary ameliorative and maintenance care poses many of the same issues as simply refusing to provide them with care. While appropriate euthanasia is not itself cruelty, the unnecessary killing of animals certainly frustrates the purpose both of animal cruelty law and those who work in the field of animal care and protection. A defendant-owner who ultimately retains ownership of a seized animal will no doubt expect to receive the animal in a live state – and being told that the animal was euthanized for reasons of convenience is unlikely to put the custodial agency in an enviable position. Moreover, depending on the specific cruelty code of the jurisdiction in question, there may be a statutory policy preference against convenience euthanasia.[4]

Nor are the costs of providing care to seized animals limited to the fiscal. Even in jurisdictions whose budgets could in theory absorb the needs of any number of seized animals,[5] the logistical resources implicated by animal care are by nature limited. Custodial agencies have only so much space within which to house animals; staff have only so much time to provide animals with care.

---

3 See Chiesa, L. (2008). Why is it a crime to stomp a goldfish? – Harm, victimhood, and the structure of anti-cruelty offenses. *Mississippi Law J.* 78: 1 (discussing the development of modern cruelty law and its aims).

4 See, e.g., Annotated California Codes, Penal Code, Pt 1, title 14, s 599d 1998 (CA). ("It is the policy of the state that no adoptable animal should be euthanized if it can be adopted into a suitable home. . . It is the policy of the state that no treatable animal should be euthanized.")

5 The author remains dubious that any such jurisdiction exists in practice.

This is particularly true when resources are strained by the seizure of large numbers of animals, animals with needs beyond those the custodial agency usually encounters, or both.

15.2 The Impact of Seizure Expenses – and Responsive Solutions

These unavoidable costs associated with providing seized animals with care have historically posed a hurdle to the justice system responding effectively to animal cruelty cases. On the law enforcement side, the prospect of unexpected costs can perversely incentivize animal cruelty to go underinvestigated. In the courtroom, attempts to recover costs expended on caring for seized animals can spawn further rounds of litigation, even after conclusion of the core criminal case. From a public-policy perspective, this also gives rise to an economic free-rider problem: defendant-owners can shift the expense of providing their animals with ameliorative and maintenance care to governments and charitable organizations, while still retaining ownership of the animal – who is being cared for at someone else's expense. This issue is particularly pointed in the case of maintenance care. As an animal's owner, the defendant has already implicitly agreed to be responsible for ensuring the animal is provided with care at a level that meets the statutory minimum set by cruelty law. When the costs of that minimum care are shifted to the custodial agency, the defendant-owner effectively avoids meeting the most basic obligations they took on when they decided to become an animal owner.[6]

In response to these challenges, lawmakers and practitioners have developed various legal strategies to provide seized animals with necessary care, ensure that the costs of that care are appropriately allocated in a timely fashion, and fairly resolve both ownership of the animal and where the animal ultimately ends up. While details vary across jurisdictions, these legal approaches generally fall into the following categories (Box 15.1):

Box 15.1 Legal Approaches		
	Stage of case	**Result**
Voluntary relinquishment	Any	Defendant-owner knowingly gives up property interest in the animal
Animal as contraband	After seizure	Upon showing that it is not possible for defendant-owner to lawfully possess animal, defendant-owner's property interest in animal is extinguished
Preconviction forfeiture	Prior to verdict	Civil hearing determines whether defendant-owner continues to have property interest in animal and/or requires defendant-owner to pay reasonable costs of care
Restitution	Sentencing	As part of sentence stemming from criminal conviction, defendant-owner reimburses for cost of animal's reasonably necessary care
Forfeiture via sentencing	Sentencing	Defendant-owner's property interest in animal is extinguished as a part of sentence stemming from criminal conviction
Cost-of-care lien	Varies (requires care to have been provided, and costs incurred)	Defendant-owner pays animal's cost of care or animal can be foreclosed upon

---

6 Owners who are unable to meet their minimum obligation to their animals – or who simply decide that they are no longer interested in the responsibilities that come with animal ownership – have the option of surrendering the animal, selling the animal, or otherwise giving the animal to someone who is willing to meet the minimum obligations of animal ownership.

Each of these strategies may be more or less effective in addressing the different issues implicated by animal seizure. For example, voluntary relinquishment – where the defendant-owner knowingly and freely surrenders the animal – resolves animal ownership with a high degree of finality (thus also enabling the custodial agency to determine the animal's disposition without impediment). Voluntary relinquishment, however, largely leaves unaddressed the cost of providing for the animal's care. Conversely, restitution often directly addresses costs of care, while remaining silent on ownership.

15.3   Voluntary Relinquishment

This is essentially the same as the familiar process by which members of the public surrender animals to animal control agencies, rescues, or shelters. The critical ingredients of such a surrender are that (i) the owner knows that they are giving up all ownership rights to the animal; and (ii) the owner is not being coerced into doing so by the custodial agency or law enforcement.[7] The surrender paperwork to be signed by the owner should note both of those factors. Upon relinquishment, the animal becomes property of the custodial agency,[8] who may then treat the animal as they would any other animal surrendered to them – e.g. placing the animal in a foster or permanent home.[9] Voluntary surrender resolves the question of ownership, but does not block progress on the cruelty charges the animal was seized pursuant to, and may not necessarily impede extracting cost-of-care restitution from the defendant (particularly for costs connected to treating injuries caused by the defendant). It is important to document each animal relinquished with specificity. In a scenario where a dozen ferrets have been seized, simply noting that the defendant-owner has decided to surrender two of them may, for example, lead to later litigation regarding which ferrets those are.

15.4   The Seized Animal as Contraband

When the government seizes contraband – property the defendant is simply not legally allowed to own – the government is generally under no obligation to give that contraband back, regardless of whether the defendant is found guilty or not guilty. This is, to take a non-animal example, why law enforcement does not return illegal drugs to defendants – regardless of how the defendant's criminal case turns out, it is not lawful for the defendant to have the drugs in question. For animals, then, the key question is: why can this animal not legally be owned by this defendant? The two most common answers are either:

---

7 *King vs. Montgomery Cty., Tennessee*, 797 F. App'x 949, 956, (2020) ("Property voluntarily surrendered . . . is not 'seized' within the meaning of the Fourth Amendment when recovered by law enforcement. . . Because the dogs at issue here were surrendered to MCAC . . . they were not unreasonably seized for Fourth Amendment purposes.") (citations omitted).

8 Assuming there are no other people who have a property interest in the animal. Voluntary relinquishment amounts to the person surrendering the animal giving up their claim – if there are others who have an ownership stake in the animal, their stakes will need to be addressed separately.

9 Note, while the surrendered animal becoming property of the custodial agency provides the agency with authority to decide on animal disposition, this decision should be made in consultation with law enforcement and prosecutors, as there may be additional factors at play (such as having access to the animal for evidentiary exam purposes).

1) The species of animal is one that the defendant cannot legally own; For example, in various jurisdictions it simply is not lawful for a private individual to own certain primates or great cats.[10] If one of those animals were seized from a defendant-owner in one of those jurisdictions, the animal would be contraband.

2) The way the defendant is using the animal makes owning them legally impossible. In certain jurisdictions, for example, it is not lawful to own chickens meant for cockfighting.[11] While this would not make all chickens contraband, it would mean that roosters seized pursuant to a cockfighting operation are contraband.

Scenarios where there simply is no basis for lawful ownership or possession of an animal – such as the great cat example given above – are instances where the animal constitutes contraband per se – i.e. property that it is simply not lawful to possess. Establishing the animal's contraband status in a contraband per se case is (relatively) straightforward. For example, in Washington State it is unlawful to possess a nonhuman primate unless the possessor falls into a specific exemption category [1]. Therefore, if an orangutan is seized in Washington, showing that the animal is contraband per se is simply a matter of establishing that orangutans are primates, and that the defendant is not someone (such as an accredited zoo) [2] explicitly allowed to possess primates. There are other, less frequently invoked circumstances where the animal in question constitutes derivative contraband – which is to say, property that only becomes unlawful to own as result of the property being sufficiently involved in perpetrating criminal conduct.[12] Because animals are property, when an animal is involved in the crime of animal cruelty – as the animal is if they themselves are the victim of that cruelty – a potential arises that the animal may be classifiable as derivative contraband.[13]

Under any contraband theory, resolving ownership of an animal requires a legal finding that the animal in question is indeed contraband – at which point the defendant's ownership interest in the animal is extinguished. Much like voluntary relinquishment, terminating the defendant's ownership of an animal under a contraband argument does not interfere with any associated cruelty case, nor does it necessarily block cost-of-care recovery.

---

10 Primates: e.g. Alaska Administrative Code, title 5, Pt 3, chapter 92, article 3, ss 92.029(a)–(b) 1985 (AK); California Fish and Game Code, article 7, chapter 2, s 2118(b) 2004 (CA); Colorado Revised Statutes Annotated, title 35, article 80, s 35-80-108(j) (II) (A) 2014 (CO); Connecticut General Statutes Annotated, title 26, chapter 490, Pt III, ss 26-40a(a)–(b) 2013 (CT); Annotated Code of Maryland, title 10, subtitle 6, s 10-621(b) (1) (vii) 2014 (MD); Massachusetts General Laws Annotated, Pt I, title XIX, chapter 131A, s 2 (2010). Great cats: e.g. Haw. Code R. s 4-71-6 (LexisNexis 2019); Louisiana Administrative Code, title 76, Pt V, chapter 1, s 115(C) (1) 2006 (LA); Oregon Revised Statutes Annotated, title 48, chapter 609, ss 609.305(2), 609.319 2010 (OR); Revised Code of Washington Annotated, title 16, chapter 16.30, ss 16.30.010, 16.30.030 2007 (WA).

11 See Annotated California Codes, Penal Code, Pt 1, title 14, s 597j 2006 (CA), making it illegal for a person to, inter alia, own or possess birds intended to be used in fighting.

12 *Allen vs. Pennsylvania Soc. for Prevention of Cruelty to Animals*, 488 F. Supp. 2d 450, 457, (2007). quoting a nonprecedential Pennsylvania Superior Court ruling concerning a Rule 588 decision regarding horses seized pursuant to allegations of neglect: "we conclude that the animals seized did, in fact, constitute derivative contraband, in that they were the subject of an unlawful act under 18 Pa.C.S.A. § 5511(c)."

13 See, e.g. *Commonwealth vs. Kuhns*, WL 5869451, (2016). "While the trial court noted that there was no proof about how the puppy was injured, preventing Appellant's conviction for maiming or torturing or disfiguring the animal . . . [there] was sufficient proof to support the trial court's conclusion that Appellant wantonly failed to seek immediate, and necessary, veterinary care for the pit bull [constituting unlawful neglect under state law]. . . Consequently, there was a sufficient nexus between the dog and Appellant's transgression so as to render the dog derivative contraband." See also Brief of Amicus Curiae Animal Legal Defense Fund in Opposition to Appellant's Motion for Return of Property, *Commonwealth vs. Kuhns*, WL 5869451, (2016) setting forth in greater detail application of derivative contraband theory to an animal subject to unlawful cruelty.

15.5   Preconviction Forfeiture

Present in 43 states and Washington DC [3], animal preconviction forfeiture statutes are designed to address the cost and ownership issues implicated by animal seizure.[14] During preconviction forfeiture proceedings, the court will determine whether the case meets a statutorily defined threshold (e.g. "the animal was subject to unlawful cruelty," "the animal was seized pursuant to a cruelty case," etc.) – if the court finds that threshold is met, the result will address payment of care costs, ownership, or – most frequently – both. While each jurisdiction's individual animal preconviction forfeiture statute is unique, three key attributes are shared by preconviction forfeiture statutes in general:

1) *Preconviction forfeiture proceedings are distinct from criminal prosecution.* While connected to the criminal case giving rise to the animal's seizure, preconviction forfeiture is a civil process – and in nearly every instance relies upon a civil standard of proof (e.g. "more likely than not," "preponderance of the evidence," etc.) rather than a criminal standard (i.e. "beyond a reasonable doubt"). Similarly, the constitutional right to a jury trial in criminal cases does not apply to preconviction forfeiture hearings, because preconviction forfeiture is not a criminal matter. Likewise, because preconviction forfeiture and the criminal case are not separate proceedings, but sound in two different areas of law (one of which is not criminal) no double jeopardy issue is implicated.[15] This also means that the outcome of the parallel criminal case generally has no bearing on preconviction forfeiture. An animal properly forfeited through this process remains forfeited, regardless of whether the defendant is found guilty, found not guilty, has the criminal case overturned on appeal, etc.

2) *Preconviction forfeiture due process is met via notice and opportunity to be heard.* As a matter of due process, defendants should be provided with notice of the preconviction forfeiture hearing, and an opportunity to be heard at the hearing. Depending on the details of the specific statute at play, providing the defendant-owner with written information about the preconviction forfeiture process during the search and seizure process can be helpful in meeting this due process requirement.[16]

3) *"Preconviction forfeiture" is not synonymous with "civil asset forfeiture."* While the fact that in both scenarios the defendant forfeits property may cause animal preconviction forfeiture proceedings to look akin to civil asset forfeiture schemes from a distance, the two are critically different in both their purpose and structure. Civil asset forfeiture laws set their sights on a wide variety of conduct, property, and purposes – aiming to address issues as disparate as nuisance abatement, victim compensation, unjust enrichment, deterrence of criminality, and

---

14 The phrase "preconviction forfeiture statute" does not imply any predicted outcome for the defendant's criminal trial. Rather, the language refers to the reality that these laws can be invoked at any stage of a case between the point of seizure and a verdict (or plea). As such, other descriptive phrases would be inaccurate: "postseizure forfeiture" fails to acknowledge that these proceedings must generally take place before the criminal case, and "pretrial forfeiture" obfuscates the fact that these proceedings can run concurrent with the trial itself.

15 See, e.g. *State vs. Tarnavsky*, 84 Wash. App. 1056, (1996). "The imposition of a remedial civil sanction is not punishment for purposes of double jeopardy. The Legislature's use of preponderance of the evidence as the applicable burden of proof indicates its intent that the forfeiture of abused animals is a civil action. The provision for forfeiture, based on death of any of the animals, prior conviction of the person convicted of animal cruelty, or upon finding cruel treatment is likely to reoccur, demonstrates the remedial purpose of the forfeiture, namely, to protect the animals. The forfeiture provisions of the animal cruelty statutes do not violate double jeopardy."

16 This sort of approach is particularly appropriate where the jurisdiction's forfeiture process puts the onus of requesting a hearing upon the owner-defendant.

contraband. As a result, the range of property vulnerable to civil asset forfeiture is significant in scope. Civil asset forfeiture laws also frequently are designed in a manner that allows the state to profit from forfeited property (whether through sale or by simply retaining the property for state use). This has given rise to civil liberty arguments that civil asset forfeiture schemes overreach or may improperly incentivize seizure. In contrast, animal preconviction forfeiture statutes focus narrowly on animal cruelty victims – specifically their reasonable costs of care, and ultimate disposition. In doing so, animal preconviction forfeiture does not implicate other property owned by the defendant. Similarly, in the event that a given jurisdiction's preconviction forfeiture statute provides a mechanism by which defendants can be asked to pay reasonable costs of care, the custodial agency is typically not able to retain funds beyond those actually spent on the animal's reasonable care. The concerns invoked by traditional civil asset forfeiture are, therefore, inapplicable to animal preconviction forfeiture: the statutory scope is narrow, and there is no profit to be realized through the animal preconviction forfeiture process.

15.6 Preconviction Forfeiture: Bond-or-Forfeit Statutes

The majority of jurisdictions have adopted a specific type of preconviction forfeiture as a best-practice model: a bond-or-forfeit statute.[17] Bond-or-forfeit statutes require the owner of a seized animal to post a bond covering the animal's reasonable costs of care. If the owner fails to do so, the animal is forfeited. The logic behind this legal mechanism is straightforward. Had the animal not been seized, the owner would have been legally obliged to provide that animal with certain basic necessities. Meeting this legal responsibility naturally entails commensurate expenses that the owner would bear. A bond-or-forfeit statute simply creates a mechanism whereby the animal owner provides the agency that is actually spending money to give the seized animal reasonable care with the funds the owner should be spending to ensure the animal has necessary food, water, shelter, medical care, and so forth. In the alternative, the defendant-owner may choose to forfeit the animals by declining to post bond – just as the owners of unseized animals may divest themselves of the responsibilities that come with animal ownership by (appropriately) transferring the animal to someone else. In this fashion, bond-or-forfeit statutes neatly address the real-world challenges posed by animal seizure: resolving ownership and costs of care, with less need for future litigation.

These statutes generally lay out who may petition the court for a bond-or-forfeiture hearing, what the time window between petition and hearing is, and – if a bond is required – how much time the owner has to post the bond before the animals are forfeited. Bond-or-forfeiture statutes also typically include a mechanism – either explicitly or implicitly – where the defendant-owner is required to repost bond when the original bond amount runs out (or forfeit the animal, should they decline to repost bond).

---

17 Bond-or-forfeit statutes can be found in Alaska, Arizona, Arkansas, Colorado, Connecticut, Delaware, Hawaii, Idaho, Illinois, Indiana, Iowa, Kansas, Louisiana, Maine, Massachusetts, Michigan, Minnesota, Mississippi, Missouri, Montana, Nebraska, New Hampshire (for appeals), New Mexico, New York, North Carolina, Ohio, Oklahoma, Oregon, Pennsylvania, Rhode Island, Tennessee, Texas (for appeals), Virginia, Washington, West Virginia, Wisconsin, and Wyoming (for cases involving livestock).

15.7   Bond-or-Forfeit Statute Examples

Several states have built on this basic bond-or-forfeit core by adding components that explicitly speak to the condition of the animals involved. Oregon's s 167.347 and Washington's RCW 16.52.085 are illustrative (Figures 15.1 and 15.2):

Oregon's statute is triggered when an animal is properly seized pending outcome of a criminal animal cruelty case. Under such circumstances, the prosecutor or custodial agency may file a bond-or-forfeit petition with the court, giving appropriate notice to the defendant. The court will hold a hearing within 14 days, at which the defendant has an opportunity to be heard. If, at the conclusion of the hearing, the court does not find probable cause that the animal in question was subject to unlawful cruelty, then the animal is returned to the defendant. If, on the other hand, the court does find probable cause that the animal was subject to unlawful cruelty, then the court will order the defendant to post a bond covering reasonable costs of care within 72 hours. If the defendant fails to post the bond, then the animal is forfeited. If the defendant does post bond, the court will require the defendant to renew the bond amount, as necessary to provide for the animal's reasonable anticipated care costs [4].

Like Oregon, Washington's bond-or-forfeit statue requires that the animal in question has been properly seized pursuant to a violation of the state's animal cruelty law, which also triggers the defendant-owner being provided with written notice outlining the bond-or-forfeit process. Washington, however, places the onus on the defendant-owner to request a hearing – if the defendant-owner does not request a hearing or post a bond covering at least one month's worth of care within 15 business days from the date of seizure, then the animal is effectively forfeited to the custodial agency.[18] If the defendant-owner posts this cost-of-care bond, then the animal continues in the possession of the custodial agency, while remaining the defendant's property.[19] If, instead, the defendant-owner requests a hearing, then they have the burden of showing by a

E.g. Oregon § 167.347 | Cruelty Showing + Bond-or-Forfeit

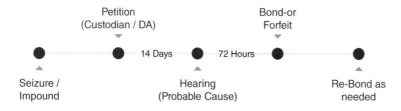

Figure 15.1   A simplified depiction of the bond-or-forfeit process in Oregon.

---

18 See Revised Code of Washington Annotated, title 16, chapter 16.52, 16.52.085 (4) 2020 (WA). "The agency having custody of the animal may euthanize the animal or may find a responsible person to adopt the animal not less than fifteen business days after the animal is taken into custody. A custodial agency may euthanize severely injured, diseased, or suffering animals at any time. An owner may prevent the animal's destruction or adoption by [initiating the bond-or-forfeit process] * * *."

19 Note, should the cost-of-care bond run out, the court may either order the bond extended or the animal is forfeited to the custodial agency. Revised Code of Washington Annotated, title 16, chapter 16.52, 16.52.085 (4) 2020 (WA).

Washington RCW 16.52.085 | Bond or Forfeit / Safety Showing

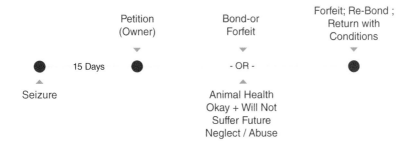

Figure 15.2 A simplified depiction of the bond-or-forfeit process in Washington.

preponderance of the evidence that the animal is currently healthy and will not suffer future cruelty if returned to the defendant.[20]

15.8 Bond-or-Forfeit Statutes Are Constitutionally Compliant

While there is relatively little case law litigating the particulars of animal preconviction forfeiture procedures at an appellate level, such cases tend to involve bond-or-forfeit statutes (hardly surprising, given that most preconviction forfeiture laws take the form of bond-or-forfeit statutes). In these cases, courts have consistently upheld bond-or-forfeit statutes as a legitimate, nonpunitive[21] way to solve the "obvious practical problem[s] that arise when animals are impounded" [5]. Constitutional arguments typically raised against bond-or-forfeiture statutes are answerable by underscoring the civil nature and remedial purpose of the bond-or-forfeiture process:[22]

In a bond-or-forfeiture hearing, does the defendant enjoy the criminal rights to trial by jury or proof beyond a reasonable doubt? No.

———

20 Revised Code of Washington Annotated, title 16, chapter 16.52, 16.52.085 (6) 2020 (WA). Specifically, "[T]he burden is on the owner to prove by a preponderance of the evidence that the animal will not suffer future neglect or abuse and is not in need of being restored to health." Given that Washington does not define specific crimes of "neglect" or "abuse," this is best read as encompassing the scope of conduct prohibited by Washington title 16, chapter 52, e.g. animal cruelty, animal fighting, animal sexual assault, etc

21 See, e.g. *People vs. Koy*, 13 N.E.3d 1267, 1267, (2014). "Koy has not demonstrated why the forfeiture of the horses under section 3.04(a) was a punishment that resulted from a criminal proceeding. Because the forfeiture proceeding was civil, the sixth amendment was not implicated * * *." See also *State vs. Tarnavsky*, 84 Wash. App. 1056, (1996). "[T]he overriding purpose of the statute is remedial protection of the animals. A fine cannot be excessive for Eighth Amendment purposes if it serves a purely remedial purpose. A forfeiture which serves primarily to protect abused animals from further abuse by a person convicted of having abused them is likewise not excessive."

22 To the extent that these arguments may be raised against preconviction forfeiture laws more broadly, many of the answers here remain applicable.

A bond-or-forfeiture hearing, like preconviction forfeiture proceedings more generally, is a fundamentally civil matter – no criminal rights are implicated:[23] ". . . although a [bond-or-forfeit proceeding] takes place in the criminal action, it does not arise from that action, is entirely separate from it, and, necessarily, is not governed by the rules that apply to criminal prosecutions" [6].

Does the requirement that the defendant either post a cost-of-care bond or forfeit the animal amount to an excessive fine, forbidden by the Eighth Amendment? Does this analysis change if the defendant is acquitted of criminal animal cruelty charges? No, and no.

Fines are a form of punishment. In contrast, the purpose of bond-or-forfeit statutes is ". . . not to punish . . . but, rather . . . to ensure the well-being and continued recovery of the injured animals" [7]. That the defendant might not *enjoy* the choice between paying for their animal's care or forfeiting the animal does not transmute the proceeding from remedial to punitive – the legal system asks people to do any number of things they may not be thrilled about, without that rising to the level of a criminal sanction.[24] By the same token, if the defendant is acquitted of animal cruelty charges at criminal trial, the bond-or-forfeiture process remains unscathed: "It is irrelevant to forfeiture under [Oregon's bond-or-forfeit statute] whether the owner is innocent or guilty of the criminal charge, because the purpose of the forfeiture is to pay for the care of the animals, not to punish the owner" [6].

15.9 Restitution

If a defendant is found guilty of animal cruelty (whether through trial or plea), the available sentencing options may include requiring the defendant to pay restitution covering the reasonable cost of treating injuries the defendant caused. While fines and restitution are superficially similar (both, after all, involve the defendant being sentenced to pay someone money), they bear critical distinctions. Fines go to the government, and typically the amount of the fine keys off the severity of the charge – e.g. misdemeanor or felony. Restitution, in contrast, goes to victims (or those who have spent money on victim care), and the amount of restitution is connected to what it costs to reasonably address the injury caused by the defendant. In the case of seized animals, costs expended to provide those animals with reasonably necessary care can often be framed in terms of restitution. Note, that because restitution is a part of the defendant's criminal sentence, if the case is later overturned on appeal, the restitution – like the rest of the criminal sentence – will be imperiled.

---

23 See, e.g. *State vs. Tarnavsky*, 84 Wash. App. 1056, (1996). "[W]e hold that a hearing on the forfeiture of companion animals before trial, pursuant to section 3.04(a) of the Act, is not a criminal proceeding and therefore does not implicate the sixth amendment right to a jury trial."

24 See *People vs. Koy*, 13 N.E.3d 1267, (2014). "Every sanction, civil or otherwise, produces some punitive effect."

15.10   Forfeiture via Sentencing

A defendant found guilty of animal cruelty (whether through trial or plea) may be required to forfeit specific animals as part of their sentence. Some jurisdictions have made forfeiture mandatory upon conviction [3]; in others, forfeiture may be permissive or unaddressed in statute [3]. Note that a sentence involving forfeiture is not the same as a sentence involving a possession ban. The former sentence results in the defendant's ownership interest in a particular animal (or animals) being extinguished. The latter is a sentence that forbids the defendant from possessing animals (whether specific animals, certain types of animals, or all animals) but may provide the defendant with some latitude in terms of determining where animals they possessed at the time of sentence go. Like restitution, because forfeiture via sentence is part of a criminal sentence following a guilty verdict, if the case is later overturned, so too is the forfeiture order [8]. Forfeiture via sentence resolves who owns the animal but does not address costs of care.

15.11   Cost-of-Care Liens

Closely related to a standard veterinary or boarding lien,[25] cost-of-care liens set out a process allowing the custodial agency to foreclose on a seized animal they have been providing care to. This involves the agency providing the defendant with notice that if they fail to pay for care costs by a certain date the animal will be eligible to be foreclosed upon. Should the defendant not have paid care costs by that date, the agency may begin legal foreclosure proceedings – the result of which is typically either ownership of the animal being transferred to the custodial agency, or the animal being sold at public auction, with proceeds going to the custodial agency.[26] The process of foreclosing on a cost-of-care lien is civil and operates separately from the resolution of the defendant's criminal case. See Appendices B and C for checklists and templates for animal lien foreclosure.

15.12   Conclusion

The question we began this chapter with was "after you have seized the animal in a cruelty case, what do you *do* with that animal?" In any given case, the answer may slot neatly into one of the options discussed here, or the best approach may be to pursue several of those options at once, or to consider a solution that combines elements of these approaches. Regardless, the fundamental goal remains the same: ensuring that seized animals receive necessary care and treatment, that costs for that care and treatment are fairly borne, and that there is clarity regarding the animal's ownership. Keeping these fundamentals in mind will help ensure an animal-forward approach to resolving these issues – both improving outcomes for the animal victims in current cases, and also reducing barriers for future case response.

_____

25 Indeed, in some scenarios a standard veterinary or animal boarding lien may serve the same function as a more specific lien focused on animals seized in the course of a criminal case.

26 Should the animal be auctioned for an amount greater than care costs, the left-over money is returned to the defendant.

References

1 Revised Code of Washington Annotated, title 16, chapter 16.30, ss 16.30.010, 16.30.020, 16.30.030 2007 (WA).

2 Revised Code of Washington Annotated, title 16, chapter 16.30, s 16.30.020 2007 (WA).

3 Animal Legal Defense Fund. (2020). 2020 U.S. state animal protection laws rankings. https://aldf.org/project/us-state-rankings. (accessed 30 May 2021).

4 Oregon Revised Statutes Annotated, title 16, chapter 167, s 167.347 2018 (OR).

5 *State vs. Branstetter*, 181 Or. App. 57, 63, (2002).

6 *State vs. Branstetter*, 181 Or. App. 57, 64, (2002).

7 *People vs. Koy*, 13 N.E.3d 1267, (2014).

8 City of Lebanon vs. Milburn, 398 P.3d 486, (2017).

16

Trial

Jake Kamins

If you investigate animal cruelty, there is a decent chance that you will have to testify in a trial. You have probably seen *Law & Order*, *Ally McBeal*, *Perry Mason*, or similar shows. Imagining a trial may conjure images of impeccably dressed attorneys calling surprise witnesses and vigorously cross-examining them, cracking their case wide open in front of an impressed jury (also, for some reason the judge always says, "I'll allow it . . . but watch yourself, Counselor" after objections).

Trials are not really like that (for one thing, our suits are not that well-tailored). Trials are a formal legal process with complex rules, traditions, and nuance. By design, drama in trials is minimized. Everything must be prepared and presented properly, or everybody's time and effort could end up wasted.

Here is a jury instruction given in every criminal trial in Oregon: "Generally, the testimony of any witness whom you believe is sufficient to prove any fact in dispute." If you are a witness, *your testimony* may prove to be the key piece in proving the prosecution's case.

When you find yourself involved in a trial, it is critical to take the process seriously and prepare in advance for your part.

This chapter is designed for nonattorneys involved in animal cruelty investigations, to give an idea of how the legal system brings cases to – and through – trial. There are also some tips for prosecutors in animal cruelty cases at the end of the chapter.

16.1 Trials: An Overview

A trial in the criminal justice system is the process by which a prosecutor attempts to prove beyond a reasonable doubt that a defendant committed a crime and to hold them accountable, while at the same time, a defense attorney fights for their client's rights and freedom.

The long road to trial starts when an investigator presents reports and evidence to a prosecutor, who must then determine whether and how to bring charges. If criminal charges are brought, the defendant is informed of the charges, and they get a defense attorney.

Next, the prosecutor and defense attorney attempt to negotiate a plea bargain. If negotiation fails, trial is the only remaining option for holding a criminal defendant accountable.

Animal Cruelty Investigations: A Collaborative Approach from Victim to Verdict™, First Edition.
Edited by Kris Otteman, Linda Fielder, and Emily Lewis.
© 2022 John Wiley & Sons, Inc. Published 2022 by John Wiley & Sons, Inc.
Companion website: www.wiley.com/go/otteman/victimtoverdict

The trial itself is preceded by pretrial matters, where questions of evidence, law, and court procedure are decided by a judge. A jury will then be selected to decide the facts of the case, unless the defendant requests the judge decide the facts rather than a jury.

The actual trial begins with the prosecutor and the defense attorney making opening statements that outline what they believe the evidence will show. The prosecutor then presents witnesses and other evidence. Since the prosecution must prove the case, they put on their case first (their "case-in-chief").

Next, the defendant has an opportunity to present their case. After the defendant's case, the prosecution typically will be allowed to put on a "rebuttal case," responding to evidence from the defendant's case.

Once both sides are done presenting their cases and making legal motions, both attorneys make closing arguments, asking the fact finder to rule in their favor. If there is a jury, the judge gives them instructions about the rules governing their deliberations and verdict. If the defendant is found guilty, the defendant is sentenced. Posttrial, a convicted defendant may file an appeal.

This is a simplified outline. Many other things can happen during a criminal trial, including motions, rulings, appeals, and other delays. The entire process can take hours, days, weeks, or even months. If you include the investigation, negotiations period, and the posttrial appeals process, a case can easily take years to resolve. If you are involved in this process, even tangentially, it is important to understand how it works, so that you can be best prepared to assist in any way you can.

16.2   The Players

A trial has many participants, each with a specific role to play. Most of these participants will have significant trial experience. If you are involved in a trial, it is vital to familiarize yourself with how these roles interact, so you know what is going on and understand the basic "chain of command" in a courtroom.

16.2.1   The Prosecutor

> The great joy of being a prosecutor is that you don't take whatever case walks in the door. You evaluate the case; you make your best judgment. You only go forward if you believe that the defendant is guilty.
>
> *Merrick Garland, at his confirmation hearing to the*
> *US Court of Appeals for the District of Columbia*

A prosecutor is the attorney who represents the government in a criminal trial. Trial prosecutors are typically deputies or assistants of an elected or appointed official: A county District Attorney, a United States Attorney, the state Attorney General, etc. The jurisdiction a prosecutor represents is used as shorthand for the prosecutor's "side" in a trial: "The State alleges," or "The Commonwealth will prove. . ."

Although the details of trials vary from jurisdiction to jurisdiction, there will always be a government represented on the prosecution side.

Prosecutors are familiar with criminal law and local court procedures. They can be invaluable resources for people who are not typically involved in the court system. When seeking advice from a prosecutor, do not take it personally if they are brusque. They are typically busy, with many other cases on their docket, and they are not allowed to give legal advice to people and agencies they do not represent.

Unfortunately, there are a few things that make most prosecutors imperfect fits for animal cruelty cases. First, with few exceptions, prosecutors handle a variety of criminal cases. The same prosecutor who had a domestic violence trial last week may be prosecuting your animal cruelty case today. Since animal cruelty is such a difficult crime to spot, investigate, and prosecute, most prosecutors will have significantly less experience with these offenses than with, for example, drunk driving cases.

To make things worse, prosecutors are often seen by court systems as fungible. If one prosecutor is not available on the day of trial, that will not be seen by judges as a reason to set the trial over to a new date. Therefore, you may end up in trial with a prosecutor who is less familiar with your case's facts than you would like (as an attorney who has been handed a case file and given 10 minutes to prepare for jury selection: they are not thrilled about it either!).

Take these challenges as opportunities. Offer your assistance to prosecutors in understanding animal cruelty generally and the facts of your case specifically. The average prosecutor does not know what body condition score is, how to read an animal's blood panel, or the tell-tale signs of an animal fighting ring. Reach out to their offices and offer to train them or answer any questions they have about your investigation.

16.2.2 The Judge

> Judges and Justices are servants of the law, not the other way around. Judges are like umpires. Umpires don't make the rules, they apply them. The role of an umpire and a judge is critical. They make sure everybody plays by the rules, but it is a limited role. Nobody ever went to a ball game to see the umpire.
>
> *John G. Roberts, Jr., at his confirmation hearing*
> *for Chief Justice of the United States*

In criminal trials, judges are gatekeepers of evidence, deciding what the jury is allowed to see and hear. This work is done both pretrial, through deciding on motions, and in the middle of trial, through ruling on objections raised by the attorneys. Judges also instruct the jury on how they are to consider evidence and reach their verdict. In many jurisdictions, sentencing is left to the judge's discretion.

Like prosecutors and defense attorneys, it is likely that you will have a judge that is less educated on animal cruelty than other areas of law. Do not be surprised or frustrated by incorrect references (calling neglect charges "animal abuse" is many judges' favorite thing to do) or lack of knowledge of the statutes and case law. Be patient and establish yourself through your presentation as the subject matter expert in the room.

The most important thing to know is that the judge is in control of the courtroom. When they talk, listen. When they instruct, obey. Be unfailingly polite and deferential. Even though they may not be the ultimate decider in the case, judges have power to influence the way a case goes. Nothing will make your case go sideways faster than a judge deciding that a prosecution witness is not heeding them.

16.2.3 The Fact Finder

> Twelve people go off into a room. Twelve different minds, twelve different hearts and twelve different walks of life. Twelve sets of eyes, ears, shapes and sizes and these twelve people are asked to judge another human being as different from them as they are from each other and in their judgment, they must become of one mind. Unanimous. That's one of the miracles of man's disorganized soul that they can do it and most instances, do it right well. God bless juries.
>
> *Anatomy of a Murder*

Deciding what happened ("fact finding") is usually the province of the jury, a group of individuals from the community chosen to hear the facts of the case and decide whether the prosecution has met its burden (a defendant may waive the right to have a jury, in which case the judge will serve as the fact finder). When dealing with animal cruelty in front of a jury, it is critical to understand how animal cruelty is seen and felt in the community.

Potential jurors from more rural areas may see their relationship to animals differently than those in more urban areas. I have prosecuted animal cruelty cases in both rural and urban communities, and have found that no matter where they live, jurors tend to be firmly on the side of justice against animal cruelty. However, that dedication manifests differently in communities that rely on agriculture for their livelihood versus communities that mostly see animals as cute and furry life companions.

One dismaying trend is people trying to "get out of" jury duty. Serving on juries is a rare duty and a privilege, one that can give a person insight into how their fellow community members evaluate information and come to a decision. If you are in a position where you may end up testifying in trial, I can think of few better prep opportunities than sitting as a juror yourself.

16.2.4 The Defendant

No person . . . shall be compelled in any criminal case to be a witness against himself, nor be deprived of life, liberty, or property, without due process of law.

Amendment V, The US Bill of Rights

The defendant in a criminal trial is the person accused by the prosecution of having committed a crime. During the trial, a defendant has a relatively limited role. They sit with their attorney and may or may not testify on their own behalf. If they are convicted, a defendant will have a right to make a statement to the court prior to sentencing (Box 16.1).

16.2.5 The Defense Attorney

Uh ... Everything that guy just said is bullshit. Thank you.

Vinny Gambini's entire opening statement in State of Alabama vs.
Gambini and Rothenstein, My Cousin Vinny

A defense attorney represents a defendant in trial (defendants have a constitutional right to defend themselves, but they must be aware of – and acknowledge – the significant risks that come along with self-representation). If a defendant cannot afford an attorney, the court will appoint an attorney to defend them.

It is a defense attorney's job to get the best outcome possible for their client. They can do this by casting doubt on the prosecution's case; either through vigorous cross-examination of prosecution witnesses (including you), or by presenting defense witnesses and evidence. Remember though, that since the burden of proof is entirely on the prosecution, the fact finder cannot hold silence on the part of the defense attorney against the defendant.

Defense attorneys can seem cold or indifferent to the suffering of animal victims of neglect and abuse. They may come off as hostile to you and the important work you do investigating these crimes. Keep in mind that defense attorneys are doing their job, a vital piece of the criminal justice puzzle that keeps everybody (not just individual defendants) safe from potential government

---

Box 16.1 Sidebar

Defendants' Rights

The criminal justice system puts defendants in a difficult position. They have been publicly accused by the government of committing a crime. The accusation itself is often enough for the average social media consumer to declare them guilty (this is particularly true in animal cruelty cases, where reactions in the "comments" typically range from calls for inhumane punishments to calls for summary execution). Even stalwart friends and family members may turn their backs on an accused person.

Defendants did not choose to be investigated, arrested, and prosecuted. They are often caught off-guard by the process, which can involve the seizure of their money and property. They may even be jailed pending trial. All of this hampers a defendant's ability to defend themselves and puts them at a significant disadvantage right away.

Regardless of how the case ultimately turns out, defendants face punishments ranging from fines to probation requirements, loss of money or property, and incarceration. Those punishments dangling over a person's head can take a toll. If they choose to fight the charges, trials take time, energy, and often significant amounts of money to defend. And, most important of all, a defendant may have a legitimate defense or be innocent of the crime altogether.

Given these disadvantages built into the process, many of the laws and rules governing criminal trials are designed to help defendants fight back. These are just a few of the rights that defendants have in a criminal trial:

- Defendants are innocent until proven guilty. This is not just a slogan but a bedrock principle of our criminal justice system. The fact that the government has brought charges is not evidence of guilt. The prosecution must prove that the defendant committed the charged crime, in the way the prosecutor said they did it, beyond a reasonable doubt.
- Defendants have the right to be represented by an attorney, regardless of their ability to afford one. Their attorney may cross-examine prosecution witnesses and may call their own witnesses to testify.
- Defendants have an absolute right to testify or not testify on their own behalf. If they choose not to testify, they can have the jury instructed that they are not to hold their decision not to testify against them in reaching their verdict.

If these rights are violated, (or the prosecution fails to prove their case beyond a reasonable doubt) the prosecution may lose. It can be extremely frustrating when pretrial rulings do not go your way, or a defendant "gets off on a technicality," or a case ends in acquittal. However, these outcomes can be learning experiences, and are a vital part of protecting a fair system for everybody.

---

overreach. In many cases, defense attorneys do not choose their clients, and a personal distaste for something like animal cruelty does not mean that an ethical defense attorney will give their client anything less than a zealous defense.

Also remember: when prosecution witnesses are openly hostile or dismissive of defense attorneys, that helps them win. That kind of behavior will make the judge and jury think that you have an agenda. Kill them with kindness, and the jury will see that you are not "out to get" anybody.

16.2.6   The Witnesses

> And now, my star witness – Shep, the Wonder Dog[1] – will spell out the clue that will convict this defendant!
>
> *Mr. District Attorney, Issue 53 of the Mr. District Attorney comic book*

A witness is a person who – through processes called examination and cross-examination – tells the fact finder what they know about the case. In animal cruelty cases, the prosecution is always at a disadvantage in that their star witness – the animal victim – cannot testify.

Most witnesses in a criminal trial testify based only on their personal observations of the facts of the case. These are "fact witnesses." Fact witnesses are typically prohibited from testifying about information they got from somebody else (hearsay), their own personal opinions, and speculation. In animal cruelty cases, examples of fact witnesses include neighbors, friends, family members, and investigators. They may not be allowed to testify to an ultimate legal conclusion ("This dog was neglected"), but they can share what they saw/heard/smelled, letting the fact finder put those pieces together.

There are also "expert witnesses." These are witnesses who can demonstrate to the court that they have sufficient expertise in a particular field. This allows them to testify to their opinions, answer hypothetical questions, and speculate about information they did not themselves observe. A witness can be both a "fact witness" *and* an "expert witness," such as a veterinarian who personally treated an animal in a neglect case.

(See more about witnesses in Sections 16.5.2 and 16.6.3.)

16.2.7   The Burden of Proof

> Reasonable doubt is doubt based on common sense and reason. Reasonable doubt means an honest uncertainty as to the guilt of the defendant.
>
> *Oregon Uniform Criminal Jury Instruction 1001, "Introduction"*

The burden of proof is a concept, not a person. Nevertheless, it plays a huge part in every criminal trial. It tells the fact finder how sure they must be to find the defendant guilty. In the US legal system, there are two main burdens of proof. In a civil trial (when somebody is suing somebody else) or in a trial about a traffic or other noncriminal violation, the burden of proof is typically "a preponderance of the evidence." In these cases, a fact is proved if one side shows that – more likely than not – it happened.

In a criminal trial, the burden of proof is "beyond a reasonable doubt." This is the highest burden of proof in the American court system. The fact finder can only vote guilty if they are left with no reasonable doubt that the defendant did what the prosecutor said he did. If they have any reasonable doubts, the fact finder must vote not guilty.

This burden is entirely on the prosecution. So how do we meet it? Through conducting confident and competent investigations and presenting testimony and other evidence reflecting the strength of those investigations and the facts they uncovered.

16.3   How a Typical Criminal Case Gets to Trial

Here is a simplified outline of the steps that precede trial (Box 16.2).

---

1 Shep, the Wonder Dog was not actually a witness (except on the cover). He was the star of a children's television show, à la Lassie. Mr. District Attorney used Shep's stand-in, Sandy, to catch a group of bank robbers after they had shot Shep, mistakenly believing that he could read their license plate and communicate it to the police.

Box 16.2   Case Flow Chart

How a Typical Criminal Case Gets to Trial

1) *Complaint.*

   A *complainant* contacts a law enforcement or animal services agency with a report of animal neglect or abuse. The details of the report are forwarded to the appropriate agency, which begins an investigation.

2) *Investigation.*

   An *investigator* with the agency reviews the complaint and gathers additional evidence, which may include speaking to the complainant/other witnesses, requesting/reviewing documents and other evidence, and interviewing suspects. The investigator then writes reports about all the information they have collected. If they have established probable cause to believe a crime has been committed, they may arrest or cite suspects. The reports are then sent to the prosecutor.

3) *Review by prosecutor.*

   A *prosecutor* (see Section 16.2.1) reviews the reports to determine what, if any, criminal charges are appropriate.

4)

   a) *Declined for prosecution.*

      There is either a legal, factual, or policy-based reason why the case will not be prosecuted. Typically, prosecutors will write a memo explaining this decision to the investigator.

   b) *Returned for further investigation.*

      Additional information is needed (evidence, witness statements, etc.) before going forward. The case will be returned to the investigator for further investigation.

   c) *Defendant is charged with a crime.*

      i) Information

         Misdemeanor-level crimes can typically proceed with a simple charging instrument called an "*Information*." These documents set forth the charges and are sworn by the prosecutor. No additional review is required. The reports establish probable cause that a crime occurred. Further investigation is not needed to begin prosecution.

      ii) Indictment (grand jury or preliminary hearing)

         For felony-level crimes, prosecutors are required to bring the charges through an additional process to determine that there is sufficient evidence. First, they list the charges, in a document called an *indictment*. Then they must present the indictment to a *grand jury*, a group of individuals from the community who meet and hear evidence to decide this issue. In some circumstances, the prosecutor may have to present evidence to a judge in a *preliminary hearing* to obtain an indictment.

5) *Initial appearance.*

   Now that charges have been filed, the defendant is told what the charges are against them. They are given the opportunity to hire a *defense attorney*, or to apply for a court-appointed defense attorney if they are indigent. In many jurisdictions, a "not guilty" plea is entered at this time. If a defendant is going to remain out of jail pending trial (very common in animal cruelty cases), *release conditions* are established. In animal cruelty cases, requested release conditions can include:

   - Restrictions on the defendant's ability to possess and control animals.
   - Restrictions on buying and selling animals.
   - No contact orders with abused animals and their owners.

   If a defendant violates these release conditions, they run the risk of being put in jail pending trial.

6) *Discovery.*

The prosecution divulges all reports, evidence, and statements from witnesses in their possession to the defense. Prosecutors – and all persons involved in prosecution – have constitutional, statutory, and ethical obligations to ensure that no discoverable information (good or bad) is hidden or otherwise kept from the defense.

If you are involved in creating this material, it is essential that you ensure that the prosecution has accurate, up-to-date information as soon as it becomes available.

Note: There also are (limited) discovery obligations on the defense attorney as well.

7) *Plea bargain negotiation.*

The attorneys for the prosecution and defense negotiate to try to resolve the case without a trial. Negotiated resolutions consider several factors:

- The severity of the underlying crime
- The defendant's criminal history
- Aggravating factors
- Mitigating factors
- How other, similarly situated defendants were treated

Most criminal cases resolve with a defendant agreeing to change their plea on one or more charges from "not guilty" to "guilty" or "no contest," in exchange for the prosecutor agreeing to dismiss other charges and/or recommend a specific sentence.

8) a) *Deferred sentencing/diversion.*

A *deferred sentencing* or *diversion* is a resolution to a criminal case where a defendant makes certain admission or pleas to the court, but the court does not enter them as a matter of record. Instead, the defendant is ordered to comply with conditions (e.g. paying restitution or costs of care, surrendering animals, agreeing not to possess animals, taking an animal welfare class) for a certain period.

If the defendant successfully completes the conditions, the case is dismissed without conviction. If they do not, they can be convicted and sentenced.

b) *Guilty/no contest plea and sentencing.*

The defendant appears in front of the judge to change their plea and be *sentenced*. Before a judge accepts a plea, they will ask questions of the defendant and the defense attorney to make sure their plea is knowing, intelligent, and voluntary.

Sentencing can be negotiated in advance, or the attorneys may argue what the appropriate sentence will be (this is called *open sentencing*). Most animal cruelty cases with a plea end with the defendant on probation. So, one of the main areas of disagreement will be what the conditions of that probation will be. Standard conditions of probation include:

- Some form of supervision
- Obeying all laws
- Engaging in full-time work or school
- Keeping the court notified of address changes

Special conditions of probation in animal cruelty cases may include
- Jail time
- Community service
- Paying restitution and/or costs of care
- Forfeiture of abused/neglected animals
- No possession of (some or all) animals
- Enrolling in and completing an animal welfare class

16.4   Pretrial Matters

16.4.1   Motions

Before the trial begins, the prosecutor and defense attorney may bring motions asking the judge to make legal rulings on how the trial will proceed. Investigators are often called as witnesses for hearings on these motions. If you are called to testify, it is important to know what topics will be covered in advance, so you can prepare.

A few examples of these motions:

16.4.1.1   Motions Related to Release Conditions

Depending on how serious a crime is alleged and how dangerous a defendant is considered to be, the court may order the defendant to be held in jail pending trial. If not, the court may impose release conditions designed to prevent further harm while a case heads to a resolution. These conditions usually have to do with staying in the jurisdiction, reporting to a pretrial release agency, and having no contact with victims and co-defendants. If a defendant is accused of animal cruelty, they may be ordered not to possess animals.

16.4.1.2   Motion to Forfeit/Return Seized Property

The prosecution (especially in animal cruelty cases) may wish to get a pretrial ruling forfeiting seized evidence (including the animal victim). Conversely, a defendant (or another party) whose property was seized may file a motion demanding the return of that property (see Chapter 15 for more on this topic).

16.4.1.3   Demurrer/Motion to Dismiss

The defense may argue either that the charges as stated in the charging instrument are insufficient or unlawful. If this motion is granted, the case may be over, or it may just need to be brought in a different manner.

16.4.1.4   Motion for Change of Venue

This is an attempt by the defense attorney to move the trial from one jurisdiction to another, typically because of local media attention resulting in an unfair jury pool (see Section 14.1.4 Risks in Media Coverage).

16.4.1.5   Motion to Exclude/Sequester Witnesses

This is a common motion to keep subpoenaed witnesses out of the courtroom while the trial is being heard, and to keep them from discussing the case while the trial is ongoing. Expect to be excluded from the courtroom and unable to watch the trial if you are a witness.

Expert witnesses (those with special training/education) are often exempt from the motion to exclude since they may analyze and respond to evidence they did not witness.

16.4.1.6   Motion in Limine/Motion to Suppress

All evidence presented to a fact finder in a criminal trial must be *admissible* according to complex rules of evidence. In many cases, the prosecutor and/or the defense attorney know that the other side wants to present evidence that they think may violate these rules. They use these motions to keep this evidence out.

Most often, a motion to suppress evidence is brought because the defense attorney believes that certain evidence was obtained illegally by the police. When police obtain evidence illegally, the law often requires that the evidence be kept out of trial.

If you are a witness, you may not be allowed to testify about some evidence due to these motions. Mentioning suppressed evidence in front of a jury, even inadvertently, can result in a mistrial or a complete dismissal of the case.

16.4.2 Jury Selection

Through a process called voir dire, the prosecution and defense attorneys question prospective jurors to attempt to seat a fair jury. Both sides can ask the judge to strike jurors "for cause," meaning that they believe that the juror cannot be fair. Additionally, each side may use a set number of "peremptory strikes," keeping prospective jurors off of the jury for (almost) any reason.

16.5 The Trial

We have reached the main event. The rules are established, and everybody (hopefully!) knows their part. If you are not accustomed to this process, I always recommend carving out a few hours to watch a trial you are not involved in. Most trials are open to the public; you can just walk into a courtroom and watch. Watching a real-life trial is the best way to understand the rules and rhythms of the system (Box 16.3).

16.5.1 Opening Statements

Both the prosecutor and the defense attorney have an opportunity to tell the fact finder how they believe the evidence will play out. If the attorneys seem subdued compared to what you are used to on television, remember that these are opening *statements*, as opposed to closing *arguments*. Attorneys are not supposed to argue their case in opening.

Box 16.3   Sidebar

Coming to Court: Behavior and Demeanor

If you are subpoenaed you should check in with the attorney a day or two before the court date to make sure your appearance is still on the schedule (court hearings and trials get set over or canceled all the time, due to more urgent matters, plea bargains, global pandemics, etc.). The attorney may also narrow down the time of your appearance so you are not waiting around all day to testify.

Dress professionally. If you are an officer or agent of the government, you should wear your uniform. Veterinarians and veterinary technicians should avoid showing up to trial in scrubs.

As soon as you are in sight of the courthouse, behave as if everything you say and do will be played back in court. The other people in and around the courthouse may be jurors, reporters, judges, defense attorneys, defense witnesses, or defense investigators.

Do not talk to the other witnesses about the case. Do not roll your eyes at defendants or give any impression that you are bored or annoyed with the proceedings.

Trials are unpredictable and can be an exercise in "hurry up and wait." Bring work you can do or a book or electronic device to occupy your time (don't forget your chargers!).

16.5.2   Presentation of Evidence

Evidence comes in two forms: testimony from witnesses and physical items, such as photos, videos, records, and other objects. Since it bears the burden of proof, the prosecution presents its evidence first. Then the defense presents its case (if it chooses to). If the defense has put on a case, the prosecution may put on a rebuttal case, responding to the evidence in the defense case.

Most of evidence is testimony from witnesses. Testimony is not like what you have seen on television. It is not like casual conversation, or even like any other kind of question-and-answer situation. Testifying in court is a skill, and just like any skill, the only way to become good at it is to practice and prepare. Before the day of trial, reread your reports and study any pictures, videos, or diagrams you have. Make a friend or co-worker quiz you on your reports. Practice making eye contact, sitting up confidently, and speaking loudly and clearly (Box 16.4).

16.5.3   Motion for a Judgment of Acquittal

When the prosecution finishes presenting its case, the defense may move for a judgment of acquittal, arguing that the prosecutor did not present enough evidence for any reasonable factfinder to convict. If the judge grants the motion, the case is dismissed. This decision is not appealable.

16.5.4   Closing Arguments

After both parties have completed presenting their evidence, the attorneys for the prosecution and the defense have an opportunity to argue their case to the fact finder. At this point, all witnesses will have been released, so if you were a witness, this may be your only chance to go into the courtroom and watch (here is also where you will see the attorneys' theater-kid backgrounds come out).

16.5.5   The Verdict

The judge will announce the jury's verdict (another thing television gets wrong!). Here is another opportunity to show your self-control and professionalism. Do not show emotion at the verdict, no matter how excited or disappointed you may be.

16.5.6   Sentencing

If a defendant is convicted on some or all charges, they will be sentenced. Sentencing may take place right away, or it may be set over for days or weeks. In most cases, judges will decide what the sentence is, although they may get input from the jury, or they may order what is called a "presentencing investigation."

Criminal sentencing typically is based on a combination of the seriousness of the underlying offense and the individual defendant's criminal history. The judge may consider aggravating and mitigating factors.

In an animal cruelty case, sentencing may include an order that the defendant pay restitution and/or costs of care for abused or neglected animals. Testimony from a representative of the animal care agency may be needed to establish those costs.

Box 16.4 Tips

More Tips For Testifying

The Golden Rule: Tell The Truth!

All witnesses take the same oath: *To tell the truth, the whole truth, and nothing but the truth.* If you are a witness, you must take this oath seriously. This is not only to protect yourself, but also to protect the case, the prosecutor, and every agency involved in the case.

What could go wrong if you lie under oath:

1) <u>Personal consequences *if you lie under oath.*</u>
   a) Lying under oath is a crime, so you may be prosecuted. Depending on the context, it could even be a felony, carrying a potential prison sentence.
   b) Even if you are not charged with a crime, the fact that you have lied under oath means your credibility will be forever called into question, both in court and out.
   c) You may lose any professional certifications you have.
   d) If your agency regularly depends on you to provide testimony, or simply believes that you can no longer be trusted, you could be fired for cause.
   e) With this sort of mark against you, finding other work could be difficult or impossible (try to think of a job for which you would feel comfortable hiring a proven liar!).
2) *Case consequences if a prosecution witness lies under oath.*
   a) The case may be declared a mistrial, meaning the entire process would need to start over.
   b) If a mistrial is declared, the case may be dismissed with prejudice (meaning that the case would be completely over).
   c) Convictions obtained and sentences imposed based on false testimony may be thrown out.
   d) If animals have been seized and rehomed as part of a case, a dismissal could mean that victimized animals must be given back to the alleged abuser/neglecter.
3) *Agency consequences if an agency employee lies under oath.*
   a) The agency will come under public scrutiny. Media and social media criticism will follow.
   b) Agencies can have their public safety certification pulled, possibly permanently. If they can reapply, they may be required to undergo training prior to getting recertified.
   c) Other agencies may be hesitant to work with the tainted agency. This could result in cases not being pursued.
   d) The defendant in the underlying case may be able to sue the agency for damage to their reputation, or deprivation of their rights and their property. A valid lawsuit can easily bankrupt an agency.

The Three Answers

Testifying in a trial can be nerve wracking. It combines two of our biggest fears: public speaking and test-taking. It may help you to remember three answers that you can always give (*as long as they are true*; see "The Golden Rule").

1) "<u>I don't know.</u>" You may be asked questions to which you do not know the answer. Do not guess! If the prosecutor is asking you the question, they will have to figure out a different way to get that information out. If you believe somebody else knows the answer, it is okay to suggest that.
2) "<u>I don't remember.</u>" Trials take place months or even years after the investigation. Your memory may have faded. If you are asked a question and you do not remember the answer,

do not guess! Attorneys have a lot of options for "refreshing" a witness's memory. If they need you to testify to information that is not fresh in your mind, it is better to take a pause and read through your report than fumble around with, "I think it's..." or "I guess it was..." If your memory needs to be refreshed by a report you wrote, do not just look down and start reading from your report. Testimony (with very few exceptions) is supposed to come from memory. The judge will not allow you to read your report verbatim.

3) "Can you repeat/rephrase the question?" As a witness testifies, questions may occur to the attorneys that they had not prepared in advance. This can lead to confusing questions. Other times, attorneys (particularly defense attorneys) intentionally ask adverse witnesses complicated questions in the hopes of getting them to trip up. Do not be afraid to (politely) ask for clarification.

Know Your Exhibits

Exhibits (physical objects) can only be admitted into evidence if a qualified witness first identifies the object and vouches for its authenticity. Additionally, the judge must agree to "admit" the exhibit before it is shown to the fact finder. In animal cruelty cases, this can include pictures or videos of animals, lab reports, and animal cost sheets.

1) If you are going to be identifying an exhibit at trial, make sure that you are not seeing it for the first time on the witness stand.
2) You do not generally need to be the person who took a picture or a video to identify it. It will be enough that you can testify that the exhibit is "a fair and accurate representation" of what it purports to show.
3) Be careful before holding up exhibits to display them to the jury. Remember, the jury cannot see an exhibit unless and until it is admitted by a judge.

Listen to the Question, Pause, Answer the Question

Unlike conversation or interrogation, testimony in court follows strict rules and patterns. This helps the judge keep witnesses from bringing up suppressed information and keeps the record clearer for appeals. When testifying, wait until the question has been completely asked until you begin to respond. It is also helpful to establish a routine where you take a brief pause before answering any question.

Direct Examination vs. Cross-Examination vs. Redirect vs. Recross

There are several steps in a witness's testimony. Initially, the side that called the witness gets to ask them open-ended questions. This is called direct examination. When a prosecutor does it, it sounds a lot like this:

How are you employed? What kind of training have you received? What did you do on the date in question? What happened next? What happened next? What happened next?

You get the idea. Sometimes there are specific pieces of information prosecutors need to draw out, but even those questions must be asked in an open manner:

What was the body condition score of the horse? [Note how this question does not suggest a yes or no answer.]

Since these are open-ended questions, answer them openly, but be cautious that you are only answering the question that was asked and not wandering into other territory.

Once direct examination of a prosecution witness is done, the defense attorney gets to cross-examine the witness. On cross-examination, an attorney may ask leading questions. These are questions that suggest a "yes or no" answer. The classic start to a leading question is "Isn't it true that..."

When you are asked a leading question by a hostile defense attorney, it is not the time to argue that the question is flawed. It is fine to say that something is complicated, or that you cannot answer yes or no, but do not argue.

Keep in mind that after cross-examination, the prosecutor will have an opportunity to ask you more questions. This is called redirect examination. In redirect, you only cover topics that were brought up by the defense attorney, but (if you have a competent prosecutor) you will be able to further explain the answers you gave on cross-examination.

Objection!
When you hear either attorney say this, it is your signal as a witness to stop talking. It does not matter if you are halfway through a sentence or halfway through a syllable. "Objection" is a signal to the judge that either what was just said – or what is about to be said – is not allowed. Do not react; attorneys may use objections to try and rattle witnesses. Listen to and follow the judge's instructions.

If a judge sustains an objection, do not try to find a clever way around it. If evidence that was successfully objected to is brought up again, that could cause a mistrial.

Release of Witnesses/Rebuttal Witnesses
When a witness is finished testifying, the court will ask the parties if the witness can be "released" from their subpoena and can come and go as they please. Note that this does not give the witness permission to speak to unreleased witnesses about the content of their testimony. If you are released and choose to watch the rest of the trial, keep your emotions and thoughts about the proceedings internal (no big sighs or eye rolls in court, and no nodding or fist-pumping either).

If a witness is not released, it could be because one of the parties is reserving the right to recall the witness to testify later in the case.

16.5.7 Appeals

A defendant can appeal rulings that were made throughout their trial, including the ultimate finding of guilty. Appeals typically take months or years to resolve. If a case is reversed on appeal, there is a chance that it will need to be retried.

16.6 Topics for Prosecutors

Res ipsa loquitor . . . void for vagueness . . . rule against perpetuities . . . Okay, now that all the investigators have left, let us attorneys talk among ourselves.

Animal cruelty cases are technical, scientific, and highly emotional. Your trials will likely end up in the media and social media, and nobody will be happy with their outcome no matter what. Your best jurors will immediately disqualify themselves, your victim cannot testify, and your witnesses do not testify regularly. You cannot rely on the police crime lab to test your evidence.

Animal cruelty cases should be specially assigned to an individual prosecutor, so they get the time and attention they deserve. If you *are* that attorney, get working on these cases early. Here are a few major issues I have flagged working on these cases exclusively.

16.6.1 The Training Gap

This is the key issue that prevents animal cruelty from getting full investigation and prosecution. The "training gap" is this: because of a lack of training, patrol officers do not understand animal cruelty cases, and animal services officers do not understand criminal investigation. In seven years, I have reviewed multiples cases where patrol officers:

- Released neglected animals back to their neglecter.
- Destroyed dead animal bodies without forensic testing.
- Referred charges without asking a veterinary witness their impression of the evidence.

From animal services officers, I have seen reports that are indecipherable walls of text, questionable readings of criminal law, and terrible interviewing techniques.

Occasionally, you will find somebody who bridges the gap, but it is very much the exception, not the rule.

How have I worked to bridge the gap? Patience and education for animal services officers and training for the patrol officers. Everybody wants to get these cases right; as an attorney you can give them the tools to make that possible. Reach out to agencies on both sides of the gap and try to bridge it.

16.6.2 Private Lab Problems

In an animal cruelty case, the likelihood that your state police crime lab will help you with forensics is basically zero. If you have a case where biological evidence is tested, it is likely you will have a difficult time figuring out who your lab witness is. Rarely, a veterinarian will do their own lab work. More often, labs will be run by a veterinary technician, another veterinary staff member, or they will be sent to an outside lab. Labs can even be sent out of state. These private companies often batch samples together, and rarely include the name of the individual technician responsible for running the lab on the report.

This makes business sense and practical sense for most veterinary work but (for obvious reasons) can be disastrous in trying to prepare a criminal case for trial.

If you are on an animal cruelty case in the investigation stages, impress upon your witnesses the importance of keeping their lab work traceable and admissible.

Also keep in mind that there is not a lot of upside in defense attorneys forcing your hand and making you produce lab witnesses for trial. Assuming there was not anything egregiously wrong with the process, it would just be another technical, science-minded witness on the stand bolstering the prosecution. Figure out exactly who the lab witness is, make sure they are available and willing to come to trial, then try to get a stipulation from the defense allowing your veterinary witness to testify about the lab results without producing the lab witness.

16.6.3 Questioning Experts

If you have any kind of animal care expert on your witness list, obtain and discover their CV and gather all the information you need to establish their bona fides. Touch base with them well in advance of trial to ensure you have their reports, pictures, invoices, etc. Prepare them for the possibility of being cross-examined on scholarly articles. Remind them to review their reports and materials before trial. Remember, by the time they are on the stand, they will have seen thousands of other animals.

Animal care witnesses come across very well on the stand; most of your jurors will have had personal and positive associations with veterinarians and animal shelters. However, they can fall into a few traps: first, they can (understandably) be very emotional about these cases. They spent time and effort saving these animals (and in some cases, watching them die) and they have dedicated their lives to animal well-being. Remind them to rein in their emotions – a witness who has clearly chosen a "side" does not help.

On the other side of the spectrum, a lot of veterinarians fall into the "doctor/scientist" trap, where they do not want to nail anything down 100%. Talk to them in advance about the burden of proof not being "beyond all doubt."

16.6.4   Jury Selection

Your best prospective jurors will disqualify themselves as soon as the judge tells them it is an animal cruelty trial. From the remaining pool, you should focus on positive associations with animal care agencies and experiences with animal ownership. Find out if jurors have adopted/purchased pets or have worked with livestock. In my experience, both types of animal ownership inspire strong, positive feelings about animal welfare.

Overall, make sure that all jurors you seat agree with the general proposition that animal cruelty should be prosecuted. Your best jurors are those who agree that animals are sentient beings that can feel pain, and that pain should be avoided.

16.6.5   Sentencing

When arguing at sentencing, remember that any live seized animals will have accrued costs. Many statutory schemes allow for "costs of care" rather than "restitution" on animal cruelty cases, which makes for a much more significant bill.

Defense attorneys will often argue that animal care agencies can offset their expenses through adoption fees and donations; here in Oregon we have codified that a sentencing judge may not take outside donations or funding into account when setting costs of care (ORS 167.350 (1) (b)).

Check for statutory bans on animal possession that come with an animal cruelty conviction. Everybody in the proceeding should be clear what legal prohibitions exist for the defendant, regardless of what the sentencing judge ultimately does. Announcing the particulars of such a statutory ban in open court also creates a good record if the defendant later violates that statute.

When asking for community service, keep in mind that most animal care organizations do not want people accused or convicted of animal cruelty to volunteer with them. Stick with court-ordered options or non-animal-related nonprofit agencies.

There are some options for animal care classes online, like the classes people take when they get traffic tickets. One that I have used recently is BARCeducation.org. I audited the course before recommending it, and though it is generic (not state-specific) in its approach, it has a lot of positive aspects. I like that it is a nonprofit, that the class covers both abuse and neglect, and that the program tracks who is taking the class using the student's webcam.

16.6.6 Animal Legal Defense Fund

(Note: Animal Legal Defense Fund [ALDF] has funded my position since 2013, but I take no instruction from them on my casework.)

If you ever have issues that need funding or specialized briefing, contact the ALDF's Criminal Justice Program, which provides free legal assistance to agencies in the criminal justice system in investigation and prosecution of animal cruelty cases. Their website is: https://aldf.org.

16.7 Conclusion

Law enforcement, humane agents, and animal care workers all work hard on the investigation of animal cruelty and protection of its victims. Trial can be the culmination of that hard work. To many in animal cruelty prevention, trials are intimidating and unfamiliar. To be successful, everybody involved in a trial must *know their part* and *prepare*. A few things to keep in mind as the trial approaches:

- Fully disclose all written and recorded material well in advance of the trial.
- If you have questions about the process, do not be afraid to ask.
- Before testifying, review your reports and know your exhibits.
- Practice testifying to reduce "stage fright."
- Behave yourself in and around the courthouse.
- When testifying, *tell the truth*, and leave emotions out of it.

If you prepare and educate yourself, trial will become a routine part of your successful fight against animal cruelty.

Introduction to the Appendix

Appendix A

Acknowledging that the investigation and prosecution of differing animal cruelty offenses present unique hallmarks or challenges, Appendix A: Specific Case Protocols is included as a quick reference source. Each protocol is organized by the discipline involved (investigator, animal care entities, veterinarian and prosecutor), and provides in-the-moment advice and reminders specific to that type of animal cruelty case, while cross-referencing recommended forms, checklists, agreements, templates, and resources provided in Appendices B–D. Your purchase of this book includes access to our companion website, which makes these resources available for download and customization. The materials provided in this appendix are not intended to, and do not, constitute legal advice; they are provided for informational purposes and as a reference.

Appendices B–D

These appendices contain forms, templates, resources, and checklists designed to support and enhance the work of investigators, veterinarians, animal care entities, and prosecutors from the initial investigation through adjudication. Many of these resources were developed after a need was identified for standardization of processes, or thorough collection and organization of information. You may find all or some of them useful in your work, but remember these are resources meant to make your work more manageable and serve as reminders of important information to collect or processes to consider. The forms themselves are not intended to add additional steps that may be unrealistic due to staffing or resources. They are also meant to be amendable, so we encourage you to adapt and transform them to fit your specific needs. Your purchase of this book includes access to our companion website, which makes these resources available for download and customization. The materials provided in these appendices are not intended to, and do not, constitute legal advice; they are provided for informational purposes and as a reference.

Animal Cruelty Investigations: A Collaborative Approach from Victim to Verdict™, First Edition.
Edited by Kris Otteman, Linda Fielder, and Emily Lewis.
© 2022 John Wiley & Sons, Inc. Published 2022 by John Wiley & Sons, Inc.
Companion website: www.wiley.com/go/otteman/victimtoverdict

Appendix A: Specific Case Protocols

Type of Case

Animal Cruelty Investigations: A Collaborative Approach from Victim to Verdict™, First Edition.
Edited by Kris Otteman, Linda Fielder, and Emily Lewis.
© 2022 John Wiley & Sons, Inc. Published 2022 by John Wiley & Sons, Inc.
Companion website: www.wiley.com/go/otteman/victimtoverdict

Case: Failure to Provide Veterinary Care

An animal cruelty charge may arise from the medical or behavioral ailments and the suffering an animal endures due to the owner's failure to provide timely and appropriate veterinary care. The owner may have neglected to seek veterinary care for a number of reasons, such as a lack of resources or failure to understand the duties of an owner, or the withholding of care may have been intentional. Research indicates that inability to provide adequate financial resources is a top barrier to veterinary care for pet owners. However, the inability to pay for services does not excuse criminal neglect. When investigating cases in which veterinary care will improve the health or save the life of the animal, responders may have the opportunity to apply education, resources, and incremental care to a situation. This may result in preservation of the human animal bond and prevent circumstances from escalating to criminal neglect.

In cases in which the investigator opts to educate the owner and monitor their compliance, the veterinarian can play an important role in formulating a treatment plan that is within the owner's means to provide, educating the owner of their role in following through with the prescribed treatment plan, and partnering with the investigator to communicate progress.

In order for the case to be closed, the owner must demonstrate their ability to provide adequate veterinary care as required by law. The animal must be brought to a state of relative comfort and recovery through treatment and other husbandry changes as outlined in the action notice and confirmed through veterinary treatment and rechecks. Investigators should document the animal's condition through photos to record progress and improvement.

Investigator

Actions that Apply to All Cases
- Interview owner, witnesses, and neighbors
- Collect all relevant veterinary records
- Consider trying a pretext phone call to the suspect to get their version of events documented early on
- Preserve evidence: victim animals, records, photos, medication; see Appendix D for comprehensive evidence list
- Engage veterinarian to assist with examination of the evidence and the investigation
- Plan for live animal evidence holding and care
- Apply for a search warrant when appropriate. Include diagnostic tests and collection of samples. See Appendix D for comprehensive evidence list
- Determine ownership status of victim animals and keep partnering agencies apprised of any changes to the status

Specific Case Actions
- Determine who is responsible for the animal(s) care
- Inform of local resources available to owner to get veterinary care when appropriate
- Interview neighbors
- Interview veterinarians who have provided previous care
- Recheck for compliance with veterinary visits and treatments
- Issue action notices (Appendix B) and follow up (depending on severity of the case)

VICTIM TO VERDICT™

Specific Case Considerations
- ☐ In some cases, education and resources can resolve the issues
- ☐ The suspect's financial situation is directly relevant to this offense
- ☐ Compliance plans must be clear and specific, follow-up and recheck schedule must be maintained

Questions
- ☐ Is there any previous history of vet care?
- ☐ Who was in charge of the animal's care?
- ☐ Are other animals in poor condition?
- ☐ How long has the condition been present and what home remedies or resources has the owner tried or explored?
- ☐ Is the condition likely to resolve with treatment or is the condition chronic and requires ongoing veterinary management to keep the animal comfortable?
- ☐ If the suspect is the owner, are they open to considering surrendering the animal for treatment and rehoming?

Forms
- ☐ Investigations Triage Matrix
- ☐ Minimum Care Checklist
- ☐ Evidence In Animal Cruelty Cases
- ☐ Action Notice

Veterinarian

Actions that Apply to All Cases
- ☐ Review all records related to the case
- ☐ Ask the investigator questions that would further your assessment of the evidence presented to you
- ☐ Exam ideally within 24 hours
- ☐ Follow photography and forensic exam protocols
- ☐ Complete written report
- ☐ Finalize diagnostic plan and create treatment and care plan
- ☐ Determine who is the follow-up contact for supplemental case reports or emergency updates (typically this will be the investigator, law enforcement, or the prosecutor)
- ☐ Examine animal and records for previous/chronic injuries or pattern of injuries
- ☐ Document euthanasia decision process if necessary.

Specific Case Actions
- ☐ Select diagnostics that are necessary to confirm physical exam findings and create a treatment plan
- ☐ Provide incremental care when possible
- ☐ Avoid unnecessary confirmatory diagnostics when finances are at issue
- ☐ If the animal dies or is euthanized proceed with forensic necropsy

Specific Case Considerations
- ☐ Review legal standards of veterinary care, degree of injury to the animal and cause of the neglect. Take this information into consideration when formulating a plan

VICTIM TO VERDICT™

Questions
- ☐ Does your knowledge of animal behavior factor into what you are seeing with the issues you are investigating?
- ☐ Is the breed, socialization, temperament, or species challenging to care for?
- ☐ Does the animal require hospitalization or veterinary care?
- ☐ Where was the animal found? Or how was it presented?
- ☐ Is this a single animal incident or multiple?
- ☐ Was veterinary care initiated if deceased? If so, review records

Forms
- ☐ Veterinary Forensic Exam Form
- ☐ Nonliving Evidence Tracking Form
- ☐ Evidence Placard
- ☐ Summary Vet Report
- ☐ Animal Cruelty Case Relinquishment Form
- ☐ Protective Custody Foster Care Agreement
- ☐ Laboratory Submission Forms with chain of custody

Animal Care

Actions that Apply to All Cases
- ☐ Confirm ownership status of victim animals
- ☐ Maintain chain of custody of animal evidence in a secure location
- ☐ Carry out veterinary treatment plan as directed
- ☐ Make sure you have the ability to provide the care necessary. If not, facilitate outside or referral care
- ☐ Create and post an emergency vet care plan and contact list
- ☐ Facilitate recheck appointments with the vet
- ☐ Provide behavior support and training to live evidence animals
- ☐ Place animals in Protective Custody (PC) foster if appropriate
- ☐ Start tracking and documenting costs of care for individual animals on intake

Specific Case Actions
- ☐ Implement PC secure housing and tracking for each animal
- ☐ Provide care at the direction of the lead veterinarian
- ☐ Make sure you have the ability to provide the care necessary
- ☐ Document improvements
- ☐ Facilitate recheck appointments with the vet
- ☐ Provide enrichment
- ☐ Start documenting restitution costs

Specific Case Considerations
- ☐ Have a plan for emergency veterinary care if necessary
- ☐ Prepare for long recovery and/or potential for humane euthanasia as an outcome
- ☐ Must provide all care directed by the veterinarian
- ☐ Do not perform medical procedures that will permanently alter the animal unless medically necessary or ownership has been transferred

VICTIM TO VERDICT™

Forms
- ☐ Protective Custody Foster Care Agreement
- ☐ Nonliving Evidence Tracking Form
- ☐ Live Animal Evidence Tracking Form
- ☐ Evidence Placard
- ☐ Case Animal Intake Checklist

Prosecutor

Actions that Apply to All Cases
- ☐ Request additional investigation, where appropriate, before declining to prosecute
- ☐ Consider long-term impact or permanent injury to the animal(s) when making charging decisions
- ☐ File a charge on each victim animal and/or each criminal incident – do not group victims/conduct into one count
- ☐ A condition of release should include no contact with victim animal or other animals as appropriate
- ☐ Pursue preconviction forfeiture without delay if the victim animal is alive and if the state has laws in place to do so
- ☐ Sign off on disposition of animal evidence when evidence collection is complete and ownership has been resolved
- ☐ Schedule pretrial meetings with veterinary expert and other witnesses
- ☐ Request continued medical discovery from veterinarian and/or animal care agency if necessary
- ☐ Request up-to-date amount of costs of care for animal care agency

Specific Case Actions
- ☐ Check your case law on the issue of not providing vet care to determine if an appellate decision discusses the issue
- ☐ Review the case documents to determine if the suspect made any admissions to the veterinarian
- ☐ Bring out the veterinarian's recommendations to the suspect and whether the recommendations were followed
- ☐ If the suspect provided some veterinary care, address that

Specific Case Considerations
- ☐ There is potential for a sympathetic jury
- ☐ Consider whether evidence of recovery will be impactful or inspire leniency by the jury/judge

Forms
- ☐ Example Forfeiture Hearing Checklist
- ☐ Forfeiture Petition Template
- ☐ Example Jury Instructions
- ☐ Forfeiture Order Template

Resources and References

AVMA (n.d.). Veterinary care for all. https://www.avma.org/javma-news/2019-09-01/veterinary-care-all (accessed 7 August 2021).

Balkin, D., Blomquist, M., Bowman, S., et al. (2019). Animal cruelty issues: What juvenile and family court judges need to know. https://www.ncjfcj.org/wp-content/uploads/2019/07/NCJFCJ_ALDF_Animal-Cruelty-TAB_Final.pdf (accessed 8 June 2021).

Governor's Commission on the Humane Treatment of Animals (2020). Animal cruelty investigation and prosecution: A user manual for New Hampshire law enforcement. http://neacha.org/resources/animal-cruelty-manual-2020.pdf (accessed 8 June 2021).

National Sheriff's Association (2019). *Sheriff & Deputy*: 2019 special issue animal cruelty. https://www.sheriffs.org/sites/default/files/2019_SD_AA.pdf (accessed 8 June 2021).

Phillips, A. and Lockwood, R. (2013). Investigating and prosecuting animal abuse. https://nationallinkcoalition.org/wp-content/uploads/2013/09/Investigating-Prosecuting-AA-Phillips-Lockwood.pdf (accessed 8 June 2021).

Case: Emaciation, Starvation

An animal may be found in emaciated condition due to starvation, a serious illness or disease process, or a combination. These cases may involve one animal or many, and in some cases a group of animals may be found in normal body condition while only one or a few are emaciated.

The veterinarian is key to diagnosing the cause of weight loss and low body condition score in emaciated animals and is able to rule out causes such as cancer, kidney disease, or dental issues and help the investigative team determine the owner's culpability and next steps for the animal. State laws require animal owners to provide adequate nutrition for their animals as well as veterinary care for medical issues that can contribute to or cause emaciation.

It is common to find emaciated animals in hoarding conditions or in a herd of livestock as a result of inadequate feed offered, or because the group competes for the available food and older or more timid animals are kept from the food by stronger or more aggressive animals. It is the responsibility of the animal caregiver(s) to be aware of and responsive to this type of situation in order to maintain the health of the animals in their custody. Livestock on pasture may receive adequate nutrition through grazing while others restricted to pens or stalls may not. In some cases, the owner is not able to provide the amount of food necessary for the number of animals in their possession.

Owners faced with financial, health, or mental health crises may struggle to properly provide for their animals. Cases of intentional starvation may be related to particular disdain for an animal, or a domestic violence scenario in which neglecting the animal is utilized as a form of control or punishment of a human victim. Severely emaciated animals require immediate care and a refeeding plan that is overseen by a veterinarian.

Investigator

Actions that Apply to All Cases
- ☐ Interview owner, witnesses, and neighbors
- ☐ Collect all relevant veterinary records
- ☐ Consider trying a pretext phone call to the suspect to get their version of events documented early on
- ☐ Preserve evidence: victim animals, records, photos, medication; see Appendix D for comprehensive evidence list
- ☐ Engage veterinary expertise to assist with examination of the evidence and the investigation
- ☐ Plan for live animal evidence holding and care
- ☐ Apply for a search warrant when appropriate. Include diagnostic tests and collection of samples. See Appendix D for comprehensive evidence list
- ☐ Determine ownership status of victim animals and keep partnering agencies apprised of any changes to the status

Specific Case Actions
- ☐ Make observations on scene that are relevant to veterinary evaluation
- ☐ For livestock – interview neighbors, feed suppliers, renderers
- ☐ Social media research may provide images of animal's prior condition
- ☐ Photograph animal on scene
- ☐ Collect food samples if possible
- ☐ Offer food to animal and record interest in eating

☐ Request full veterinary exam and bloodwork within 24 hours of intake
☐ Issue action notices and follow up (depending on severity of the case)

Specific Case Considerations
☐ Consider dental condition as possible barrier to maintaining adequate food intake
☐ Old age is not a blanket excuse for emaciation
☐ The financial situation of the suspect is relevant to this investigation
☐ Determine whether the emaciated body condition is related to starvation or a disease process Either scenario could result in criminal charges. Veterinary care should be provided to an animal suffering from a disease process that results in emaciation
☐ Consider other aspects of minimum care such as shelter, environment, vet care, access to water

Questions
☐ What was the animal eating and how much each day?
☐ Who was responsible for the care of the animal?
☐ Is there access to water and how much is available?
☐ Are there other animals, children, or seniors at risk in the home?

Forms
☐ Body Condition Score Charts
☐ Minimum Care Checklist
☐ Nonliving and Live Evidence Tracking Forms
☐ Evidence Placard

Veterinarian

Actions that Apply to All Cases
☐ Review all records related to the case
☐ Exam ideally within 24 hours
☐ Follow photography and forensic exam protocols
☐ Complete written report
☐ Ask the investigator questions that would further your assessment of the evidence presented to you
☐ Finalize diagnostic plan and create treatment and care plan
☐ Determine who is the follow-up contact for supplemental case reports or emergency updates (typically this will be the investigator, law enforcement, or the prosecutor)

Specific Case Actions
☐ Photograph and video water and food consumption immediately
☐ Collect samples for baseline: fecal, urinalysis, complete blood count, creatine kinase, and electrolytes panel
☐ Rule out gastrointestinal tract foreign bodies
☐ Collect first fecal to look for nonnutritive substances the animal(s) may have consumed out of hunger such as dirt, wood, or other items
☐ Reference a standardized body condition chart
☐ Complete other diagnostics as needed
☐ Create a feeding plan
☐ Record progress of weight gain and condition
☐ Illustrate via timeline

VICTIM TO VERDICT ™

Specific Case Considerations
- ☐ In equine cases, explain dental care. Horses with inadequate dentition may become emaciated on excellent feed due to lack of ability to chew food
- ☐ Speak to the pain, trauma, and timeline involved (i.e. how long it would take for the animal to lose that amount of weight)
- ☐ Rule out other causes of poor body condition
- ☐ Case is decided based on evidence collected at time of finding and veterinarian's opinion, and rarely does reported progress of animal (weight and condition improvement) come into consideration as to the legal outcome
- ☐ If animal is deceased, dies, or is euthanized, proceed with necropsy to determine cause of death

Questions
- ☐ What is the condition of other animals with the same owner/property?
- ☐ What is the medical history of the animal?
- ☐ Where was the animal found? Or how was it presented?

Forms
- ☐ Summary Vet Report
- ☐ Veterinary Forensic Exam Form
- ☐ Evidence Placard
- ☐ Nonliving and Live Evidence Tracking Forms
- ☐ Animal Observation Chart
- ☐ Body Condition Score Chart
- ☐ Laboratory Submission Forms with chain of custody

Animal Care

Actions that Apply to All Cases
- ☐ Confirm ownership status of victim animals
- ☐ Maintain chain of custody of animal evidence in a secure location
- ☐ Carry out veterinary treatment plan as directed
- ☐ Make sure you have the ability to provide the care necessary. If not, facilitate outside or referral care
- ☐ Create and post an emergency veterinary care plan and contact list
- ☐ Facilitate recheck appointments with the veterinarian
- ☐ Provide behavior support and training to live evidence animals
- ☐ Place animals in Protective Custody foster if appropriate
- ☐ Start tracking and documenting costs of care for individual animals on intake

Specific Case Actions
- ☐ Follow veterinarian's treatment and feeding plan
- ☐ Tare scale and weigh every four days at same time of day. Record weights
- ☐ Follow up with photography and video as instructed
- ☐ Maintain chain of custody
- ☐ Provide enrichment
- ☐ Prevent volunteers from feeding outside the scope of the refeeding plan
- ☐ Assess whether animal(s) are candidates for protective custody foster and initiate process for foster placement where appropriate

Specific Case Considerations
- ☐ Strictly adhere to refeeding and vet care plan

Forms
- ☐ Protective Custody Foster Care Agreement
- ☐ Evidence Placard
- ☐ Nonliving and Live Evidence Tracking Forms
- ☐ Case Animal Intake Checklist
- ☐ Animal Observation Chart

Prosecutor

Actions that Apply to All Cases
- ☐ Request additional investigation, where appropriate, before declining to prosecute
- ☐ Consider long-term impact or permanent injury to the animal(s) when making charging decisions
- ☐ File a charge on each victim animal and/or each criminal incident – do not group victims/conduct into one count
- ☐ A condition of release should include no contact with victim animal or other animals as appropriate
- ☐ Pursue preconviction forfeiture without delay if the victim animal is alive and if the state has laws in place to do so
- ☐ Sign off on disposition of animal evidence when evidence collection is complete and ownership has been resolved
- ☐ Schedule pretrial meetings with veterinary expert and other witnesses
- ☐ Request continued medical discovery from veterinarian and/or animal care agency if necessary
- ☐ Request up-to-date amount of costs of care for animal care agency

Specific Case Actions
- ☐ Contact the lead veterinarian with questions about severity of condition
- ☐ If relevant, introduce the position of the doghouse or kennel where the owner saw the animal every day but did not provide adequate food. Seeing the animal every day as the emaciated condition develops without providing food is intentional

Specific Case Considerations
- ☐ Consider starvation as torture and/or serious bodily injury, despite animal's ability to recover eventually
- ☐ Consider whether evidence of recovery will be impactful or inspire leniency by the jury/judge

Forms
- ☐ Example Forfeiture Hearing Checklist
- ☐ Forfeiture Petition Template
- ☐ Example Jury Instructions
- ☐ Forfeiture Order Template

Resources and References

Body condition scoring examples and charts: https://vet.tufts.edu/wp-content/uploads/tacc.pdf and https://oregonvma.org/files/Purina-Dog-Condition-Chart.pdf

VICTIM TO VERDICT™

Balkin, D., Blomquist, M., Bowman, S., et al. (2019). Animal cruelty issues: What juvenile and family court judges need to know. https://www.ncjfcj.org/wp-content/uploads/2019/07/NCJFCJ_ALDF_Animal-Cruelty-TAB_Final.pdf (accessed 8 June 2021).

Governor's Commission on the Humane Treatment of Animals (2020). Animal cruelty investigation and prosecution: A user manual for New Hampshire law enforcement. http://neacha.org/resources/animal-cruelty-manual-2020.pdf (accessed 8 June 2021).

Miller, L. and Zawistowski, S.L. (eds.) (2013). *Shelter Medicine for Veterinarians and Staff*, 2e. Ames, IA: Iowa State University Press.

National Sheriff's Association (2019). *Sheriff & Deputy*: 2019 special issue animal cruelty. https://www.sheriffs.org/sites/default/files/2019_SD_AA.pdf (accessed 8 June 2021).

Phillips, A. and Lockwood, R. (2013). Investigating and prosecuting animal abuse. https://nationallinkcoalition.org/wp-content/uploads/2013/09/Investigating-Prosecuting-AA-Phillips-Lockwood.pdf (accessed 8 June 2021).

Case: Animal Hoarding

Animal hoarding cases are complex and challenging. They involve large numbers of animals and, at their center, one or more individuals living with complex mental health problems. By the time a case is reported, caregivers may have been engaging in hoarding behaviors for years, accumulating not only animals, but objects and debris, which can make crime scenes difficult and dangerous to maneuver. Animals living in these conditions suffer from serious and chronic health issues, many related to the squalid conditions of their confinement. While one may think of a houseful of cats when picturing a hoarding scenario, any species or combination of species may be discovered in these cases.

Animal hoarding cases are best addressed through a cooperative multi-agency response. Mental health agencies are valuable partners in addressing the stress and anxiety caregivers experience when faced with the loss of their animals. These individuals rarely possess a realistic understanding of the conditions their animals suffer, and often will go to any length to prevent their removal, including hiding or relocating animals and evading investigators. Many are so connected to their animals that attempts by authorities to address the problem can trigger suicidal thoughts and behaviors.

In addition to considering the inclusion of a mental health response for the suspect, investigators must address and report any other vulnerable adults or children within the home. These environments present serious human health risks from high levels of ammonia, mold, and structural and fire hazards, including the risk presented by hoarded objects falling on or preventing individuals from exiting or entering the home in an emergency. Code enforcement and fire marshals should be included as scene responders.

Removal of live and deceased animals through the authority of a search warrant is preferred. Caregivers who are cooperative initially often panic and shut down removal efforts once underway. Scene processing is complicated by the amount of debris and objects in homes and outbuildings, making animals difficult to locate and capture.

While the processing of the scene itself may take hours, don't be tempted to skip thorough documentation of the conditions through video and photography and the creation of a map and record of where animals were contained. Seizures require animal handlers equipped with humane capture equipment and personal protective gear including thick gloves and respirators. A veterinarian on scene can help triage animal care, address any medical emergencies, as well as provide identification of related evidence and opinions on environmental conditions and their effect on animal health.

Plans for animal protective custody must consider the number of animals and a thorough veterinary plan for treatment and rehabilitation. Plan for pregnant animals and nursing litters and provide comprehensive vaccination, deworming, and quarantine for infectious disease for all animals upon shelter entry. Animals may be poorly socialized but often respond to behavioral rehabilitation efforts and become candidates for adoption, albeit some will have ongoing special needs. Foster homes are valuable in providing socialization and specialized care.

Prosecutors should consider all available avenues for forfeiture and/or foreclosure to reduce the length of stay for the population. Suspects may elicit sympathy and concern, but it is important to remember that hoarding has a very high recidivism rate, and criminal charges may be most effective at preventing reoffending and in some cases may be a gateway to professional mental health counseling. Cases involving large numbers of seized animals are costly. Agencies should have policies in place to prevent the offender from readoption of the animals and explore grants and other options for funding shelter and medical care.

VICTIM TO VERDICT™

Investigator

Actions that Apply to All Cases

☐ Interview owner, witnesses, and neighbors

☐ Collect all relevant veterinary records

☐ Consider trying a pretext phone call to the suspect to get their version of events documented early on

☐ Preserve evidence: victim animals, records, photos, medication; see Appendix D for comprehensive evidence list

☐ Engage veterinarian to assist with examination of the evidence and the investigation

☐ Plan for live animal evidence holding and care

☐ Apply for a search warrant when appropriate

☐ Include diagnostic tests and collection of samples. See Appendix D for comprehensive evidence list

☐ Determine ownership status of victim animals and keep partnering agencies apprised of any changes to the status

Specific Case Actions

☐ Build rapport with suspect

☐ Make note of the property and the outside of the residence and look for indicators of animals being contained inside such as shredded blinds, fly dirt on the windows, the bottom of the door is rusted or eroded from urine, animal crates littered around the property, or empty bags of pet food or litter

☐ Coordinate multidisciplinary response

☐ Plan seizure

☐ Coordinate care and housing

☐ Secure personal protective equipment (PPE), proper capture equipment

☐ Recruit and identify expert handlers

☐ Ensure scene safety and security

☐ Document each area housing animals as a separate crime scene

☐ Photograph each animal at the scene even if it is through the crate gaps

☐ Dig to find out if the animals have been seen in multiple veterinary practices, as these cases often travel between clinics

Specific Case Considerations

☐ Try to avoid having the suspect witness the process of capturing the animals at the scene

☐ Assisting animal care agency will need as much notice as possible to prepare for intake of many animals

Forms

☐ Minimum Care Checklist

☐ Multi-Animal Site Visit Report

☐ On Scene Habitat Evaluation

☐ Large Animal Premises Inspection Report

☐ Evidence Tracking Forms

☐ Evidence Placard

☐ Nonliving and Live Evidence Tracking Forms

☐ Animal Cruelty Case Relinquishment Form

☐ Action Notice

Veterinarian

Actions That Apply To All Cases
- ☐ Review all records related to the case
- ☐ Ask the investigator questions that would further your assessment of the evidence presented to you
- ☐ Exam ideally within 24 hours
- ☐ Follow photography and forensic exam protocols
- ☐ Finalize diagnostic plan and create treatment and care plan
- ☐ Determine who is the follow-up contact for supplemental case reports or emergency updates (typically this will be the investigator, law enforcement, or the prosecutor)
- ☐ Complete written report

Specific Case Actions
- ☐ Guide law enforcement if necessary in evidence collection at scene including records, food, medications, photos, and other important items
- ☐ Partner with law enforcement to establish a protocol for collection of deceased, injured, and critical animals during scene response
- ☐ Establish specific exam and screening protocol for a large volume of animals
- ☐ Incorporate behavioral assessment into the health assessment process
- ☐ Follow necropsy protocol for any deceased animals
- ☐ Establish sheltering or foster care protocol including preventative care, nutrition, and overall health care
- ☐ Conduct pregnancy screening
- ☐ Establish screening protocols for populations – Retrovirus, heartworm, fecals, complete blood count, etc. (30%) initially and as indicated by physical exam for the individual
- ☐ Complete fecal analysis for parasites prior to deworming
- ☐ Establish and oversee follow-up animal care (weight recording, behavioral plans etc.)
- ☐ Review rabies vaccination status and vaccinate as necessary

Specific Case Considerations
- ☐ Look for previous veterinary records via investigator
- ☐ Explain why some animals may be in better body condition than others (competition, hierarchy, etc.)
- ☐ Discuss stress and behavioral outcomes for the animals based on your knowledge of animal husbandry and welfare and describe the implications when living under these conditions

Questions
- ☐ Who owns the animals, are there third-party owners?

Forms
- ☐ Veterinary Forensic Exam Form
- ☐ Necropsy Exam Notes Form
- ☐ Nonliving and Live Evidence Tracking Forms
- ☐ Evidence Placard
- ☐ Summary Vet Report
- ☐ Examples of On Scene Veterinary Assessments
- ☐ Laboratory Submission Forms with chain of custody

VICTIM TO VERDICT™

Animal Care

Actions that Apply to All Cases
☐ Confirm ownership status of victim animals
☐ Maintain chain of custody of animal evidence in a secure location
☐ Carry out veterinary treatment plan as directed
☐ Make sure you have the ability to provide the care necessary. If not, facilitate outside or referral care
☐ Create and post an emergency vet care plan and contact list
☐ Facilitate recheck appointments with the vet
☐ Provide behavior support and training to live evidence animals
☐ Place animals in Protective Custody foster if appropriate
☐ Start tracking and documenting costs of care for individual animals on intake

Specific Case Actions
☐ Assist with scene documentation and assessment
☐ Assist with safe capture and transport of animals
☐ Wear appropriate PPE for scene processing
☐ Implement Protective Custody secure housing and tracking for each animal
☐ Take intake photo series/video
☐ Administer treatments as directed by the veterinarian
☐ Facilitate recheck exams
☐ Provide enrichment
☐ Report animal births/deaths to veterinarian/law enforcement/prosecutor

Specific Case Considerations
☐ Be prepared for media interest
☐ Prepare for up to double the number of animals expected
☐ Only trained animal handlers should be involved in capture
☐ Unload animals in secure area in case any got loose during transport

Questions
☐ Is there documentation of seizure or owner release?

Forms
☐ Nonliving and Live Evidence Tracking Forms
☐ Animal Observation Chart
☐ Evidence Placard

Prosecutor

Actions that Apply to All Cases
☐ Request additional investigation, where appropriate, before declining to prosecute
☐ Consider long-term impact or permanent injury to the animal(s) when making charging decisions
☐ File a charge on each victim animal and/or each criminal incident – do not group victims/conduct into one count
☐ A condition of release should include no contact with victim animal or other animals as appropriate

VICTIM TO VERDICT™

□ Pursue preconviction forfeiture without delay if the victim animal is alive and if the state has laws in place to do so

□ Sign off on disposition of animal evidence when evidence collection is complete and ownership has been resolved

□ Schedule pretrial meetings with veterinary expert and other witnesses

□ Request continued medical discovery from veterinarian and/or animal care agency if necessary

□ Request up-to-date amount of costs of care for animal care agency

Specific Case Actions

□ Charge on each victim animal

□ Show pictures of the conditions

□ Include behavior of the animals as evidence of conditions

□ Show video or photos of the PPE necessary to process the case

□ Look for statements by the suspect in the discovery materials that everything is fine

Specific Case Considerations

□ Include ongoing inspections as a part of sentencing

□ Include counseling as a part of sentencing

□ Don't concede unnecessary ground by grouping victims/conduct into one count

Forms

□ Example Forfeiture Hearing Checklist

□ Forfeiture Petition Template

□ Example Jury Instructions

□ Forfeiture Order Template

Resources and References

Animal Legal Defense Fund (n.d.). Animal hoarding facts. https://aldf.org/article/animal-hoarding-facts (accessed 8 June 2021).

Balkin, D., Blomquist, M., Bowman, S., et al. (2019). Animal cruelty issues: What juvenile and family court judges need to know. https://www.ncjfcj.org/wp-content/uploads/2019/07/NCJFCJ_ALDF_Animal-Cruelty-TAB_Final.pdf (accessed 8 June 2021).

Frost, R., Patronek, G., Arluke, A., and Steketee, G. (2015). The hoarding of animals: An update. https://www.psychiatrictimes.com/view/hoarding-animals-update (accessed 8 June 2021).

Governor's Commission on the Humane Treatment of Animals (2020). Animal cruelty investigation and prosecution: A user manual for New Hampshire law enforcement. http://neacha.org/resources/animal-cruelty-manual-2020.pdf (accessed 8 June 2021).

Levit, L., Patronek, G., and Grisso, T. (2015). *Animal Maltreatment Forensic Mental Health Issues and Evaluations*. Oxford: Oxford University Press.

Ockenden, E.M., De Groef, B., and Marston, L. (2014). Animal hoarding in Victoria Australia: An exploratory study. *Anthrozoos* 27: 33–47.

Merck, M.D., Miller, D.M., Reisman, R.W., and Miller, D.M. (2013). Animal hoarders and animal sanctuaries. In: *Veterinary Forensics: Animal Cruelty Investigations*, 2e (ed. M.D. Merck), 219–222. Hoboken, NJ: Wiley-Blackwell.

Miller, L. and Zawistowski, S.L. (eds.) (2013). *Shelter Medicine for Veterinarians and Staff*, 2e. Ames, IA: Iowa State University Press.

National Sheriff's Association (2019). *Sheriff & Deputy*: 2019 special issue animal cruelty. https://www.sheriffs.org/sites/default/files/2019_SD_AA.pdf (accessed 8 June 2021).

Phillips, A. and Lockwood, R. (2013). Investigating and prosecuting animal abuse. https://nationallinkcoalition.org/wp-content/uploads/2013/09/Investigating-Prosecuting-AA-Phillips-Lockwood.pdf (accessed 8 June 2021).

Tufts Cummings School of Veterinary Medicine (2021). Crisis intervention, counseling and case management for Hoarding of Animals Research Consortium. https://vet.tufts.edu/hoarding/crisis-intervention-counseling-and-case-management (accessed 8 June 2021).

Case: Substandard Breeding or Rescue Operation

These cases are characterized by a large number of animals, poor sanitation, and a lack of veterinary care. Puppy mills and individuals or operations that breed cats, birds, reptiles, small animals, and any number of other species for sale and/or transport may fall into this category. Rescue groups, sanctuaries, and exhibitors are also included if they own or manage a number of animals and do not provide adequate or minimum care, veterinary treatment, adequate housing, nutrition, exercise, or sanitation.

Substandard breeding or rescue operations rarely allow visitors or clients in areas where animals are kept and so these cases may reach a critical level before they are discovered or reported. Preliminary investigations should include searches of internet sites and publications where the animals may be advertised for sale and review of medical records and complaints from owners or recently acquired animals that are ill or injured. These efforts may offer a glimpse into the number and types of animals being sold; occasionally their living conditions are visible in photographs or videos. Most often, though, breeders and dealers maintain websites and social media pages that portray pristine and ideal conditions.

A veterinarian should accompany investigators and law enforcement to on-site inspections and seizures to address medical emergencies and assess the conditions on scene. Veterinarians can also be useful in examining evidence such as medications, home remedies, and records related to veterinary care, breeding, sales, and shipping of animals.

The scene should be processed methodically with care given to document, photograph, and videotape the conditions inside each enclosure or cage. Evidence identification should be assigned so that each animal can be connected later to the cage or pen it was housed in. Prepare for animals that may be poorly socialized and difficult to handle and transport. Handlers and scene-processing teams will require personal protective equipment due to the potential for zoonotic disease transmission and unsanitary conditions. Other agencies such as the United States Department of Agriculture (USDA), code enforcement, and agencies that require facilities licensing may also have laws or regulations that apply to these cases.

Animal care facilities will need time to prepare for the number of animals estimated and the population should be vaccinated immediately as well as quarantined and monitored for contagious diseases. Plan for pregnant and nursing animals with litters to enter protective custody foster care if possible, or to be housed in a quiet and low-traffic area of the shelter.

These cases can garner a huge amount of interest from the media and the public. Individuals may come forward claiming to have ownership interest in purebred animals. Former employees, suppliers, clients, volunteers, and others who have had dealings with the operation may also contact your agency as witnesses. A public information officer can be valuable to address media requests and public concern while investigators follow up with witnesses.

Investigator

Actions that Apply to All Cases
□ Interview owner, witnesses, and neighbors
□ Collect all relevant veterinary records
□ Consider trying a pretext phone call to the suspect to get their version of events documented early on
□ Preserve evidence: victim animals, records, photos, medication; see Appendix D for comprehensive evidence list

☐ Engage veterinarian to assist with examination of the evidence and the investigation
☐ Plan for live animal evidence holding and care
☐ Apply for a search warrant when appropriate
☐ Include diagnostic tests and collection of samples. See Appendix D for comprehensive evidence list
☐ Determine ownership status of victim animals and keep partnering agencies apprised of any changes to the status

Specific Case Actions
☐ Find out who is the veterinarian for the operation
☐ Check social media sites like Yelp for reviews and photos
☐ Each kennel is a separate crime scene – document it as such, and be able to connect the animal to where it was housed
☐ Search the scene and seize evidence
☐ Document supplies and feed on premises
☐ Do a full financial investigation to show how invested the suspect is in the ongoing enterprise
☐ Review euthanasia protocol and disposal methods
☐ Consider seizing records, computers, cell phones
☐ Interview previous clients
☐ Review preventive care records, breeding records, breed registry, staffing hours and duties, and veterinarians of record

Specific Case Considerations
☐ Identify third-party owners
☐ Write unborn offspring into search warrant
☐ Diverting animals to breeding community to preserve bloodline
☐ Large number of animals may overwhelm animal care partners at seizure
☐ Partner with enforcement agencies: Department of Agriculture, USDA, local or state kennel licensing, etc.
☐ Difficult to gain access to premises

Questions
☐ Are there any county regulations for breeders?
☐ Has USDA done any inspections?
☐ Have there been any complaints to the Better Business Bureau or regulatory agencies?
☐ How are the animals sold or rehomed?

Forms
☐ Minimum Care Checklist
☐ Multi-Animal Site Visit Report
☐ On Scene Habitat Evaluation
☐ Animal Cruelty Case Relinquishment Form
☐ Nonliving and Live Evidence Tracking Forms

Veterinarian

Actions that Apply to All Cases
☐ Review all records related to the case

- □ Ask the investigator questions that would further your assessment of the evidence presented to you
- □ Exam ideally within 24 hours
- □ Follow photography and forensic exam protocols
- □ Finalize diagnostic plan and create treatment and care plan
- □ Determine who is the follow-up contact for supplemental case reports or emergency updates (typically this will be the investigator, law enforcement, or the prosecutor)
- □ Complete written report

Specific Case Actions
- □ Conduct overview and assessment of facilities and evidence
- □ Review vaccination and preventive care history
- □ Establish screening protocols for populations – Retrovirus, heartworm, fecals, complete blood count, etc. (30%) initially and as indicated by physical exam for the individual
- □ Conduct fecals before deworming
- □ Scan and document ID: microchip, tattoo, etc.
- □ If taking into care, set up preventive care, nutritional plan, medical care, behavioral enrichment plan, and tracking procedures
- □ Review and inform investigator:
  - – Breeding records
  - – Breed registry
  - – Staffing hours and duties
  - – Veterinarian(s) of record
- □ Follow euthanasia, necropsy protocols

Specific Case Considerations
- □ Consider zoonotic diseases
- □ Obsessive or repetitive behaviors (i.e. circling) can be related to housing conditions and may require a specific behavioral plan.
- □ Plan for poor socialization and no house-training
- □ Review rabies vaccination status and vaccinate as needed
- □ Look for and preserve remains – necropsy if possible and relevant

Questions
- □ Are there any known congenital abnormalities or diseases in the group?

Forms
- □ Examples of On Scene Veterinary Assessments
- □ Veterinary Forensic Exam Form
- □ Nonliving and Live Evidence Tracking Forms
- □ Animal Observation Chart
- □ Laboratory Submission Forms with chain of custody

Animal Care

Actions that Apply to All Cases
- □ Confirm ownership status of victim animals
- □ Maintain chain of custody of animal evidence in a secure location
- □ Carry out veterinary treatment plan as directed

□ Make sure you have the ability to provide the care necessary. If not, facilitate outside or referral care
□ Create and post an emergency veterinary care plan and contact list
□ Facilitate recheck appointments with the veterinarian
□ Provide behavior support and training to live evidence animals
□ Place animals in Protective Custody foster if appropriate
□ Start tracking and documenting costs of care for individual animals on intake

Specific Case Actions

□ Assist with safe animal capture and transport from the scene
□ Assist with documentation of the scene
□ Assist with taking a photo of every animal before it leaves the scene
□ Assist with uniquely identifying each animal and attaching that unique identifier to the animal for future reference
□ Maintain chain of custody from scene to intake location
□ Consider foster for pregnant mothers/newborn litters
□ Documentation of daily care and treatments as prescribed

Specific Case Considerations

□ Treat each enclosure as a separate crime scene to be documented
□ Plan for highly interested adopters if purebred
□ Media interest
□ Do not perform medical procedures that will permanently alter the animal unless medically necessary or ownership has been transfered

Questions

□ Is there documentation of seizure or owner release?

Forms

□ Protective Custody Foster Care Agreement
□ Evidence Placard
□ Nonliving and Live Evidence Tracking Forms
□ Animal Cruelty Case Relinquishment Form
□ Animal Observation Chart

Prosecutor

Actions that Apply to All Cases

□ Request additional investigation, where appropriate, before declining to prosecute
□ Consider long-term impact or permanent injury to the animal(s) when making charging decisions
□ File a charge on each victim animal and/or each criminal incident – do not group victims/conduct into one count
□ A condition of release should include no contact with victim animal or other animals as appropriate
□ Pursue preconviction forfeiture without delay if the victim animal is alive and if the state has laws in place to do so
□ Sign off on disposition of animal evidence when evidence collection is complete and ownership has been resolved
□ Schedule pretrial meetings with veterinary expert and other witnesses

☐ Request continued medical discovery from veterinarian and/or animal care agency if necessary

☐ Request up-to-date amount of costs of care for animal care agency

Specific Case Actions

☐ Pursue preconviction forfeiture without delay if state includes it in the law

Specific Case Considerations

☐ Be prepared to be confronted with third-party owners

☐ Consider including the business/corporation/LLC if there is one for the breeding operation

☐ Show the suffering of all the animals and how the animals are commodities

☐ The genetic makeup of the animals can demonstrate that money is the priority

☐ Determine whether they are breeding to American Kennel Club or industry ethical standards

☐ If the conduct crossed stated lines, consider the application of the Preventing Animal Cruelty and Torture Act (PACT act)

☐ Include ongoing inspections as a part of sentencing

☐ Don't concede unnecessary ground by grouping victims/conduct into one count

Forms

☐ Example Forfeiture Hearing Checklist

☐ Forfeiture Petition Template

☐ Example Jury Instructions

☐ Forfeiture Order Template

Resources and References

Governor's Commission on the Humane Treatment of Animals (2020). Animal cruelty investigation and prosecution: A user manual for New Hampshire law enforcement. http://neacha.org/resources/animal-cruelty-manual-2020.pdf (accessed 8 June 2021).

Kaminski Leduc, J.L. (2013). Standards of care for dog and cat breeders. www.cga.ct.gov/2013/rpt/2013-R-0309.htm (accessed August 7, 2021).

Miller, L. and Zawistowski, S.L. (eds.) (2013). *Shelter Medicine for Veterinarians and Staff*, 2e. Ames, IA: Iowa State University Press.

National Sheriff's Association (2019). *Sheriff & Deputy*: 2019 special issue animal cruelty. https://www.sheriffs.org/sites/default/files/2019_SD_AA.pdf (accessed 8 June 2021).

Phillips, A. and Lockwood, R. (2013). Investigating and prosecuting animal abuse. https://nationallinkcoalition.org/wp-content/uploads/2013/09/Investigating-Prosecuting-AA-Phillips-Lockwood.pdf (accessed 8 June 2021).

Case: Blunt Force Trauma: Victim Dies

Nonaccidental fatal injuries involving blunt force trauma must always be on the rule-out list as a cause of injury and death among companion animals particularly, with dogs and cats most most commonly. Because young dogs and cats are known to display destructive behaviors such as chewing and house soiling, abuse events may be related to the owner's anger, frustration, or inappropriate methods of training and discipline.

Upon receipt of the body, a comprehensive necropsy should be performed as soon as possible before postmortem changes and decomposition alter evidence of trauma beneath the skin.

Often, the suspect's account of how the animal became injured does not match the veterinarian's findings upon necropsy. Investigators should utilize the veterinarian's findings when considering what may have been used to strike and kill the animal as well as the force used and length of time of the abuse event.

Fatal injuries may be the culmination of a series of abuse events. In addition to examining the animal remains for evidence of prior injury, such as healed or healing fractures, it is prudent to collect previous veterinary records and statements from neighbors and other people associated with the suspect.

Intentional animal abuse often co-occurs alongside domestic violence, so always consider other animals and humans in the home who might also be victims of abuse.

Investigator

Actions that Apply to All Cases
- ☐ Interview owner, witnesses, and neighbors
- ☐ Collect all relevant veterinary records
- ☐ Consider trying a pretext phone call to the suspect to get their version of events documented early on
- ☐ Preserve evidence: records, photos, medication; see Appendix D for comprehensive evidence list
- ☐ Preserve the body as evidence. Do not freeze the body, if possible
- ☐ Request a forensic necropsy
- ☐ Engage veterinarian to assist with examination of the evidence and the investigation
- ☐ Apply for a search warrant when appropriate
- ☐ Include diagnostic tests and collection of samples. See Appendix D for comprehensive evidence list

Specific Case Actions
- ☐ Protect other vulnerable entities in the home – other pets, children, elderly, partners (cross-reporting)
- ☐ Search for and seize evidence (weapons, blood spatter, cell phone records, etc.)
- ☐ Map and photograph the scene and animal as found

Specific Case Considerations
- ☐ Use knowledge gained from veterinary report to interview suspect and question about events that occurred
- ☐ Create a media plan
- ☐ Review medical history looking for the animal having been seen by multiple practices as these cases often travel between clinics

VICTIM TO VERDICT™

Questions
- ☐ Who had access to the animal in the timeframe of the injury(s)?
- ☐ If the victim is buried, should you excavate it?
- ☐ Any previous pet deaths and, if so, what were the causes?

Forms
- ☐ Nonliving Evidence Tracking Forms
- ☐ Evidence Placard
- ☐ Animal Cruelty Case Relinquishment Form
- ☐ Animal Cruelty Case Consent to Search Form

Veterinarian

Actions that Apply to All Cases
- ☐ Review all records related to the case including previous medical history. Refrigerate the remains until necropsy
- ☐ Necropsy ideally within 24 hours
- ☐ Follow photography and forensic necropsy protocols
- ☐ Shave the animal to look for bruising or wounds
- ☐ Perform full-body radiographs and an examination of the external areas of the animal's body, looking for evidence of current and previous injury such as healed fractures and scars as well as any wound patterns
- ☐ Photograph each finding
- ☐ Submit samples for histopathology of tissues and other organs that appear to have evidence of traumatic injury
- ☐ Complete written report

Specific Case Actions
- ☐ Examine head for signs of trauma: sclera, intraocular hemorrhage, external ear canals, dental, split palate, skull, and soft tissue
- ☐ Examine for cutaneous, subcutaneous, and deep bruising, and shave to assist visualization. Include all relevant areas. Most common areas of bruising: neck, thorax, ventral abdomen
- ☐ Review radiographs for healed fractures: most commonly ribs, facial bones, radius, ulna, and teeth
- ☐ Look for intrathoracic or abdominal injury with hemorrhage, abdominal wall bruising, hernia, fractures of liver or spleen, and broken ribs
- ☐ Evaluate and report the type or amount of force required for injuries and, when possible, determine if history and the cause reported aligns with injury
- ☐ Create rule-out list and include or exclude possible causes

Specific Case Considerations
- ☐ Create a media plan

Questions
- ☐ Ask the investigator questions that would further your assessment of the evidence presented to you such as:
- ☐ Where was the animal found? How was it presented?
- ☐ Is this a single animal incident or multiple?
- ☐ Was veterinary care initiated if deceased? If so, review records

VICTIM TO VERDICT™

□ Does your knowledge of animal behavior factor into what you are seeing with any of the injuries and the existing crime reports?

□ Does the history make sense?

Forms

□ Necropsy Exam Notes Form

□ Nonliving Evidence Tracking Forms

□ Evidence Placard

□ Summary Vet Report

□ Laboratory Submission Forms with chain of custody

Animal Care

Actions that Apply to All Cases

□ Maintain chain of custody of animal and associated evidence in a secure location

□ Freeze or refrigerate remains at the direction of the veterinarian

□ Facilitate forensic necropsy

Specific Case Considerations

□ Create media plan

Forms

□ Nonliving Evidence Tracking Forms

□ Evidence Placard

Prosecutor

Actions that Apply to All Cases

□ Request additional investigation, where appropriate, before declining to prosecute

□ File a charge on each victim animal and/or each criminal incident – do not group victims/conduct into one count

□ A condition of release should include no contact with animals as appropriate

□ Sign off on disposition of animal evidence when evidence collection is complete and ownership has been resolved

□ Schedule pretrial meetings with veterinarian and other witnesses

Specific Case Actions

□ Instruct law enforcement on additional investigation if needed

□ Use the veterinarian to address possible explanations/defenses

Specific Case Considerations

□ Include restriction from possessing animals as a condition of release

□ Facilitate disposition of the body once evidence has been gathered and defense has had opportunity to examine (or waived)

Questions

□ Are there any relevant charging enhancements?

□ Are there other relevant charges in addition to abuse, i.e. neglect for failure to seek care for injured animal?

Resources and References

Balkin, D., Blomquist, M., Bowman, S., et al. (2019). Animal cruelty issues: What juvenile and family court judges need to know. https://www.ncjfcj.org/wp-content/uploads/2019/07/NCJFCJ_ALDF_ Animal-Cruelty-TAB_Final.pdf (accessed 8 June 2021).

Colorado LINK Project (2013). The relevance of the link for prosecutors. https://coloradolinkproject. com/prosecutor-toolkit (accessed June 8, 2021).

Employment Division vs. Smith, 494 U.S. 872, (1990). "We have never held that an individual's religious beliefs excuse him from compliance with an otherwise valid law prohibiting conduct that the State is free to regulate . . . the right of free exercise does not relieve an individual of the obligation to comply with a 'valid and neutral law of general applicability on the ground that the law proscribes (or prescribes) conduct that his religion prescribes (or proscribes).'"

Governor's Commission on the Humane Treatment of Animals (2020). Animal cruelty investigation and prosecution: A user manual for New Hampshire law enforcement. http://neacha.org/resources/ animal-cruelty-manual-2020.pdf (accessed 8 June 2021).

Merck, M.D., Miller, D.M., Reisman, R.W., and Miller, D.M. (2013). Animal hoarders and animal sanctuaries. In: *Veterinary Forensics: Animal Cruelty Investigations*, 2e (ed. M.D. Merck), 219–222. Hoboken, NJ: Wiley-Blackwell.

Miller, L. and Zawistowski, S.L. (eds.) (2013). *Shelter Medicine for Veterinarians and Staff*, 2e. Ames, IA: Iowa State University Press.

National Sheriff's Association (2019). *Sheriff & Deputy*: 2019 special issue animal cruelty. https://www. sheriffs.org/sites/default/files/2019_SD_AA.pdf (accessed 8 June 2021).

Norris, P. (2020). Blunt force trauma. In: *Veterinary Forensic Medicine and Forensic Sciences* (eds. J.H. Byrd, P. Norris and N. Bradley-Siemens), 129–144. London: CRC Press.

Phillips. A. (2014). Understanding the link between violence to animals and people. https:// nationallinkcoalition.org/wp-content/uploads/2014/06/Allies-Link-Monograph-2014.pdf (accessed June 8, 2021).

Phillips, A. and Lockwood, R. (2013). Investigating and prosecuting animal abuse. https:// nationallinkcoalition.org/wp-content/uploads/2013/09/Investigating-Prosecuting-AA-Phillips-Lockwood.pdf (accessed 8 June 2021).

Stern, A.W. and Sula, M.-J. (2021). Blunt force trauma. In: *Veterinary Forensics: Investigation, Evidence Collection, and Expert Testimony* (eds. E. Rogers and A.W. Stern), 208–211. London: CRC Press.

IVFSA (2020). Veterinary forensic postmortem examination standards. https://www.ivfsa.org/ wp-content/uploads/2020/12/IVFSA-Veterinary-Forensic-Postmortem-Exam-Standards_ Approved-2020_with-authors.pdf (accessed August 7, 2021).

Case: Blunt Force Trauma: Victim Lives

Time is of the essence when examining live animals for signs of blunt force trauma. While blunt force injuries may result in visible bruising or expression of pain such as limping or reluctance to move, other times no external evidence of the trauma will be found. In some cases, even though no visible injury is noted, internal injuries including fractures, damage to organs, and internal hemorrhage may be discovered through imaging, blood chemistry panels, and other diagnostics. Always check for petechiae, scleral hemorrhage, injuries to the head and teeth, torn nails, and bruising at the tail base and abdomen. Shave fur to look for evidence of wounds, scars, and bruising. Always perform and review full-body radiographs looking for both acute and chronic fractures.

The investigator must prioritize speedy examination by a veterinarian. Investigators should look for evidence of implements that may have been used to strike the animal, record witness statements regarding kicking or striking the animal, and present their findings to the veterinarian. Because young dogs and cats often display destructive behaviors such as chewing and house soiling, abuse events may be related to the owner's anger, frustration, or inappropriate training methods in cases involving puppies and kittens. Often, the suspect's account of how the animal became injured does not match the veterinarian's findings upon physical examination. The investigator should utilize the veterinarian's expertise in determining if the narrative matches the degree and type of injury the animal sustained.

Intentional animal abuse often co-occurs alongside domestic violence, so always consider other animals and humans in the home who might also be victims of abuse.

Investigator

Actions that Apply to All Cases
- ☐ Interview owner, witnesses, and neighbors
- ☐ Collect all relevant veterinary records
- ☐ Consider trying a pretext phone call to the suspect to get their version of events documented early on
- ☐ Preserve evidence: victim animals, records, photos, medication; see Appendix D for comprehensive evidence list
- ☐ Engage veterinary expertise to assist with examination of the evidence and the investigation
- ☐ Plan for live animal evidence holding and care
- ☐ Apply for a search warrant when appropriate
- ☐ Include diagnostic tests and collection of samples. See Appendix D for comprehensive evidence list
- ☐ Determine ownership status of victim animals and keep partnering agencies apprised of any changes to the status

Specific Case Actions
- ☐ Interview suspect and witnesses
- ☐ Assess risk to other animals in the home and seize where appropriate
- ☐ Assess risk to humans in the environment
- ☐ Gather previous vet history
- ☐ Take photos
- ☐ Attempt to view scene and document
- ☐ Facilitate vet exam

Specific Case Considerations

- □ Be aware of other potential victims in the environment – human and animal
- □ Refer to human services as appropriate
- □ Seize cell phones and surveillance video footage if available

Questions

- □ Is there anyone else who might have seen or heard the incident?
- □ Were there any previous pet deaths and what were the causes?
- □ Who had access to the animal in the timeframe of the injury?

Forms

- □ Nonliving and Live Evidence Tracking Forms
- □ Animal Cruelty Case Consent to Search Form
- □ Evidence Placard
- □ Animal Cruelty Case Relinquishment Form
- □ Laboratory Submission Forms with chain of custody

Veterinarian

Actions that Apply to All Cases

- □ Review all records related to the case
- □ Exam ideally within 24 hours
- □ Follow photography and forensic exam protocols
- □ Complete full-body imaging
- □ Ask the investigator questions that would further your assessment of the evidence presented to you
- □ Finalize diagnostic plan and create treatment and care plan
- □ Complete written report
- □ Determine who is the follow-up contact for supplemental case reports or emergency updates (typically this will be the investigator, law enforcement, or the prosecutor)

Specific Case Actions

- □ Review for chronic, healed, and acute injuries or patterns of injuries
- □ Shave to reveal bruising, document, and photograph
- □ Examine for petechiae and scleral, intraocular, cranial, inner ear hemorrhage
- □ Treat injuries and document progress
- □ Submit blood chemistry including creatine kinase
- □ Compare findings to alleged cause
- □ Speak to long-term damage or permanent injury in report

Specific Case Considerations

- □ Be aware of other potential victims in the environment – human and animal
- □ Interview clients with witness present and take detailed notes when possible
- □ Refer to human services as appropriate
- □ Dig to find out if the pet has been seen elsewhere as these cases often travel between practices

Questions

- □ Where was the animal found? Or how was it presented?
- □ Is this a single-animal incident or multiple?
- □ Does the narrative fit the injury?
- □ How could this injury occur? What people have access to the animal?

VICTIM TO VERDICT™

Forms
- ☐ Veterinary Forensic Exam Form
- ☐ Animal Cruelty Case Relinquishment Form
- ☐ Animal Observation Chart
- ☐ Nonliving and Live Evidence Tracking Forms

Animal Care

Actions that Apply To All Cases
- ☐ Confirm ownership status of victim animals
- ☐ Maintain chain of custody of animal evidence in a secure location
- ☐ Carry out veterinary treatment plan as directed
- ☐ Make sure you have the ability to provide the care necessary. If not, facilitate outside or referral care
- ☐ Create and post an emergency veterinary care plan and contact list
- ☐ Facilitate recheck appointments with the veterinarian
- ☐ Provide behavior support and training to live evidence animals
- ☐ Place animals in Protective Custody foster if appropriate
- ☐ Start tracking and documenting costs of care for individual animals on intake

Specific Case Actions
- ☐ Intake the animal(s) through standard intake procedures
- ☐ Implement Protective Custody secure housing and tracking for each animal
- ☐ Take intake photo series/video
- ☐ Administer treatments as directed by the veterinarian
- ☐ Facilitate recheck exams
- ☐ Provide enrichment
- ☐ Deliver and document treatment plan if in-house

Specific Case Considerations
- ☐ Assess risk if the suspect is likely to show up at your facility
- ☐ Notify organization if necessary and have trespass protocol in place

Questions
- ☐ Who is the current owner of the animal?
- ☐ Is there documentation of seizure or owner release?
- ☐ What is the veterinary treatment plan?
- ☐ Is the suspect aware of where the animal is being held?

Forms
- ☐ Evidence Placard
- ☐ Case Animal Intake Checklist
- ☐ Protective Custody Foster Care Agreement
- ☐ Animal Observation Chart
- ☐ Nonliving and Live Evidence Tracking Forms

Prosecutor

Actions that Apply to All Cases
- ☐ Request additional investigation, where appropriate, before declining to prosecute
- ☐ Consider long-term impact or permanent injury to the animal(s) when making charging decisions

VICTIM TO VERDICT™

☐ File a charge on each victim animal and/or each criminal incident – do not group victims/conduct into one count

☐ A condition of release should include no contact with victim animal or other animals as appropriate

☐ Pursue preconviction forfeiture without delay if the victim animal is alive and if the state has laws in place to do so

☐ Sign off on disposition of animal evidence when evidence collection is complete and ownership has been resolved

☐ Schedule pretrial meetings with veterinary expert and other witnesses

☐ Request continued medical discovery from veterinarian and/or animal care agency if necessary

☐ Request up-to-date amount of costs of care for animal care agency

Specific Considerations

☐ Include no contact with animals as a condition of release

☐ Consider whether evidence of recovery will be impactful or inspire leniency by the jury/judge

Questions

☐ Are there any relevant enhancement statutes (i.e. in the presence of a minor or prior domestic violence convictions)?

☐ Are there other relevant charges in addition to abuse, i.e. neglect for failure to seek care for injured animal?

Forms

☐ Example Forfeiture Hearing Checklist

☐ Forfeiture Petition Template

☐ Example Jury Instructions

☐ Forfeiture Order Template

Resources and References

Merck, M.D., Miller, D.M., Reisman, R.W., and Maiorka, P.C. (2013). Blunt force trauma. In: *Veterinary Forensics: Animal Cruelty Investigations*, 2e (ed. M.D. Merck), 97–121. Hoboken, NJ: Wiley-Blackwell.

Norris, P. (2020). Blunt force trauma. In: *Veterinary Forensic Medicine and Forensic Sciences* (eds. J.H. Byrd, P. Norris and N. Bradley-Siemens), 129–144. London: CRC Press.

Stern, A.W. and Sula, M.-J. (2021). Blunt force trauma. In: *Veterinary Forensics: Investigation, Evidence Collection, and Expert Testimony* (eds. E. Rogers and A.W. Stern), 208–211. London: CRC Press.

Case: Sharp Force Injuries

Sharp force injuries consist of wounds by any sharp implement that are the result of cutting, stabbing, or chopping. They may cause or contribute to the death of an animal through blood loss, organ damage, or accompanying infection. Victim animals may be presented as living or deceased.

Investigators may have evidence of a weapon or the weapon may have yet to be discovered when the animal is presented for forensic exam. Veterinarians should thoroughly examine the entire animal for deep and superficial wounds. Shaving can uncover wounds not visible with the hair coat intact. Blunt force trauma from a heavy implement may result in splitting of the skin and appear as a sharp force injury. Wounds should be examined for size, depth, and other characteristics that may rule in or out a certain implement as a weapon. While knives come to mind immediately, other implements can cause sharp force injuries such as axes, pointed sticks or rods, glass, and sheet metal. Examination of the body for trace evidence and collection of DNA may prove useful in linking a weapon or a suspect to the injuries at a later time. Photograph all wounds using a photo scale to measure and illustrate length, width, and depth of each wound.

Investigators should search the crime scene for not only knives but other instruments that could have caused cutting or stabbing wounds, as well as blood spatter. Look for defensive wounds such as bites and scratches when interviewing suspects.

Investigator

Actions that Apply to All Cases
- ☐ Interview owner, witnesses, and neighbors
- ☐ Collect all relevant veterinary records
- ☐ Consider trying a pretext phone call to the suspect to get their version of events documented early on
- ☐ Preserve evidence: records, photos, medication; see Appendix reference for comprehensive evidence list
- ☐ Preserve the body as evidence. Do not freeze the body, if possible
- ☐ Request a forensic necropsy
- ☐ Engage veterinarian to assist with examination of the evidence and the investigation
- ☐ Apply for a search warrant when appropriate. Include diagnostic tests and collection of samples. See Appendix reference for comprehensive evidence list

Specific Case Actions
- ☐ Search scene for weapons, signs of struggle, blood spatter
- ☐ Collect any item that may have been used as a weapon
- ☐ Map, photograph, and video the scene

Questions
- ☐ Were there any witnesses?
- ☐ Is this a domestic violence scenario with other people or animals at risk?

Forms
- ☐ Animal Cruelty Consent to Search Form
- ☐ Animal Cruelty Case Relinquishment Form
- ☐ Nonliving and Live Evidence Tracking Forms
- ☐ Evidence Placard

Veterinarian

Actions that Apply to All Cases
☐ Review all records related to the case
☐ Ask the investigator questions that would further your assessment of the evidence presented to you
☐ Necropsy ideally within 24 hours
☐ Follow photography and forensic necropsy protocols
☐ Complete full-body radiographs
☐ Collect samples for pathology
☐ Complete written report

Specific Case Considerations
☐ Testify to the pain, fear, and suffering the animal experienced

Questions
☐ Does the given explanation for the injury align with the wounds and damage found?
☐ Where was the animal found? Or how was it presented?
☐ Is this a single- or multiple-animal incident?
☐ Was veterinary care initiated if deceased? If so, are there records?

Forms
☐ Necropsy Exam Notes Form
☐ Veterinary Forensic Exam Form
☐ Nonliving and Live Evidence Tracking Forms
☐ Evidence Placard
☐ Animal Cruelty Case Relinquishment Form
☐ Summary Vet Report
☐ Laboratory Submission Forms with chain of custody

Animal Care

Actions That Apply To All Cases
☐ Maintain chain of custody of animal and associated evidence in a secure location
☐ Freeze or refrigerate remains at the direction of the veterinarian
☐ Facilitate forensic necropsy

If victim survives:

☐ Confirm ownership status of victim animals
☐ Carry out veterinary treatment plan as directed
☐ Make sure you have the ability to provide the care necessary. If not, facilitate outside or referral care
☐ Create and post an emergency vet care plan and contact list
☐ Facilitate recheck appointments with the vet
☐ Provide behavior support and training to live evidence animals
☐ Place animals in protective custody foster if appropriate
☐ Start tracking and documenting costs of care for individual animals on intake

VICTIM TO VERDICT™

Specific Case Actions

☐ Intake the animal(s) through standard intake procedures

☐ Implement Protective Custody secure housing and tracking for each animal

☐ Take intake photo series/video

☐ Administer treatments as directed by the veterinarian

☐ Facilitate recheck exams

☐ Provide enrichment

☐ Assess whether animal(s) are candidates for Protective Custody foster and initiate process for placement where appropriate

Specific Case Considerations

☐ Assess risk if the suspect is likely to show up at your facility

☐ Notify organization if necessary and have trespass protocol in place

☐ Give the animal a different name when making it available for adoption

Questions

☐ Who is the current owner of the animal?

☐ Is there documentation of seizure or owner release?

☐ What is the vet treatment plan?

☐ Is the suspect aware of where the animal is being held?

Forms

☐ Nonliving and Live Evidence Tracking Forms

☐ Animal Observation Chart

☐ Protective Custody Foster Care Agreement

Prosecutor

Actions that Apply to All Cases

☐ Request additional investigation, where appropriate, before declining to prosecute

☐ File a charge on each victim animal and/or each criminal incident; do not group victims/conduct into one count

☐ A condition of release should include no contact with animals as appropriate

☐ Sign off on disposition of animal evidence when evidence collection is complete and ownership has been resolved

☐ Schedule pretrial meetings with veterinarian and other witnesses

Specific Case Actions

☐ Include counseling as part of sentencing

☐ Use the veterinarian's testimony to inform the jury/judge about the extent of the injuries and the pain and suffering associated

☐ Determine if the victim animal suffered serious or permanent injury (or death) as a result of the conduct and charge accordingly

Specific Case Considerations

☐ Consider whether evidence of recovery will be impactful or inspire leniency by the jury/judge

Questions

☐ Are there any relevant enhancement statutes (i.e. in the presence of a minor or prior domestic violence record)

☐ Are there other relevant charges in addition to abuse, i.e. neglect for failure to seek care for injured animal?

Forms
☐ Example Forfeiture Hearing Checklist
☐ Forfeiture Petition Template
☐ Example Jury Instructions
☐ Forfeiture Order Template

Resources and References

Balkin, D., Blomquist, M., Bowman, S., et al. (2019). Animal cruelty issues: What juvenile and family court judges need to know. https://www.ncjfcj.org/wp-content/uploads/2019/07/NCJFCJ_ALDF_Animal-Cruelty-TAB_Final.pdf (accessed 8 June 2021).

Colorado LINK Project (2013). The relevance of the link for prosecutors. https://coloradolinkproject.com/prosecutor-toolkit (accessed June 8, 2021).

De Siqueira, A. and Norris, P. (2020). Sharp force trauma. In: *Veterinary Forensic Medicine and Forensic Sciences* (eds. J.H. Byrd, P. Norris and N. Bradley-Siemens), 145–156. London: CRC Press.

Doheny, S.L. (2006). Free exercise does not protect animal sacrifice: The misconception of *Church of Lukumi Babalu Aye v. City of Hialeah* and constitutional solutions for stopping animal sacrifice. *J. Animal L* 2: 121.

Governor's Commission on the Humane Treatment of Animals (2020). Animal cruelty investigation and prosecution: A user manual for New Hampshire law enforcement. http://neacha.org/resources/animal-cruelty-manual-2020.pdf (accessed 8 June 2021).

Merck, M.D., Miller, D.M., and Maiorka, P.C. (2013). Sharp force injuries. In: *Veterinary Forensics: Animal Cruelty Investigations, 2nd edn, 123–137*. Hoboken, NJ: Wiley-Blackwell.

National Sheriff's Association (2019). *Sheriff & Deputy*: 2019 special issue animal cruelty. https://www.sheriffs.org/sites/default/files/2019_SD_AA.pdf (accessed 8 June 2021).

Phillips. A. (2014). Understanding the link between violence to animals and people. https://nationallinkcoalition.org/wp-content/uploads/2014/06/Allies-Link-Monograph-2014.pdf (accessed June 8, 2021).

Phillips, A. and Lockwood, R. (2013). Investigating and prosecuting animal abuse. https://nationallinkcoalition.org/wp-content/uploads/2013/09/Investigating-Prosecuting-AA-Phillips-Lockwood.pdf (accessed 8 June 2021).

Zannin, A. (2021). Bloodstain pattern analysis. In: *Veterinary Forensics: Investigation, Evidence Collection, and Expert Testimony* (eds. E. Rogers and A.W. Stern), 73–108. London: CRC Press.

Case: Gunshot Wounds

Projectiles such as bullets, pellets, and BBs may be found in both living and deceased animal victims. Examination and analysis of evidence can provide information such as the type of weapon used, the distance and angle from which shots were fired, and whether an animal was advancing or retreating from the shooter when the incident occurred. Gunshot wounds must be examined carefully so that trace evidence, points of entry and exit, and path of trajectory are not altered. Full-body and specific imaging assists in identifying the location of projectiles in an animal's body and can determine if the projectile passed through. Imaging will also assist in revealing evidence of damage caused by projectiles including soft tissue, skeletal injury or old, healed fractures.

Documentation through photography, drawings, and the use of photo scales and trajectory rods helps illustrate findings. All projectiles and fragments must be collected and preserved as evidence when possible.

Investigators should search the crime scene for bullets and casings, weapons and blood spatter, or patterns that show the animal's movements during the incident. Crime lab analysis can prove helpful in these cases.

Investigator

Actions That Apply To All Cases
- ☐ Interview owner, witnesses, and neighbors
- ☐ Collect all relevant veterinary records
- ☐ Consider trying a pretext phone call to the suspect to get their version of events documented early on
- ☐ Preserve evidence: victim animals, records, photos, medication; see Appendix D for comprehensive evidence list
- ☐ Engage veterinarian to assist with examination of the evidence and the investigation
- ☐ Plan for live animal evidence holding and care
- ☐ Apply for a search warrant when appropriate
- ☐ Include diagnostic tests and collection of samples. See Appendix D for comprehensive evidence list
- ☐ Determine ownership status of victim animals and keep partnering agencies appraised of any changes to the status

Specific Case Actions
- ☐ Make a reward offer for people with information if you do not have a suspect
- ☐ Draw map of scene
- ☐ Video and photograph scene
- ☐ Search for blood spatter, bullet casings, and weapons
- ☐ Contact neighbors who may have heard or seen an incident
- ☐ Consider other vulnerable animals or people in the home

Questions
- ☐ Do suspect statements (self defense claims) match the veterinary findings?

Forms
- ☐ Animal Cruelty Consent to Search Form
- ☐ Animal Cruelty Case Relinquishment Form

□ Nonliving and Live Evidence Tracking Forms
□ Evidence Placard

Veterinarian

Actions That Apply To All Cases
□ Review all records related to the case
□ Ask the investigator questions that would further your assessment of the evidence presented to you
□ Exam ideally within 24 hours
□ Follow photography and forensic exam protocols
□ Complete written report
□ Complete full-body imaging or radiographs
□ Finalize diagnostic plan and create treatment and care plan
□ Determine who is the follow-up contact for supplemental case reports or emergency updates (typically this will be the investigator, law enforcement, or the prosecutor)

Specific Case Actions
□ Review map and any other evidence available from the scene
□ Follow up on medical progress and continue documentation

Specific Case Considerations
□ Determine whether findings align with the suspect's account of the incident
□ Determine whether knowledge and history of animal behavior reveal or contribute to assessment of how and why injuries resulted
□ If the animal dies or is deceased proceed with necropsy

Questions
□ Where was the animal found? Or how was it presented?
□ Is this a single- or multiple-animal incident?
□ Was veterinary care initiated and are records available?
□ Is permanent injury or death a result of this event?
□ Are any tissue samples or residue samples relevant to this case or diagnostic?

Forms
□ Necropsy Exam Notes Form
□ Veterinary Forensic Exam Form
□ Nonliving and Live Evidence Tracking Forms
□ Evidence Placard
□ Animal Cruelty Case Relinquishment Form
□ Summary Vet Report
□ Laboratory Submission Forms with chain of custody

Animal Care

Actions That Apply To All Cases
□ Confirm ownership status of victim animals
□ Maintain chain of custody of animal evidence in a secure location
□ Carry out veterinary treatment plan as directed

VICTIM TO VERDICT™

- ☐ Make sure you have the ability to provide the care necessary. If not, facilitate outside or referral care
- ☐ Create and post an emergency veterinary care plan and contact list
- ☐ Facilitate recheck appointments with the veterinarian
- ☐ Provide behavior support and training to live evidence animals
- ☐ Place animals in Protective Custody foster if appropriate
- ☐ Start tracking and documenting costs of care for individual animals on intake

Specific Case Actions
- ☐ Intake the animal(s) through standard intake procedures
- ☐ Implement Protective Custody secure housing and tracking for each animal
- ☐ Take intake photo series/video
- ☐ Administer treatments as directed by the veterinarian
- ☐ Facilitate recheck exams
- ☐ Provide enrichment
- ☐ Delivering and documenting treatment plan if in house

Specific Case Considerations
- ☐ If animal is deceased:
  - Maintain chain of custody of animal and associated evidence in a secure location
  - Freeze or refrigerate remains at the direction of the veterinarian
- ☐ Facilitate forensic necropsy

Questions
- ☐ Who is the current owner of the animal?
- ☐ Is there documentation of seizure or owner release?
- ☐ Is the suspect aware of where the animal is being held?

Forms
- ☐ Nonliving and Live Evidence Tracking Forms
- ☐ Animal Observation Chart
- ☐ Protective Custody Foster Care Agreement

Prosecutor

Actions that Apply to All Cases
- ☐ Request additional investigation, where appropriate, before declining to prosecute
- ☐ Consider long-term impact or permanent injury to the animal(s) when making charging decisions
- ☐ File a charge on each victim animal and/or each criminal incident – do not group victims/conduct into one count
- ☐ A condition of release should include no contact with victim animal or other animals as appropriate
- ☐ Pursue preconviction forfeiture without delay if the victim animal is alive and if the state has laws in place to do so
- ☐ Sign off on disposition of animal evidence when evidence collection is complete and ownership has been resolved
- ☐ Schedule pretrial meetings with veterinary expert and other witnesses
- ☐ Request continued medical discovery from veterinarian and/or animal care agency if necessary
- ☐ Request up-to-date amount of costs of care for animal care agency

Victim to Verdict™

Specific Case Actions

☐ Determine whether other criminal offenses have occurred (e.g. probation violation for firearm use, unlawful discharge of a firearm, coercion)

☐ File different charges as appropriate if the animal was permanently injured or killed

☐ Use the veterinarian to address defenses

Specific Case Considerations

☐ If the suspect was attempting to euthanize their animal, have the veterinarian testify to the pain and suffering that occurred

Questions

☐ If the animal is deceased, did the animal suffer and for how long?

Forms

☐ Example Forfeiture Hearing Checklist

☐ Forfeiture Petition Template

☐ Example Jury Instructions

☐ Forfeiture Order Template

Resources and References

Balkin, D., Blomquist, M., Bowman, S., et al. (2019). Animal cruelty issues: What juvenile and family court judges need to know. https://www.ncjfcj.org/wp-content/uploads/2019/07/NCJFCJ_ALDF_Animal-Cruelty-TAB_Final.pdf (accessed 8 June 2021).

Bradley-Siemens, N. (2020). Gunshot wounds and wound ballistics. In: *Veterinary Forensic Medicine and Forensic Sciences* (eds. J.H. Byrd, P. Norris and N. Bradley-Siemens), 157. London: CRC Press.

Colorado LINK Project (2013). The relevance of the link for prosecutors. https://coloradolinkproject.com/prosecutor-toolkit (accessed June 8, 2021).

Governor's Commission on the Humane Treatment of Animals (2020). Animal cruelty investigation and prosecution: A user manual for New Hampshire law enforcement. http://neacha.org/resources/animal-cruelty-manual-2020.pdf (accessed 8 June 2021).

Merck, M.D. and Miller, D.M. (2013). Burn-, electrical-, and fire-related injuries. In: *Veterinary Forensics: Animal Cruelty Investigations*, 2e (ed. M.D. Merck), 140–153. Hoboken, NJ: Wiley-Blackwell.

National Sheriff's Association (2019). *Sheriff & Deputy*: 2019 special issue animal cruelty. https://www.sheriffs.org/sites/default/files/2019_SD_AA.pdf (accessed 8 June 2021).

Phillips. A. (2014). Understanding the link between violence to animals and people. https://nationallinkcoalition.org/wp-content/uploads/2014/06/Allies-Link-Monograph-2014.pdf (accessed June 8, 2021).

Phillips, A. and Lockwood, R. (2013). Investigating and prosecuting animal abuse. https://nationallinkcoalition.org/wp-content/uploads/2013/09/Investigating-Prosecuting-AA-Phillips-Lockwood.pdf (accessed 8 June 2021).

Zannin, A. (2021). Bloodstain pattern analysis. In: *Veterinary Forensics: Investigation, Evidence Collection, and Expert Testimony* (eds. E. Rogers and A.W. Stern), 73–108. London: CRC Press.

Case: Mutilated or Skinned Animal

Reports of mutilated or skinned animals can send shockwaves through a community and garner considerable media attention. While mutilation can be attributed to intentional abuse by humans, absent a witness, the investigators and veterinarians will usually start by ruling out other causes of death, primarily predation or motor vehicle trauma. Coyotes, wolves, and cougars, as well as domestic dogs roaming singly or in packs, are known to track and kill companion animals and may not ingest all or even part of the remains. Scavenger animals including canids, raptors, opossum, rodents, birds, foxes, and raccoons may spread remains and further damage the body after the initial death, which may have been accidental. Livestock animals are also prey for coyotes, wolves, bears, and large cats, as well as animals who scavenge their remains.

The investigator can begin by thoroughly documenting the scene, taking photos of the body's position and proximity to the roadway, forested areas, and developed housing or businesses. Animal control agencies as well as departments of fish and wildlife may keep a record of coyote, large cat, or other predatory animal sightings, which can inform a conclusion. If owners or neighbors identify a suspect in the area who has harmed or threatened harm to neighborhood animals, these leads should be followed. Neighbors may also provide investigators access to property surveillance video that may have recorded the event or wildlife activity.

Small- to medium-sized companion animals may be found in a condition that leads one to believe the animal has been skinned, with large portions of dermis and fur over the back and sides seemingly removed by a sharp implement. Again, these cases are horrifying, and while they may be the work of an individual, certain raptors and other predators can inflict such large injuries when seizing and pulling at their prey with their teeth or talons. The veterinarian should examine the margins of these wounds carefully for evidence of cut hairs, which one would expect to find if the skin were removed by a blade or scissors. When the wound is a result of a pulling or tearing force, the absence of cut hairs along the margin can be confirmatory. Predator DNA may also be identified through laboratory testing.

When initially assessing and investigating an animal cruelty case where religion may be a factor (animal sacrifice, for example) – either with respect to the conduct or the reason for the conduct – law enforcement should focus their investigation on whether the elements of the animal cruelty statutes or other state and local laws (such as inhumane slaughter, public safety regulations, and zoning requirements) are being met. Investigators should focus on collecting the evidence related to the offense(s) and remain undeterred from carrying out their duties even if religion is implicated. It is the role of the prosecutor to assess the evidence and the laws to determine whether and how to proceed with the case.

Investigator

Actions that Apply to All Cases
- ☐ Interview owner, witnesses, and neighbors
- ☐ Collect all relevant veterinary records
- ☐ Consider trying a pretext phone call to the suspect to get their version of events documented early on
- ☐ Preserve evidence: records, photos, medication; see Appendix D for comprehensive evidence list
- ☐ Preserve the body as evidence. Do not freeze the body, if possible
- ☐ Request a forensic necropsy
- ☐ Engage veterinarian to assist with examination of the evidence and the investigation

☐ Apply for a search warrant when appropriate. Include diagnostic tests and collection of samples. See Appendix D for comprehensive evidence list

Specific Case Actions
☐ Record and review scene photos
☐ Coordinate with wildlife officials who have knowledge of predation and scavenging based on the region
☐ Search and document scene
☐ Collect remains
☐ Search for weapons (blunt and sharp force)
☐ Assess likelihood of surveillance video
☐ Check with wildlife services and animal control to confirm predator (coyote, fox, raptors, cougar) sightings in that area

Specific Case Considerations
☐ Explore the possibility of a domestic violence component
☐ Be prepared to respond to media inquiries

Questions
☐ Are there other vulnerable entities in the home?
☐ Can the veterinarian tell you what kind of implements to search for if you execute a warrant?
☐ Is there any religious or cult-related activity to consider?

Forms
☐ Animal Cruelty Consent to Search Form
☐ Animal Cruelty Case Relinquishment Form
☐ Nonliving and Live Evidence Tracking Forms
☐ Evidence Placard

Veterinarian

Actions that Apply to All Cases
☐ Review all records related to the case
☐ Ask the investigator questions that would further your assessment of the evidence presented to you
☐ Exam or necropsy ideally within 24 hours
☐ Follow photography and forensic necropsy protocols
☐ Full-body radiographs
☐ Collect samples for laboratory and pathology
☐ Complete written report

Specific Case Actions
☐ Victim may be alive with moderate to severe skin loss or deceased and presented for necropsy. Help define circumstances of an event based on discussion with the investigator
☐ Review scene photos
☐ Determine cause of death if possible – rule out the animal being hit by a car
☐ Look for hallmarks of predation: tooth marks on bones, removal of organs of small domestic animal (thorax) and abdomen, bowel intact with omentum mostly missing, patches of skin missing

VICTIM TO VERDICT™

□ Examine margins of skin tear for sharp, blunt, or tearing force trauma, collect a sample for histopath and save sample for DNA

Specific Case Considerations
□ Rule out predation and scavenger behaviors
□ Consider coyote or wolf attack if a large amount of skin is pulled from dorsum of animal
□ Sample collection from the victim and DNA analysis may link perpetrator to case

Questions
□ Where was the animal found?
□ Is this a single- or multiple-animal incident?
□ Was veterinary care initiated if deceased? If so are there records?

Forms
□ Necropsy Exam Notes Form
□ Veterinary Forensic Exam Form
□ Nonliving and Live Evidence Tracking Forms
□ Evidence Placard
□ Animal Cruelty Case Relinquishment Form
□ Summary Vet Report
□ Laboratory Submission Forms with chain of custody

Animal Care

Actions that Apply to All Cases
□ Maintain chain of custody of animal and associated evidence in a secure location
□ Freeze or refrigerate remains at the direction of the veterinarian
□ Facilitate forensic necropsy

Specific Case Considerations
□ Create a media plan

Questions
□ Is there documentation/paperwork transferring the custody of the animal?

Forms
□ Nonliving and Live Evidence Tracking Forms
□ Animal Observation Chart
□ Protective Custody Foster Care Agreement

Prosecutor

Actions that Apply to All Cases
□ Request additional investigation, where appropriate, before declining to prosecute
□ File a charge on each victim animal and/or each criminal incident; do not group victims/conduct into one count
□ A condition of release should include no contact with animals as appropriate
□ Sign off on disposition of animal evidence when evidence collection is complete and ownership has been resolved
□ Schedule pretrial meetings with veterinarian and other witnesses

Specific Case Considerations
□ Include counseling in sentencing.
□ Are there any relevant enhancements (i.e. domestic violence convictions or minors present)
□ Be prepared to respond to freedom of religion defenses

Forms
□ Example Forfeiture Hearing Checklist
□ Forfeiture Petition Template
□ Example Jury Instructions
□ Forfeiture Order Template

Resources and References

Balkin, D., Blomquist, M., Bowman, S., et al. (2019). Animal cruelty issues: What juvenile and family court judges need to know. https://www.ncjfcj.org/wp-content/uploads/2019/07/NCJFCJ_ALDF_Animal-Cruelty-TAB_Final.pdf (accessed 8 June 2021).

Doheny, S.L. (2006). Free exercise does not protect animal sacrifice: The misconception of *Church of Lukumi Babalu Aye v. City of Hialeah* and constitutional solutions for stopping animal sacrifice. *J. Animal L.* 2: 121.

Colorado LINK Project (2013). The relevance of the link for prosecutors. https://coloradolinkproject.com/prosecutor-toolkit (accessed June 8, 2021).

Governor's Commission on the Humane Treatment of Animals (2020). Animal cruelty investigation and prosecution: A user manual for New Hampshire law enforcement. http://neacha.org/resources/animal-cruelty-manual-2020.pdf (accessed 8 June 2021).

Levitt, L., Patronek, G., and Grisso, T. (eds.) (2015). *Animal Maltreatment: Forensic Mental Health Issues and Evaluations*. New York, NY: Oxford University Press.

Nation, P.N. and St Clair, C.C. (2019). A forensic pathology investigation of dismembered domestic cats: Coyotes or cults? *Vet Pathol* 56 (3): 444–451. https://journals.sagepub.com/doi/full/10.1177/0300985819827968.

National Sheriff's Association (2019). *Sheriff & Deputy*: 2019 special issue animal cruelty. https://www.sheriffs.org/sites/default/files/2019_SD_AA.pdf (accessed 8 June 2021).

Phillips. A. (2014). Understanding the link between violence to animals and people. https://nationallinkcoalition.org/wp-content/uploads/2014/06/Allies-Link-Monograph-2014.pdf (accessed June 8, 2021).

Phillips, A. and Lockwood, R. (2013). Investigating and prosecuting animal abuse. https://nationallinkcoalition.org/wp-content/uploads/2013/09/Investigating-Prosecuting-AA-Phillips-Lockwood.pdf (accessed 8 June 2021).

Webb, K.M. (2021). DNA evidence collection and analysis. In: *Veterinary Forensics: Investigation, Evidence Collection, and Expert Testimony* (eds. E. Rogers and A.W. Stern), 295–312. London: CRC Press.

Case: Burned Animal: Victim Dies

Burns may be caused by heat or fire (thermal burns), electricity, liquids (scalding wounds from boiling water), electromagnetic radiation (exposure to microwave ovens), or chemicals (acids or other corrosives). While an animal may be accidentally injured in some instances, other cases, such as an animal entrapped in an oven or burned multiple times by a cigarette, are more easily identified as malicious in intent.

In the case of a deceased animal, it is important that the veterinarian and investigator attempt to determine if the burn was inflicted before the animal died, if the burn was the primary cause of death, or if the burn occurred after the animal was deceased. Forensic necropsy should include examination for traumatic injury, determination and mapping of burn and traumatic injury patterns, as well as physical and radiologic examination for history of previous or recent skeletal injuries. Examination and histopathology of airway tissue and lungs can be helpful in determining if an animal died of smoke inhalation. Analysis of fur or skin samples may identify chemical compounds or accelerants. Specialized testing to determine cause and time of death may include blood for carboxyhemoglobin analysis.

Investigators should carefully examine the crime scene for chemicals, restraints, and accelerants such as lighter fluid or gasoline. In cases where the animal struggled against the suspect, the investigator might notice scratch or bite wounds on a suspect's face, arms, hands, and torso. Work directly with the examining veterinarian to formulate interview questions, consider the suspect's explanation of how the injuries occurred when compared to the necropsy findings, and plan next steps.

A11.1   Investigator

Actions that Apply to All Cases
- ☐ Interview owner, witnesses, and neighbors
- ☐ Collect all relevant veterinary records
- ☐ Consider trying a pretext phone call to the suspect to get their version of events documented early on
- ☐ Preserve evidence: records, photos, medication; see Appendix D for comprehensive evidence list
- ☐ Preserve the body as evidence. Do not freeze the body, if possible
- ☐ Request a forensic necropsy
- ☐ Engage veterinarian to assist with examination of the evidence and the investigation
- ☐ Apply for a search warrant when appropriate. Include diagnostic tests and collection of samples. See Appendix D for comprehensive evidence list

Specific Case Actions
- ☐ Document previous veterinary care
- ☐ Create a map of how/where found
- ☐ Take photos of scene
- ☐ Interview witness/suspects/firefighters
- ☐ Look for indication animal was restrained or confined

Specific Case Considerations
- ☐ Do not throw the body away
- ☐ Crime scene may be dangerous or impossible to examine due to fire damage
- ☐ Ask questions to understand if the fire was premeditated fire

Questions

☐ Are there other animals who may have escaped the fire?
☐ Is surveillance or other security video available?
☐ Are there other victims?
☐ Is there motivation for fire starting such as a domestic violence component?

Forms

☐ Nonliving Evidence Tracking Forms
☐ Evidence Placard
☐ Animal Cruelty Case Relinquishment Form
☐ Animal Cruelty Case Consent to Search Form

Veterinarian

Actions that Apply to All Cases

☐ Review all records related to the case
☐ Request and review previous medical history
☐ Necropsy ideally within 24 hours
☐ Perform full-body imaging
☐ Ask the investigator questions that would further your assessment of the evidence presented to you
☐ Follow photography and forensic necropsy protocols
☐ Collect samples for laboratory and pathology
☐ Complete written report

Specific Case Actions

☐ Submit blood samples for carbon monoxide (carboxyhemoglobin analysis)
☐ Collect hair samples for accelerant/chemical analysis
☐ Document the pain and fear involved with the manner of injury or death

Specific Case Considerations

☐ Create a media plan

Questions

☐ Was the animal alive before the fire or dead when the fire started?
☐ Was the fire the cause of death? Smoke inhalation and carbon monoxide poisoning vs. deceased before fire (gunshot or other cause)?
☐ Where was the animal found? Or how was it presented?
☐ Is this a single- or multiple-animal incident?
☐ Was veterinary care initiated if deceased? If so, are records accessible?
☐ Are specific chemicals or accelerants a consideration? If so, consider collecting fur/skin, tissue and proactive research crime laboratory or other laboratory availability.

Forms

☐ Necropsy Exam Form
☐ Laboratory Submission Forms with chain of custody
☐ Evidence Placard
☐ Veterinary Forensic Exam Report

Animal Care

Actions that Apply to All Cases
☐ Maintain chain of custody of animal and associated evidence in a secure location
☐ Freeze or refrigerate remains at the direction of the veterinarian
☐ Facilitate forensic necropsy

Questions
☐ Ask the veterinarian how to preserve burned remains

Forms
☐ Nonliving Evidence Tracking Forms
☐ Evidence Placard

Prosecutor

Actions that Apply to All Cases
☐ Request additional investigation, where appropriate, before declining to prosecute
☐ File a charge on each victim animal and/or each criminal incident – do not group victims/conduct into one count
☐ A condition of release should include no contact with animals as appropriate
☐ Sign off on disposition of animal evidence when evidence collection is complete and ownership has been resolved
☐ Schedule pretrial meetings with veterinarian and other witnesses

Specific Case Actions
☐ Show pictures and have the veterinarian testify to the suffering

Specific Case Considerations
☐ Evaluate the case file for other crimes: arson, domestic violence, assault/battery, intimidation/coercion, or fraud

Resources and References

Balkin, D., Blomquist, M., Bowman, S., et al. (2019). Animal cruelty issues: What juvenile and family court judges need to know. https://www.ncjfcj.org/wp-content/uploads/2019/07/NCJFCJ_ALDF_Animal-Cruelty-TAB_Final.pdf (accessed 8 June 2021).

Bradley-Siemens, N. (2020). Environmental and situational injuries/death. In: *Veterinary Forensic Medicine and Forensic Sciences* (eds. J.H. Byrd, P. Norris and N. Bradley-Siemens), 226–240. London: CRC Press.

Doheny, S.L. (2006). Free exercise does not protect animal sacrifice: The misconception of *Church of Lukumi Babalu Aye v. City of Hialeah* and constitutional solutions for stopping animal sacrifice. *J. Animal L.* 2: 121.

Governor's Commission on the Humane Treatment of Animals (2020). Animal cruelty investigation and prosecution: A user manual for New Hampshire law enforcement. http://neacha.org/resources/animal-cruelty-manual-2020.pdf (accessed 8 June 2021).

Merck, M.D. and Miller, D.M. (2013). Burn-, electrical-, and fire-related injuries. In: *Veterinary Forensics: Animal Cruelty Investigations*, 2e (ed. M.D. Merck), 139–159. Hoboken, NJ: Wiley-Blackwell.

National Sheriff's Association (2019). *Sheriff & Deputy*: 2019 special issue animal cruelty. https://www.sheriffs.org/sites/default/files/2019_SD_AA.pdf (accessed 8 June 2021).

Phillips, A. and Lockwood, R. (2013). Investigating and prosecuting animal abuse. https://nationallinkcoalition.org/wp-content/uploads/2013/09/Investigating-Prosecuting-AA-Phillips-Lockwood.pdf (accessed 8 June 2021).

Stern, A.W. and Sula, M.-J. (2021). Thermal injuries. In: *Veterinary Forensics: Investigation, Evidence Collection, and Expert Testimony* (eds. E. Rogers and A.W. Stern), 216–218. London: CRC Press.

Case: Burned Animal: Victim Lives

Burns may be caused by heat or fire (thermal burns), electricity, liquids (scalding wounds from boiling water), electromagnetic radiation (exposure to microwave ovens) or chemicals (acids or other corrosives). While an animal may be accidentally injured in some instances, other cases, such as an animal entrapped in an oven or burned multiple times by a cigarette, are more easily identified as malicious in intent.

Animals suffering from burn injuries may be discovered in critical condition or may appear relatively stable. Investigators and animal welfare professionals who encounter these animals must understand that tissue damage from burns may not appear serious at first when in fact the animal has experienced life-threatening burns, and internal injuries from burns – such as damage to airways or organs – may not be immediately recognizable. For these reasons, animals at the scene of a fire must always be presented for veterinary care immediately.

The animal should be stabilized and administered emergency care as a priority. The collection of evidence by the veterinarian will include physical exam findings, full-body radiographs, and examination for history of previous injury. Analysis of fur and skin swabs for chemical compounds and accelerants can be helpful in determining the cause of the burns.

Investigators should carefully examine the crime scene for chemicals, restraints, and accelerants such as lighter fluid or gasoline. In cases where the animal struggled against the suspect the investigator might notice scratch or bite wounds on a suspect's face, arms, hands, and torso. Work directly with the examining veterinarian to formulate interview questions, consider the suspect's explanation of how the injuries occurred when compared to the examination findings, and plan next steps.

Investigator

Actions That Apply To All Cases
- Interview owner, witnesses, and neighbors
- Collect all relevant veterinary records
- Consider trying a pretext phone call to the suspect to get their version of events documented early on
- Preserve evidence: victim animals, records, photos, medication; see Appendix D for comprehensive evidence list
- Engage veterinarian to assist with examination of the evidence and the investigation
- Plan for live animal evidence holding and care
- Apply for a search warrant when appropriate
- Include diagnostic tests and collection of samples. See Appendix D for comprehensive evidence list
- Determine ownership status of victim animals and keep partnering agencies apprised of any changes to the status

Specific Case Actions
- Interview witnesses and provide information to veterinarian prior to exam if possible
- Find previous veterinary records
- Consider looking for social media posts referencing the incident
- Include exam of the animal when authoring search warrant/affidavit
- Include lead veterinarian if you search the location of the incident

□ Take photos and video of the scene
□ Search for objects that may have been used to restrain animal or used as accelerants or combustibles

Questions
□ Are there vulnerable victims in the home?
□ Is there a domestic violence component?
□ Could there be other animals hiding who fled the area of the fire?

Forms
□ Animal Cruelty Consent to Search Form
□ Animal Cruelty Case Relinquishment Form
□ Nonliving and Live Evidence Tracking Forms
□ Evidence Placard

Veterinarian

Actions that Apply to All Cases
□ Review all records related to the case
□ Request and review previous medical history
□ Examine and begin treatment immediately
□ Ask the investigator questions that would further your assessment of the evidence presented to you
□ Follow photography and forensic exam protocols
□ Complete written report
□ Finalize diagnostic plan and create treatment and care plan
□ Determine who is the follow-up contact for supplemental case reports or emergency updates (typically this will be the investigator, law enforcement, or the prosecutor)

Specific Case Actions
□ Document age and type of burn, including scarring (repetitive injury)
□ Look for other evidence of cruelty (neglect or additional injuries/wounds)
□ Report on likelihood of permanent long-term damage
□ Review the map of the scene
□ If fire or smoke are involved look for other injuries (gunshot, trauma, repetitive injury)

Specific Case Considerations
□ Testify to the pain and fear likely involved
□ Consider full-body imaging or radiographs
□ If the victim does not survive, proceed to necropsy protocol

Questions
□ Where was the animal before the burns occurred?
□ How was the animal found?
□ Are specific chemicals or accelerants a consideration?
□ Where was the animal found? Or how was it presented?
□ Is this a single- or multiple-animal incident?
□ Was veterinary care initiated elsewhere?

VICTIM TO VERDICT™

Forms
- ☐ Veterinary Forensic Exam Form
- ☐ Nonliving and Live Evidence Tracking Forms
- ☐ Evidence Placard
- ☐ Animal Cruelty Case Relinquishment Form
- ☐ Summary Vet Report
- ☐ Laboratory Submission Forms with chain of custody

Animal Care

Actions That Apply To All Cases
- ☐ Confirm ownership status of victim animals
- ☐ Maintain chain of custody of animal evidence in a secure location
- ☐ Carry out veterinary treatment plan as directed
- ☐ Make sure you have the ability to provide the care necessary. If not, facilitate outside or referral care
- ☐ Create and post an emergency veterinary care plan and contact list
- ☐ Facilitate recheck appointments with the veterinarian
- ☐ Provide behavior support and training to live evidence animals
- ☐ Place animals in Protective Custody foster if appropriate
- ☐ Start tracking and documenting costs of care for individual animals on intake

Specific Case Actions
- ☐ Ensure that improvements to burn(s) are documented on regular basis (photograph and record)
- ☐ Administer treatment as directed by the veterinarian

Questions
- ☐ Can you provide the necessary care for a victim animal with these injuries? If not, facilitate outside or referral care

Forms
- ☐ Nonliving and Live Evidence Tracking Forms
- ☐ Animal Observation Chart
- ☐ Protective Custody Foster Care Agreement

Prosecutor

Actions that Apply to All Cases
- ☐ Request additional investigation, where appropriate, before declining to prosecute
- ☐ Consider long-term impact or permanent injury to the animal(s) when making charging decisions
- ☐ File a charge on each victim animal and/or each criminal incident – do not group victims/conduct into one count
- ☐ A condition of release should include no contact with victim animal or other animals as appropriate
- ☐ Pursue preconviction forfeiture without delay if the victim animal is alive and if the state has laws in place to do so
- ☐ Sign off on disposition of animal evidence when evidence collection is complete and ownership has been resolved

□ Schedule pretrial meetings with veterinarian and other witnesses

□ Request continued medical discovery from veterinarian and/or animal care agency if necessary

□ Request up-to-date amount of costs of care for animal care agency

Specific Case Actions

□ Look to the veterinary report during charging assessment

□ Consider multiple charges for various burns if veterinarian has aged them

□ Have the veterinarian testify to the pain and suffering, and how long it took the animal to heal

□ If the suspect took video of the burning, point out the enjoyment of the act

Specific Case Considerations

□ Include counseling as part of sentence

□ Consider whether evidence of recovery will be impactful or inspire leniency by the jury/judge

Forms

□ Example Forfeiture Hearing Checklist

□ Forfeiture Petition Template

□ Forfeiture Order Template

Resources and References

Balkin, D., Blomquist, M., Bowman, S., et al. (2019). Animal cruelty issues: What juvenile and family court judges need to know. https://www.ncjfcj.org/wp-content/uploads/2019/07/NCJFCJ_ALDF_Animal-Cruelty-TAB_Final.pdf (accessed 8 June 2021).

Bradley-Siemens, N. (2020). Environmental and situational injuries/death. In: *Veterinary Forensic Medicine and Forensic Sciences* (eds. J.H. Byrd, P. Norris and N. Bradley-Siemens), 226–240. London: CRC Press.

Colorado LINK Project (2013). The relevance of the link for prosecutors. https://coloradolinkproject.com/prosecutor-toolkit (accessed June 8, 2021).

Doheny, S.L. (2006). Free exercise does not protect animal sacrifice: The misconception of *Church of Lukumi Babalu Aye v. City of Hialeah* and constitutional solutions for stopping animal sacrifice. *J. Animal L.* 2: 121.

Governor's Commission on the Humane Treatment of Animals (2020). Animal cruelty investigation and prosecution: A user manual for New Hampshire law enforcement. http://neacha.org/resources/animal-cruelty-manual-2020.pdf (accessed 8 June 2021).

Merck, M.D. and Miller, D.M. (2013). Burn-, electrical-, and fire-related injuries. In: *Veterinary Forensics: Animal Cruelty Investigations*, 2e (ed. M.D. Merck), 139–159. Hoboken, NJ: Wiley-Blackwell.

National Sheriff's Association (2019). *Sheriff & Deputy*: 2019 special issue animal cruelty. https://www.sheriffs.org/sites/default/files/2019_SD_AA.pdf (accessed 8 June 2021).

Phillips. A. (2014). Understanding the link between violence to animals and people. https://nationallinkcoalition.org/wp-content/uploads/2014/06/Allies-Link-Monograph-2014.pdf (accessed June 8, 2021).

Phillips, A. and Lockwood, R. (2013). Investigating and prosecuting animal abuse. https://nationallinkcoalition.org/wp-content/uploads/2013/09/Investigating-Prosecuting-AA-Phillips-Lockwood.pdf (accessed 8 June 2021).

Stern, A.W. and Sula, M.-J. (2021). Thermal injuries. In: *Veterinary Forensics: Investigation, Evidence Collection, and Expert Testimony* (eds. E. Rogers and A.W. Stern), 216–218. London: CRC Press.

Case: Sexual Assault of An Animal

Animal sexual assault cases are complex, whether they involve one suspect and a single animal, or a group of perpetrators who engage in organized and highly secretive bestiality activities. Bestiality is often tied to the crimes of child pornography or pornography depicting the torture or killing of animals. If at any time investigators uncover evidence that the case involves multiple suspects or locations, enacting the assistance of state and federal agencies is prudent. The sexual abuse of animals may also be perpetrated to execute control and punishment in a domestic violence scenario.

Domestic dogs as well as livestock animals are the most common victims in these cases. Investigators should search the crime scene for evidence such as supplies and equipment used to restrain, train, record, and otherwise facilitate animal sexual abuse, as well as photo or video evidence or pornography. If a larger web of participants is suspected, seizure and examination of cell phones, computers, online web search and chat history, and search for use of encrypted sites should be initiated.

The veterinary exam is conducted in a similar manner to human sexual assault examinations. The veterinarian may consider consulting with a human health expert versed in diagnosing and documenting human sexual assault cases. Time is of the essence when searching for evidence of assault on and in the victim animal. Evidence may include restraint injuries, body fluids, and DNA.

Investigator

Actions that Apply to All Cases
☐ Interview owner, witnesses, and neighbors
☐ Collect all relevant veterinary records
☐ Consider trying a pretext phone call to the suspect to get their version of events documented early on
☐ Preserve evidence: victim animals, records, photos, medication; see Appendix D for comprehensive evidence list
☐ Engage veterinarian to assist with examination of the evidence and the investigation
☐ Plan for live animal evidence holding and care
☐ Apply for a search warrant when appropriate. Include diagnostic tests and collection of samples See Appendix D for comprehensive evidence list
☐ Determine ownership status of victim animals and keep partnering agencies apprised of any changes to the status

Specific Case Actions
☐ Arrange for immediate veterinary examination and diagnostics
☐ Coordinate multi-agency response if organized activity is suspected
☐ Search social media accounts
☐ Seize cell phone and computer to search for photos/videos

Specific Case Considerations
☐ Look for evidence such as restraints, ropes, stockades, or other equipment used to facilitate the abuse
☐ Observe suspects for signs of injury inflicted by victim animal such as scratch or bite marks on arms and hands

VICTIM TO VERDICT™

□ Look for any wounds or marks on neck, ears, or abdomen of the animal from restraint or ligatures

□ Consider searching chat rooms, forums, and social media for activity and admissions there

Questions

□ Are there other vulnerable entities at risk?

□ Who had access to the animal?

Forms

□ Animal Cruelty Consent to Search Form

□ Animal Cruelty Case Relinquishment Form

□ Nonliving and Live Evidence Tracking Forms

□ Evidence Placard

Veterinarian

Actions that Apply to All Cases

□ Review all records related to the case

□ Ask the investigator questions that would further your assessment of the evidence presented to you

□ Exam ideally within hours

□ Follow photography and forensic exam protocols

□ Complete written report

□ Finalize diagnostic plan and create treatment and care plan

□ Determine who is the follow-up contact for supplemental case reports or emergency updates (typically this will be the investigator, law enforcement, or the prosecutor)

Specific Case Actions

□ Collect fecal sample in all cases, and urine sample if the animal victim is female (screening for sperm or DNA of suspect)

□ Collect hair and buccal swab from animal for identification of DNA of the animal victim that may have transferred to the suspect

□ Assist by informing law enforcement of specific items to look for as evidence

□ Examine the animal's full body with an alternative light source, looking for body fluids, fibers, and hair

□ Collect samples using wet then dry sterile cotton swabs and package for testing

□ Conduct full-body imaging to look for other signs of abuse and specific injury to tail

□ Examine for other evidence of chronic and/or repetitive abuse

□ Examine tail area for injury due to restraint or pulling

□ Examine anal and perineal area for bruising or injury

□ Examine neck region carefully for injury or damage due to restraint

Specific Case Considerations

□ Evidence is time-sensitive and fragile

□ DNA testing for human traces: include swabs of lips (exterior and interior), tongue, perineal and genital areas, vagina, and rectum

□ Consider toxicology and drug analysis of blood and urine. Collect samples and consider looking for sedatives or anesthetic agents

VICTIM TO VERDICT™

Questions

□ Where was the animal found? Or how was it presented?

□ Is this a single- or multiple-animal incident?

□ Was veterinary care initiated if deceased? If so, are there records?

Forms

□ Necropsy Exam Notes Form

□ Veterinary Forensic Exam Form

□ Nonliving and Live Evidence Tracking Forms

□ Evidence Placard

□ Animal Cruelty Case Relinquishment Form

□ Summary Vet Report

□ Laboratory Submission Forms with chain of custody

Animal Care

Actions that Apply to All Cases

□ Confirm ownership status of victim animals

□ Maintain chain of custody of animal evidence in a secure location

□ Carry out veterinary treatment plan as directed

□ Make sure you have the ability to provide the care necessary. If not, facilitate outside or referral care

□ Create and post an emergency veterinary care plan and contact list

□ Facilitate recheck appointments with the veterinarian

□ Provide behavior support and training to live evidence animals

□ Place animals in protective custody foster if appropriate

□ Start tracking and documenting costs of care for individual animals on intake

Specific Case Considerations

□ Evaluation by a behaviorist may be useful to the investigation

□ Rename animal if s/he is made available for adoption

Questions

□ Is there documentation of seizure or owner release?

Forms

□ Nonliving and Live Evidence Tracking Forms

□ Animal Observation Chart

□ Protective Custody Foster Care Agreement

Prosecutor

Actions that Apply to All Cases

□ Request additional investigation, where appropriate, before declining to prosecute

□ Consider long-term impact or permanent injury to the animal(s) when making charging decisions

□ File a charge on each victim animal and/or each criminal incident – do not group victims/conduct into one count

□ A condition of release should include no contact with victim animal or other animals as appropriate

□ Pursue preconviction forfeiture without delay if the victim animal is alive and if the state has laws in place to do so

□ Sign off on disposition of animal evidence when evidence collection is complete and ownership has been resolved

VICTIM TO VERDICT™

□ Schedule pretrial meetings with veterinarian and other witnesses
□ Request continued medical discovery from veterinarian and/or animal care agency if necessary
□ Request up-to-date amount of costs of care for animal care agency

Specific Case Considerations
□ Include counseling as part of sentencing
□ Include possession ban in sentencing
□ If the conduct crossed state lines, consider the Preventing Animal Cruelty and Torture Act (PACT act)

Forms
□ Example Forfeiture Hearing Checklist
□ Forfeiture Petition Template
□ Example Jury Instructions
□ Forfeiture Order Template

Resources and References

Balkin, D., Blomquist, M., Bowman, S., et al. (2019). Animal cruelty issues: What juvenile and family court judges need to know. https://www.ncjfcj.org/wp-content/uploads/2019/07/NCJFCJ_ALDF_Animal-Cruelty-TAB_Final.pdf (accessed 8 June 2021).

Colorado LINK Project (2013). The relevance of the link for prosecutors. https://coloradolinkproject.com/prosecutor-toolkit (accessed June 8, 2021).

Doheny, S.L. (2006). Free exercise does not protect animal sacrifice: The misconception of *Church of Lukumi Babalu Aye v. City of Hialeah* and constitutional solutions for stopping animal sacrifice. *J. Animal L.* 2: 121.

Edwards, J.M. (2019). Arrest and prosecution of animal sex abuse (bestiality) offenders in the United States, 1975–2015. *J Am Acad Psychiatry Law.* 47 (3): 335–346.

Governor's Commission on the Humane Treatment of Animals (2020). Animal cruelty investigation and prosecution: A user manual for New Hampshire law enforcement. http://neacha.org/resources/animal-cruelty-manual-2020.pdf (accessed 8 June 2021).

IVFSA (2020). Veterinary forensic postmortem examination standards. https://www.ivfsa.org/wp-content/uploads/2020/12/IVFSA-Veterinary-Forensic-Postmortem-Exam-Standards_Approved-2020_with-authors.pdf (accessed August 7, 2021).

Merck, M.D. and Miller, D.M. (2013). *Sexual abuse.* In: *Veterinary Forensics: Animal Cruelty Investigations,* 2e (ed. M.D. Merck), 233–241. Hoboken, NJ: Wiley-Blackwell.

National Sheriff's Association (2019). *Sheriff & Deputy*: 2019 special issue animal cruelty. https://www.sheriffs.org/sites/default/files/2019_SD_AA.pdf (accessed 8 June 2021).

Phillips. A. (2014). Understanding the link between violence to animals and people. https://nationallinkcoalition.org/wp-content/uploads/2014/06/Allies-Link-Monograph-2014.pdf (accessed June 8, 2021).

Phillips, A. and Lockwood, R. (2013). Investigating and prosecuting animal abuse. https://nationallinkcoalition.org/wp-content/uploads/2013/09/Investigating-Prosecuting-AA-Phillips-Lockwood.pdf (accessed 8 June 2021).

Smith-Blackmore, M. and Bradley-Siemens, N. (2020). Animal sexual abuse. In: *Veterinary Forensic Medicine and Forensic Sciences* (eds. J.H. Byrd, P. Norris and N. Bradley-Siemens), 113–128. London: CRC Press.

Stern, A.W. and Smith-Blackmore, M. (2021). Animal sexual abuse. In: *Veterinary Forensics: Investigation, Evidence Collection, and Expert Testimony* (eds. E. Rogers and A.W. Stern), 349–362. London: CRC Press.

Case: Drowning

When investigators and veterinarians are presented with a deceased animal found in a body of water or with the appearance of having been submerged in water, it can be challenging to determine a definitive cause of death. While drowning is certainly one possibility, the animal may have died of hypothermia, or other causes before being submerged in or saturated with water.

Necropsy should include full-body radiographs to look for skeletal injuries. Physical examination should also include a search for bruising, strangulation and ligature wounds, shredded nails, and other signs of struggle, although when bodies are submerged in water for a period of time tissue changes may occur that can make these findings more difficult to visualize. During necropsy veterinarians may discover changes and edema in lung tissue, although some drowning cases do not show visible signs of water inhalation. Submit lung and other tissue samples for pathology.

Investigators should search the scene where the body was found and seize any materials that may have been used to restrain or contain an animal such as bags, crates, or ropes. Interviews with witnesses and a search for any available surveillance recordings of the area may prove helpful. Suspects may be found with bite or scratch wounds from the animal struggling during a drowning event.

Investigator

Actions that Apply to All Cases
- ☐ Interview owner, witnesses, and neighbors
- ☐ Collect all relevant veterinary records
- ☐ Consider trying a pretext phone call to the suspect to get their version of events documented early on
- ☐ Preserve evidence: records, photos, medication; see Appendix D for comprehensive evidence list
- ☐ Preserve the body as evidence. Do not freeze the body, if possible
- ☐ Request a forensic necropsy
- ☐ Engage veterinarian to assist with examination of the evidence and the investigation
- ☐ Apply for a search warrant when appropriate
- ☐ Include diagnostic tests and collection of samples
- ☐ See Appendix D for comprehensive evidence list

Specific Case Actions
- ☐ Provide details to the veterinarian regarding how the animal was found
- ☐ Look for claw marks on the suspect that would occur during a struggle
- ☐ Determine if there was any veterinary care prior to death

Specific Case Considerations
- ☐ Investigate whether other implements were used in the commission of the drowning (crates, leashes, etc.) – be sure to seize those as evidence
- ☐ Note characteristics of the environment and the water characteristics such as temperature and movement

Questions
- ☐ Is there any surveillance footage that might have recorded the incident?
- ☐ Do the suspect's social media accounts provide information about the incident or events leading up to the incident and who may have been a witness?

VICTIM TO VERDICT™

Forms
- ☐ Nonliving Evidence Tracking Forms
- ☐ Evidence Placard
- ☐ Animal Cruelty Case Relinquishment Form
- ☐ Animal Cruelty Case Consent to Search Form

Veterinarian

Actions that Apply to All Cases
- ☐ Review all records related to the case
- ☐ Ask the investigator questions that would further your assessment of the evidence presented to you
- ☐ Necropsy ideally within 24 hours
- ☐ Follow photography and forensic necropsy protocols
- ☐ Perform full-body radiographs
- ☐ Collect samples for pathology
- ☐ Complete written report
- ☐ Determine who is the follow-up contact for supplemental case reports or emergency updates (typically this will be the investigator, law enforcement, or the prosecutor)

Specific Case Actions
- ☐ Avoid freezing body if possible
- ☐ Photograph animal and document any visible injury or abnormality
- ☐ Collect samples (lungs, heart, liver, kidney, other) for histopathology to rule out other causes of death and confirm drowning
- ☐ Request or create a map of the scene

Specific Case Considerations
- ☐ Document the pain and fear likely involved
- ☐ Document the time it would take for an animal to drown based on the evidence reviewed

Questions
- ☐ Was the animal dead before it was submerged in water?
- ☐ Where was the animal found? Or how was it presented?
- ☐ Is this a single- or multiple-animal incident?
- ☐ Was veterinary care initiated if deceased? If so, are there records?

Forms
- ☐ Necropsy Exam Notes Form
- ☐ Nonliving and Live Evidence Tracking Form
- ☐ Evidence Placard
- ☐ Summary Vet Report
- ☐ Laboratory Submission Forms and chain of custody

Animal Care

Actions that Apply to All Cases
- ☐ Maintain chain of custody of animal and associated evidence in a secure location
- ☐ Freeze or refrigerate remains at the direction of the veterinarian
- ☐ Facilitate forensic necropsy

VICTIM TO VERDICT™

Specific Case Actions

☐ Preserve the remains as evidence and maintain chain of custody

Specific Case Considerations

☐ Confirm that location of remains is secure

Forms

☐ Nonliving Evidence Tracking Forms
☐ Evidence Placard

Prosecutor

Actions That Apply To All Cases

☐ Request additional investigation, where appropriate, before declining to prosecute
☐ File a charge on each victim animal and/or each criminal incident – do not group victims/conduct into one count
☐ A condition of release should include no contact with animals as appropriate
☐ Sign off on disposition of animal evidence when evidence collection is complete and ownership has been resolved
☐ Schedule pretrial meetings with veterinarian and other witnesses

Specific Case Actions

☐ Use circumstantial evidence to prove the drowning if necessary
☐ Review veterinary records for any admissions to the veterinarian
☐ Consult with the veterinarian on whether circumstantial evidence is consistent with drowning

Specific Case Considerations

☐ Include restriction from possessing animals as a condition of release
☐ Include counseling as component of sentencing

Resources and References

Balkin, D., Blomquist, M., Bowman, S., et al. (2019). Animal cruelty issues: What juvenile and family court judges need to know. https://www.ncjfcj.org/wp-content/uploads/2019/07/NCJFCJ_ALDF_Animal-Cruelty-TAB_Final.pdf (accessed 8 June 2021).

Bradley-Siemens, N. (2020). Environmental and situational injuries/death. In: *Veterinary Forensic Medicine and Forensic Sciences* (eds. J.H. Byrd, P. Norris and N. Bradley-Siemens), 226–240. London: CRC Press.

Colorado LINK Project (2013). The relevance of the link for prosecutors. https://coloradolinkproject.com/prosecutor-toolkit (accessed June 8, 2021).

Governor's Commission on the Humane Treatment of Animals (2020). Animal cruelty investigation and prosecution: A user manual for New Hampshire law enforcement. http://neacha.org/resources/animal-cruelty-manual-2020.pdf (accessed 8 June 2021).

Merck, M.D. and Miller, D.M. (2013). Drowning. In: *Veterinary Forensics: Animal Cruelty Investigations*, 2e, vol. 178 (ed. M.D. Merck). Hoboken, NJ: Wiley-Blackwell.

National Sheriff's Association (2019). *Sheriff & Deputy*: 2019 special issue animal cruelty. https://www.sheriffs.org/sites/default/files/2019_SD_AA.pdf (accessed 8 June 2021).

Phillips. A. (2014). Understanding the link between violence to animals and people. https://nationallinkcoalition.org/wp-content/uploads/2014/06/Allies-Link-Monograph-2014.pdf (accessed June 8, 2021).

Phillips, A. and Lockwood, R. (2013). Investigating and prosecuting animal abuse. https://nationallinkcoalition.org/wp-content/uploads/2013/09/Investigating-Prosecuting-AA-Phillips-Lockwood.pdf (accessed 8 June 2021).

Case: Poisoning

Cases of accidental poisoning occur when an animal ingests a toxin such as rodenticide, slug bait, herbicides, pharmaceuticals, illegal drugs, algae, or poisonous plant material, or when an animal ingests a rodent that has been poisoned. Intentional poisoning events may be predated by neighbor disputes over noisy dogs or animals trespassing, and there may be a history of complaints on file with animal control or other agencies.

Antifreeze (ethylene glycol) is well known to be toxic to animals and readily available, so it may be identified in cases of intentional poisoning. Rodenticides are also readily available and may be hidden in or combined with meat or canned food left as bait for dogs or cats to ingest. Investigators should search areas accessible to the animal for any bait or treats that contain evidence of toxic substances and for any rodent bait stations or bodies of rodents that the animal may have accessed.

Some infectious diseases of cats and dogs such as parvovirus, panleukopenia, or fresh fish disease may be mistaken for poisoning, so it is prudent to review the pet's vaccination history and status, and request a veterinarian to rule out infectious disease during the exam or necropsy. Toxicology tests are specific and helpful when determining what type of toxin an animal ingested, but testing may require narrowing the list of suspected toxins, thus rule-outs are very important in these cases prior to submitting samples.

Investigator

Actions that Apply to All Cases
- ☐ Interview owner, witnesses, and neighbors
- ☐ Collect all relevant veterinary records
- ☐ Consider trying a pretext phone call to the suspect to get their version of events documented early on
- ☐ Preserve evidence: victim animals, records, photos, medication; see Appendix D for comprehensive evidence list
- ☐ Engage veterinarian to assist with examination of the evidence and the investigation
- ☐ Plan for live animal evidence holding and care
- ☐ Apply for a search warrant when appropriate. Include diagnostic tests and collection of samples. See Appendix D for comprehensive evidence list
- ☐ Determine ownership status of victim animals and keep partnering agencies apprised of any changes to the status

Specific Case Actions
- ☐ Take photos of the area where the poisoning occurred to show the veterinarian
- ☐ Search online neighborhood groups (like Nextdoor) if poisoning happened at a park
- ☐ Rule out accidental poisoning
- ☐ Collect unusual food or treats found in the area
- ☐ Interview neighbors
- ☐ Look for surveillance cameras that may have captured relevant video of the incident

Specific Case Considerations
- ☐ Investigate whether there is a domestic violence component to the situation (i.e. was the animal poisoned as a means of control or coercion?)
- ☐ Garbage pulls may uncover the poison that was used

VICTIM TO VERDICT™

Questions

☐ Any prior unusual events such as arguments with a neighbor, or complaints about animal barking or trespassing?

☐ Any problems in the area with rats or rodents such that a neighbor or other could be utilizing rodenticide for pest control in the surrounding area?

☐ Any dead rodents or wildlife found in recent days?

☐ Any history of other pets poisoned in the neighborhood?

☐ Is the pet up to date on all vaccines?

☐ Any exposure to or ingestion of raw fish?

Forms

☐ Animal Cruelty Consent to Search Form

☐ Animal Cruelty Case Relinquishment Form

☐ Nonliving and Live Evidence Tracking Forms

☐ Evidence Placard

Veterinarian

Actions that Apply to All Cases

☐ Review all records related to the case

☐ Ask the investigator questions that would further your assessment of the evidence presented to you

☐ Veterinarian should examine immediately

☐ Follow photography and forensic exam protocols

☐ Complete written report

☐ Finalize diagnostic plan and create treatment and care plan

☐ Determine who is the follow-up contact for supplemental case reports or emergency updates (typically this will be the investigator, law enforcement, or the prosecutor)

Specific Case Actions

☐ Collect samples from live animals: feces, blood, stomach contents (via vomit), serum or plasma, and hair

☐ Complete diagnostics with a broad to narrow diagnosis plan: complete blood count, serum chemistry, urinalysis, and fecal

☐ Help define circumstances of the event based on discussion with the investigator

☐ Perform full-body imaging if warranted

☐ Rule out other causes of death (trauma, disease)

☐ Collect specimens during necropsy: liver, kidney, urine, stomach, small and large bowel contents

☐ Preserve fresh samples for toxicology in refrigeration until testing is narrowed. The lab will direct whether to freeze and how to transport

Questions

☐ Where was the animal found?

☐ Is this a single- or multiple-animal incident?

☐ Was veterinary care initiated if deceased? If so, are there records?

Forms

☐ Necropsy Exam Notes Form

☐ Veterinary Forensic Exam Form

VICTIM TO VERDICT™

- ☐ Nonliving and Live Evidence Tracking Forms
- ☐ Evidence Placard
- ☐ Animal Cruelty Case Relinquishment Form
- ☐ Summary Vet Report
- ☐ Laboratory Submission Forms with chain of custody

Animal Care

Actions that Apply to All Cases

- ☐ Confirm ownership status of victim animals
- ☐ Maintain chain of custody of animal evidence in a secure location
- ☐ Carry out veterinary treatment plan as directed
- ☐ Make sure you have the ability to provide the care necessary. If not, facilitate outside or referral care
- ☐ Create and post an emergency veterinary care plan and contact list
- ☐ Facilitate recheck appointments with the veterinarian
- ☐ Provide behavior support and training to live evidence animals
- ☐ Place animals in Protective Custody foster if appropriate
- ☐ Start tracking and documenting costs of care for individual animals on intake

Specific Case Actions

- ☐ Document improvements and condition

Questions

- ☐ Are there restrictions on feeding?

Forms

- ☐ Nonliving and Live Evidence Tracking Forms
- ☐ Animal Observation Chart
- ☐ Protective Custody Foster Care Agreement

Prosecutor

Actions that Apply to All Cases

- ☐ Request additional investigation, where appropriate, before declining to prosecute
- ☐ Consider long-term impact or permanent injury to the animal(s) when making charging decisions
- ☐ File a charge on each victim animal and/or each criminal incident – do not group victims/conduct into one count.
- ☐ A condition of release should include no contact with victim animal or other animals as appropriate
- ☐ Pursue preconviction forfeiture without delay if the victim animal is alive and if the state has laws in place to do so
- ☐ Sign off on disposition of animal evidence when evidence collection is complete and ownership has been resolved
- ☐ Schedule pretrial meetings with veterinarian and other witnesses
- ☐ Request continued medical discovery from veterinarian and/or animal care agency if necessary
- ☐ Request up-to-date amount of costs of care for animal care agency

Forms

☐ Example Forfeiture Hearing Checklist
☐ Forfeiture Petition Template
☐ Example Jury Instructions
☐ Forfeiture Order Template

Resources and References

Toxicology https://www.vet.cornell.edu/animal-health-diagnostic-center/laboratories/toxicology, https://pubmed.ncbi.nlm.nih.gov/27090769/, https://journals.sagepub.com/doi/full/10.1177/0300985816641994 (all accessed August 27, 2021)

Algae poisoning https://vcahospitals.com/know-your-pet/algae-poisoning (accessed August 27, 2021)

Salmon poisoning https://vcahospitals.com/know-your-pet/salmon-poisoning (accessed August 27, 2021)

Drug toxicity in animals https://www.merckvetmanual.com/toxicology/toxicities-from-human-drugs/toxicities-from-illicit-and-abused-drugs (accessed August 27, 2021)

Governor's Commission on the Humane Treatment of Animals (2020). Animal cruelty investigation and prosecution: A user manual for New Hampshire law enforcement. http://neacha.org/resources/animal-cruelty-manual-2020.pdf (accessed 8 June 2021).

National Sheriff's Association (2019). *Sheriff & Deputy*: 2019 special issue animal cruelty. https://www.sheriffs.org/sites/default/files/2019_SD_AA.pdf (accessed 8 June 2021).

Phillips, A. and Lockwood, R. (2013). Investigating and prosecuting animal abuse. https://nationallinkcoalition.org/wp-content/uploads/2013/09/Investigating-Prosecuting-AA-Phillips-Lockwood.pdf (accessed 8 June 2021).

Case: Heat Stroke/Hyperthermia

Hyperthermia occurs when an animal's body temperature rises to a level such that it cannot be lowered by its own physiological temperature-regulating mechanisms. Animals, dogs most frequently, left in parked cars are particularly susceptible to heat stroke and likely the most common scenario in which severe injury or death occurs as a result. The temperature inside a vehicle can rise as fast as 20° Fahrenheit every 10 minutes, creating a medical emergency for the animal. In some cases this emergency is a result of a mistake or lack of accurate judgment about how the temperature can change, and in others it is a result of unreasonable and reckless behavior; either may result in tragedy for the animal.

Signs of heat stroke include nonresponsiveness or hyperactivity, shaking or seizing, heavy panting, and brick-red gums. The priority in these cases must be to remove the animal from the hot environment and begin efforts to lower the body temperature by covering the animal with a wet towel and applying cool (not cold) water to the abdominal area and feet while preparing for and transporting to emergency veterinary services if immediate improvement is not seen or the animal is nonresponsive. Allow the animal to drink if it is able. Many times the owner is unavailable and so emergency access to the animal is required.

In addition to providing emergency first aid to the animal, investigators should attempt to record the temperature inside the vehicle when the animal was removed, as well as make note of National Weather Service records of the temperature on that date and time. Gather witness information for later contact when time allows. In the case of a deceased animal, care should be taken to photograph the scene as evidence. These cases present an emergency situation such that law enforcement should be able to render aid and seize the animal. Additionally, many states have laws permitting intervention by citizens as well as law enforcement on behalf of an animal suffering in a hot vehicle (https://aldf.org/project/an-avoidable-tragedy-dogs-in-hot-cars/).

Animals confined or tied outdoors without shade or indoors without ventilation are at risk of heat stroke. Livestock and horses that have been overexercised on hot days and not cooled and watered properly may experience heat-related emergencies. Animals in poor condition, overweight animals, and those with heavy fur coats are more susceptible to overheating, as are short-nosed dog breeds such as bulldogs and pugs.

Heat stroke is life threatening and can cause permanent organ and brain damage in animals that do survive. These cases require swift veterinary response for the animal and benefit from a veterinarian's reporting and testimony at trial to explain the mechanisms of heat stroke and the risk to the animal.

Investigator

Actions that Apply to All Cases
- ☐ Interview owner, witnesses, and neighbors
- ☐ Collect all relevant veterinary records
- ☐ Consider trying a pretext phone call to the suspect to get their version of events documented early on
- ☐ Preserve evidence: victim animals, records, photos, medication; see Appendix D for comprehensive evidence list
- ☐ Engage veterinary expertise to assist with examination of the evidence and investigation
- ☐ Plan for live animal evidence holding and care
- ☐ Apply for a search warrant when appropriate. Include diagnostic tests and collection of samples. See Appendix D for comprehensive evidence list.
- ☐ Determine ownership status of victim animals and keep partnering agencies apprised of any changes to the status

Specific Case Actions

- ☐ Provide immediate first aid to the animal. Begin efforts to lower body temp on scene – apply water blankets, soak foot pads, etc.
- ☐ Call ahead to veterinary clinic so they can be ready to provide emergency care
- ☐ Transport for care
- ☐ Document the conditions and relay those to the veterinarian
- ☐ Record temperature inside vehicle or weather at scene
- ☐ Collect witness information for later interview
- ☐ Research weather, date, time, location of event. Use reliable weather sources
- ☐ Interview witnesses regarding how long the animal was subjected to the conditions when time allows

Questions

- ☐ What conditions led to the emergency? Locked in hot car with windows up, tied outside without shade?
- ☐ Did the vehicle have a mechanism for cooling that malfunctioned?

Forms

- ☐ Animal Cruelty Consent to Search Form
- ☐ Animal Cruelty Case Relinquishment Form
- ☐ Nonliving and Live Evidence Tracking Forms
- ☐ Evidence Placard

A16.2 Veterinarian

Actions that Apply to All Cases

- ☐ Review all records related to the case
- ☐ Ask the investigator questions that would further your assessment of the evidence presented to you
- ☐ Exam ideally within 24 hours
- ☐ Follow photography and forensic exam protocols
- ☐ Complete written report
- ☐ Finalize diagnostic plan and create treatment and care plan
- ☐ Determine who is the follow-up contact for supplemental case reports or emergency updates (typically this will be the investigator, law enforcement, or the prosecutor)

Specific Case Actions

- ☐ Initiate emergency care for hyperthermia if animal is alive
- ☐ Document specific necropsy characteristics: rigor, generalized autolysis of tissues, petechiae of skin, internal organs, and abdominal cavity
- ☐ Examine animal and records for previous/chronic injuries or pattern of injuries
- ☐ Collect samples for pathology – heart, lung, kidney, and others as needed
- ☐ Use "hot car calculator," available online, to approximate time in heated environment to cause injury or stroke

Specific Case Considerations

- ☐ If animal survives, document any lasting impact of incident (brain damage, chronic seizures, etc.)
- ☐ Define the circumstances of the events based on questions and the reports/records

Questions

- ☐ Where was the animal found?
- ☐ Is this a single- or multiple-animal incident?
- ☐ What was the ambient temperature at the time?
- ☐ Was veterinary care initiated if deceased? If so, are there records?
- ☐ Do physical exam or necropsy findings conclude heat exhaustion or stroke? Rule out other causes

Forms

- ☐ Necropsy Exam Notes Form
- ☐ Veterinary Forensic Exam Form
- ☐ Nonliving and Live Evidence Tracking Forms
- ☐ Evidence Placard
- ☐ Animal Cruelty Case Relinquishment Form
- ☐ Summary Vet Report
- ☐ Laboratory Submission Forms with chain of custody

Animal Care

Actions that Apply to All Cases

- ☐ Confirm ownership status of victim animals
- ☐ Maintain chain of custody of animal evidence in a secure location
- ☐ Carry out veterinary treatment plan as directed
- ☐ Make sure you have the ability to provide the care necessary. If not, facilitate outside or referral care
- ☐ Create and post an emergency veterinary care plan and contact list
- ☐ Facilitate recheck appointments with the veterinarian
- ☐ Provide behavior support and training to live evidence animals
- ☐ Place animals in Protective Custody foster if appropriate
- ☐ Start tracking and documenting costs of care for individual animals on intake

Questions

- ☐ Is there documentation of seizure or owner release?

Forms

- ☐ Nonliving and Live Evidence Tracking Forms
- ☐ Animal Observation Chart
- ☐ Protective Custody Foster Care Agreement

Prosecutor

Actions that Apply to All Cases

- ☐ Request additional investigation, where appropriate, before declining to prosecute
- ☐ Consider long-term impact or permanent injury to the animal(s) when making charging decisions
- ☐ File a charge on each victim animal and/or each criminal incident – do not group victims/conduct into one count
- ☐ A condition of release should include no contact with victim animal or other animals as appropriate
- ☐ Pursue preconviction forfeiture without delay if the victim animal is alive and if the state has laws in place to do so

☐ Sign off on disposition of animal evidence when evidence collection is complete and ownership has been resolved

☐ Schedule pretrial meetings with veterinary expert and other witnesses

☐ Request continued medical discovery from veterinarian and/or animal care agency if necessary

☐ Request up-to-date amount of costs of care for animal care agency

Specific Case Actions

☐ Use the veterinarian to discuss timeline and pain related to the incident

Specific Case Considerations

☐ Does the mental state of the offender meet the statutory requirements?

☐ Confirm whether the surviving victim animal suffered long-term permanent damage and charge accordingly

Forms

☐ Example Forfeiture Hearing Checklist

☐ Forfeiture Petition Template

☐ Example Jury Instructions

☐ Forfeiture Order Template

Estimated vehicle interior air temperature vs. elapsed time

	Outside air temperature (°F)					
Elapsed time	**70**	**75**	**80**	**85**	**90**	**95**
0 min	70	75	80	85	90	95
10 min	89	94	99	104	109	114
20 min	99	104	109	114	119	124
30 min	104	109	114	119	124	129
40 min	108	113	118	123	128	133
50 min	111	116	121	126	131	136
60 min	113	118	123	128	133	138
>1h	115	120	125	130	135	140

American Veterinary Medical Association. Pets in vehicles. https://www.avma.org/resources-tools/pet-care/pets-vehicles (accessed August 27, 2021).

Resources and References

American Veterinary Medical Association. Pets in vehicles. https://www.avma.org/resources-tools/pet-owners/petcare/pets-vehicles (accessed August 27, 2021).

Animal Legal Defense Fund (2018). Please don't leave me in the car. https://aldf.org/wp-content/uploads/2018/07/FLYER_Dog-in-hot-car.pdf (accessed August 27, 2021).

Governor's Commission on the Humane Treatment of Animals (2020). Animal cruelty investigation and prosecution: A user manual for New Hampshire law enforcement. http://neacha.org/resources/animal-cruelty-manual-2020.pdf (accessed 8 June 2021).

Merck, M.D., Miller, D.M., and Reisman, R.W. (2013). Heat stroke. In: *Veterinary Forensics: Animal Cruelty Investigations*, 2e, vol. 218 (ed. M.D. Merck). Hoboken, NJ: Wiley-Blackwell.

National Sheriff's Association (2019). *Sheriff & Deputy*: 2019 special issue animal cruelty. https://www.sheriffs.org/sites/default/files/2019_SD_AA.pdf (accessed 8 June 2021).

Phillips, A. and Lockwood, R. (2013). Investigating and prosecuting animal abuse. https://nationallinkcoalition.org/wp-content/uploads/2013/09/Investigating-Prosecuting-AA-Phillips-Lockwood.pdf (accessed 8 June 2021).

Case: Cockfighting

Cockfighting is illegal in all 50 states and the District of Columbia. In many states cockfighting is a felony and additional laws criminalize the possession of cockfighting paraphernalia or attending cockfights as a spectator. Federal laws also apply in these cases, as buying, selling, exhibiting, and shipping fighting birds is considered a misdemeanor offense under a 2002 amendment to the Animal Welfare Act of 1996.

Considered a "blood sport," trained roosters fight to the death in high-stakes matches called "derbies." During these well-organized and highly secretive events, spectators and cockfighters wager up to thousands of dollars on the matches in which birds are outfitted with 3-in. blades called "gaffs" strapped to their legs. Cockfighting roosters are conditioned for matches, and are often injected with testosterone and other steroids to enhance their performance. Their combs and wattles are removed for fighting. Cockfighting is almost always associated with other serious crimes such as gambling, drug distribution, gang activity, and human trafficking.

Cockfighting cases are challenging due to the number of birds involved as well as the lengths individuals participating in the cruel sport will go to keep their activities (both fighting and keeping of birds) secret. Cases require a multi-agency approach and should include federal, state, and local law enforcement response. Cases may include multiple suspects and several locations where birds are kept, conditioned, and fought.

Most animal shelters are not equipped to house the type and number of birds seized in cockfighting cases, thought must be given to the construction and staffing of secure and humane Protective Custody holding facilities. Birds must be housed individually and should undergo behavioral evaluation to determine if they can safely be introduced into home chicken flocks or sanctuaries upon release from evidence. Some states allow for fighting roosters to be "seized in place" which may be the only viable option when faced with a case involving hundreds of birds.

Investigator

Actions that Apply to All Cases
- ☐ Interview owner, witnesses, and neighbors
- ☐ Collect all relevant veterinary records
- ☐ Consider trying a pretext phone call to the suspect to get their version of events documented early on
- ☐ Preserve evidence: victim animals, records, photos, medication; see Appendix D for comprehensive evidence list
- ☐ Engage veterinarian to assist with examination of the evidence and the investigation
- ☐ Plan for live animal evidence holding and care
- ☐ Apply for a search warrant when appropriate. Include diagnostic tests and collection of samples. See Appendix D for comprehensive evidence list
- ☐ Determine ownership status of victim animals and keep partnering agencies apprised of any changes to the status

Specific Case Actions
- ☐ Secure a facility for holding birds
- ☐ Request and/or coordinate multi-agency response
- ☐ Create a search and seizure plan
- ☐ Set up and supervise on scene animal count

□ Research social media and enthusiast websites/chat rooms for history of breeding, selling, buying
□ Do a full financial investigation to show how invested the suspect is in the ongoing enterprise
□ Identify fighting birds by physical alterations, housing set-up
□ Identify training and treating equipment as well as evidence of breeding, fighting, altering, selling, and transporting birds
□ Map of scene, photograph enclosures with birds in place as well as evidence in place
□ Search for records of sales, supply receipts, match rosters, magazines, photos, and classified ads
□ Look for other victim animals at the location (dogs, other livestock, etc.)
□ Interview neighbors about activity at the scene

Specific Case Considerations
□ Physical hazards, personal protective equipment (PPE), handling equipment
□ May require translator for interviewing suspects or witnesses
□ Guard dogs, weapons, security fencing, etc.
□ Be aware of other criminal activity
□ Document deceased birds
□ Be prepared to respond to the excuse that the birds are showing roosters not fighting roosters
□ Animal care agency will need advance notice to adequately prepare to assist
□ Consider surveillance of fighting events

Questions
□ What does your state criminalize? Is the possession of the fighting paraphernalia a crime? Is attending a cockfight a crime?
□ Is there a federal agency that might be conducting an undercover investigation?
□ Is this location the primary location or part of a bigger ring?
□ Will you be able to seize nonfighting birds (i.e. the hens/chicks)?
□ Is seizing in place an option and what would that look like and is it safe?

Forms
□ Search Warrant Example
□ List of Evidence to Search and Seize

Veterinarian

Actions that Apply to All Cases
□ Review all records related to the case
□ Exam or evidence collection within 24 hours
□ Follow photography and forensic exam protocols
□ Complete written report
□ Finalize diagnostic plan and create treatment and care plan
□ Determine who is the follow-up contact for supplemental case reports or emergency updates (typically this will be the investigator, law enforcement, or the prosecutor)

Specific Case Actions
□ Provide information to law enforcement during service of search warrant regarding conditions of birds and nature of evidence found on scene (steroids, antibiotics, and fighting equipment such as muffs and gaffs)
□ Exam and photography of birds

VICTIM TO VERDICT™

□ Set up treatment and care plan for population
□ Determine the process for euthanasia if required

Specific Case Considerations
□ Consider zoonotic diseases and take precautions accordingly
□ Coordinate with state and federal authorities (Department of Agriculture, Department of Public Health) who may have jurisdiction and guidance related to poultry such as influenza testing, euthanasia, or other specific requirements.

Questions
□ What other agencies are involved and who is in charge of the scene?

Forms
□ Fighting Bird Exam Form
□ Evidence Placard
□ Veterinary Forensics Report
□ Summary Vet Report
□ Laboratory Submission Forms with chain of custody

Animal Care

Actions that Apply to All Cases
□ Confirm ownership status of victim animals
□ Maintain chain of custody of animal evidence in a secure location
□ Carry out veterinary treatment plan as directed
□ Make sure you have the ability to provide the care necessary. If not, facilitate outside or referral care
□ Create and post an emergency veterinary care plan and contact list
□ Facilitate recheck appointments with the veterinarian
□ Provide behavior support and training to live evidence animals
□ Place animals in Protective Custody foster if appropriate
□ Start tracking and documenting costs of care for individual animals on intake

Specific Case Actions
□ Assist with safe animal capture and transport from the scene
□ Assist with documentation of the scene
□ Assist with taking a photo of every animal before it leaves the scene
□ Assist with uniquely identifying each animal and attaching that unique identifier to the animal for future reference
□ Maintain chain of custody from scene to intake location
□ Implement Protective Custody secure housing and tracking for each animal

Specific Case Considerations
□ Large numbers of birds
□ Separation of fighting birds
□ Noisy population
□ Identification of each bird
□ Plan for ultimate disposition
□ Prepare for media interest in the case and the disposition of the birds

VICTIM TO VERDICT™

Questions
- ☐ Who owns the birds?
- ☐ What protocols are required by the state's department of agriculture?

Forms
- ☐ Evidence Placard
- ☐ Volunteer Confidentiality Forms
- ☐ Nonliving and Live Evidence Tracking Forms

Prosecutor

Actions That Apply To All Cases
- ☐ Request additional investigation, where appropriate, before declining to prosecute
- ☐ Consider long-term impact or permanent injury to the animal(s) when making charging decisions
- ☐ File a charge on each victim animal and/or each criminal incident, do not group victims/conduct into one count
- ☐ A condition of release should include no contact with victim animal or other animals as appropriate
- ☐ Pursue preconviction forfeiture without delay if the victim animal is alive and if the state has laws in place to do so
- ☐ Sign off on disposition of animal evidence when evidence collection is complete and ownership has been resolved
- ☐ Schedule pretrial meetings with veterinarian and other witnesses
- ☐ Request continued medical discovery from veterinarian and/or animal care agency if necessary
- ☐ Request up-to-date amount of costs of care for animal care agency

Specific Case Actions
- ☐ Show the housing of the animals and the trimming/dubbing of the roosters
- ☐ Show the ratio of roosters to hens and explain how that is indicative of cockfighting; circumstantial evidence of a cockfighting operation

Specific Case Considerations
- ☐ Other crimes connected: child endangerment, firearms, drugs, gambling, animal neglect, racketeer influenced and corrupt organizations (RICO), and gang activity
- ☐ Multiple defendants
- ☐ Don't concede unnecessary ground by grouping victims/conduct into one count

Questions
- ☐ Does the law permit seizing the birds in place?
- ☐ Does the state have a specific statute regarding disposition of fighting birds?

Forms
- ☐ Example Cockfighting Warrant
- ☐ Release Order Template

VICTIM TO VERDICT™

Resources and References

https://www.humanesociety.org/resources/cockfighting-fact-sheet, https://aldf.org/article/animal-fighting-facts/animal-fighting-state-laws, https://www.ncsl.org/research/agriculture-and-rural-development/cockfighting-laws.aspx (all accessed 6 September 2021).

Governor's Commission on the Humane Treatment of Animals (2020). Animal cruelty investigation and prosecution: A user manual for New Hampshire law enforcement. http://neacha.org/resources/animal-cruelty-manual-2020.pdf (accessed 8 June 2021).

Merck, M.D. (ed.) (2013). *Veterinary Forensics: Animal Cruelty Investigations*, 2e. Hoboken, NJ: Wiley-Blackwell.

National Sheriff's Association (2019). *Sheriff & Deputy*: 2019 special issue animal cruelty. https://www.sheriffs.org/sites/default/files/2019_SD_AA.pdf (accessed 8 June 2021).

Phillips, A. and Lockwood, R. (2013). Investigating and prosecuting animal abuse. https://nationallinkcoalition.org/wp-content/uploads/2013/09/Investigating-Prosecuting-AA-Phillips-Lockwood.pdf (accessed 8 June 2021).

The American Standard of Perfection, Illustrated. A Complete Description of all Recognized Varieties of Fowls, American Poultry Association, Andesite Press (August 8 2015).

Case: Dogfighting

Felony laws prohibit dogfighting in all 50 states. Dogfighting is a blood sport in which dogs are bred and conditioned to fight each other in a ring until one dog is disqualified usually due to injuries so severe it cannot continue. It is often associated with other criminal conduct such as drug use and distribution, illegal firearms, racketeering, and gang activity. Federal laws exist prohibiting dog-fighting and some states include the possession of training and fighting paraphernalia as separate criminal offenses. Reports from the public often stem from someone witnessing a dog breeding operation or individuals conditioning and training dogs. Dogfights themselves may be highly organized events carrying high stakes or may take place on a more amateur level, but are nearly always conducted in secret. These cases involve multiple suspects and animals may be co-owned by several individuals.

Cases should include a multi-agency investigation and response with federal, state, and local law enforcement involvement. Detailed planning is paramount to ensuring scene and officer safety. Veterinarian participation in warrant execution will ensure any critically ill or injured dogs are tri-aged immediately. Animal sheltering organizations involved in the handling and housing of dogs bred for fighting must engineer kenneling and exercise enclosures as well as operational plans that take the dogs' behavior into account, as animals from these cases are often aggressive to other dogs. Enclosures may need to include barriers preventing a dog from seeing the dog next to or across from it and plan for one-way movement of dogs to and from kennels and exercise yards.

Because these dogs represent a significant financial asset for their owners, facilities where they are held must be secure as suspects may be inclined to try to regain possession of their animals. Dogs from fighting cases often require behavioral rehabilitation as well as extensive veterinary care to address untreated or serious wounds and injuries.

Investigator

Actions that Apply to All Cases
☐ Interview owner, witnesses, and neighbors
☐ Collect all relevant veterinary records
☐ Consider trying a pretext phone call to the suspect to get their version of events documented early on
☐ Preserve evidence: victim animals, records, photos, medication; see Appendix D for comprehensive evidence list
☐ Engage veterinarian to assist with examination of the evidence and the investigation
☐ Plan for live animal evidence holding and care
☐ Apply for a search warrant when appropriate
☐ Include diagnostic tests and collection of samples. See Appendix D for comprehensive evidence list
☐ Determine ownership status of victim animals and keep partnering agencies apprised of any changes to the status

Specific Case Actions
☐ Do a full financial investigation to show how invested the suspect is in the ongoing enterprise
☐ Create a search warrant preparation checklist
☐ Coordinate multi-agency response
☐ Plan for handlers, animal capture and handling equipment, personal protective equipment, bolt cutters

- Plan for a veterinarian to assist with a search warrant execution and immediate veterinary exams of all seized animals
- Map and photograph/video scene
- Photograph and assign evidence ID to each animal
- Search for evidence of breeding, medical treatment, training and conditioning, fighting, buying, selling
- Search for paraphernalia such as trophies, ribbons, recordings of matches, hobby magazines, match rosters
- Search for equipment such as treadmills, break sticks, carpets and panels, harnesses and leashes, tire swings
- Establish ownership of each animal
- Be sure to seize computers and phone(s)

Specific Case Considerations
- Often connected to another criminal activity: firearms, drugs, gangs, racketeer-influenced and corrupt organizations (RICO), illegal gambling
- Understand how to interview in a way to refute weight-pulling competitions excuse
- Understand the terminology used in social media to discuss the dogs and events associated with dogfighting
- Consider applicable federal charges
- Evaluate whether fighting dog DNA database is helpful/relevant
- Search for animal remains on the property
- Be aware of other victims: children, bait animals
- Do not leave behind pregnant female dogs who do not have clear fighting wounds
- Animal care agency will need advance notice to adequately prepare to assist

Questions
- Could a federal agency be investigating undercover?
- What is criminalized in your state? Owning fighting paraphernalia? Attending a fight?
- Is the current case the primary location of the fights or is further investigation needed to uncover a larger ring?

Forms
- Multi-Animal Site Visit Report
- On Scene Habitat Evaluation
- Animal Cruelty Case Consent to Search
- Animal Cruelty Case Relinquishment Form
- Nonliving and Live Evidence Tracking Forms
- Example Dogfighting Affidavit and Search Warrant
- Evidence Placard

Veterinarian

Actions that Apply to All Cases
- Review all records related to the case
- Examination or evidence collection within 24 hours
- Follow photography and forensic exam protocols
- Complete written report

□ Finalize diagnostic plan and create treatment and care plan

□ Determine who is the follow-up contact for supplemental case reports or emergency updates (typically this will be the investigator, law enforcement, or the prosecutor)

Specific Case Actions

□ Assist law enforcement in identifying evidence related to breeding, fighting, and conditioning

□ Identify breeding, fighting, and all dogs on scene

□ Review for old injuries or pattern of injuries and conduct diagnostic imaging of the full body

□ Look for other evidence of cruelty (neglect or additional injuries/wounds)

□ Check for microchip/tags as a way to confirm ID

□ Collect samples for baseline: fecal, urinalysis, complete blood count, and chemistry panel

□ Review medical records, medications, and supplies found on scene

□ Map wounds to face, forelimbs, body

□ Document acute and chronic scars

Specific Case Considerations

□ Document the pain and fear likely involved

□ Collect DNA sample for fighting dog database

Questions

□ How many dogs are involved in the case?

□ What other agencies are involved? What are the specific roles?

Forms

□ Necropsy Exam Notes Form

□ Nonliving and Live Evidence Tracking Forms

□ Examples of On Scene Veterinary Assessments

□ Evidence Placard

□ Summary Vet Report

□ Laboratory Submission Forms with chain of custody

Animal Care

Actions that Apply to All Cases

□ Confirm ownership status of victim animals

□ Maintain chain of custody of animal evidence in a secure location

□ Carry out veterinary treatment plan as directed

□ Make sure you have the ability to provide the care necessary. If not, facilitate outside or referral care

□ Create and post an emergency veterinary care plan and contact list

□ Facilitate recheck appointments with the veterinarian

□ Provide behavior support and training to live evidence animals

□ Place animals in Protective Custody foster if appropriate

□ Start tracking and documenting costs of care for individual animals on intake

Specific Case Actions

□ Assist with safe animal capture and transport from the scene

□ Assist with documentation of the scene

□ Assist with taking a photo of every animal before it leaves the scene

VICTIM TO VERDICT™

□ Assist with uniquely identifying each animal and attaching that unique identifier to the animal for future reference

□ Maintain chain of custody from scene to intake location

□ Provide care and treatment (as directed by a veterinarian) to victim animals from the case

□ Adequately track the chain of custody of evidence animals and any other evidence related to the case in connection with the animals

□ Begin behavior enrichment and rehabilitation for victim animals

□ Document wound healing and provide to law enforcement and prosecutor

□ Protect staff and resident shelter animals from potential incident

□ Create plan for safe movement and assess risk

□ Assess whether animal(s) are candidates for Protective Custody foster and initiate process for foster placement where appropriate

Specific Case Considerations

□ Treat each enclosure as separate crime scene

□ Consider temperament of victim animals

□ Include behavior rehab as part of treatment

Questions

□ Who owns the dogs? Are they seized?

□ Who will determine outcome for the dogs?

□ What is the media plan?

Forms

□ Evidence Placard

□ Nonliving and Live Evidence Tracking Forms

□ Confidentiality Agreement

Prosecutor

Actions that Apply to All Cases

□ Request additional investigation, where appropriate, before declining to prosecute

□ Consider long-term impact or permanent injury to the animal(s) when making charging decisions

□ File a charge on each victim animal and/or each criminal incident – do not group victims/conduct into one count

□ A condition of release should include no contact with victim animal or other animals as appropriate

□ Pursue preconviction forfeiture without delay if the victim animal is alive and if the state has laws in place to do so

□ Sign off on disposition of animal evidence when evidence collection is complete and ownership has been resolved

□ Schedule pretrial meetings with veterinarian and other witnesses

□ Request continued medical discovery from veterinarian and/or animal care agency if necessary

□ Request up-to-date amount of costs of care for animal care agency

Specific Case Considerations

□ Consider other animal cruelty charges of neglect and abuse

□ Charge for each victim animal and each fight as a separate criminal incident

- ☐ Don't concede unnecessary ground by grouping victims/conduct into one count
- ☐ Include restriction from possessing animals as a condition of release
- ☐ Include ongoing inspections as a part of sentencing
- ☐ Consider other crimes such as gambling, firearms, RICO

Resources and References

Animal Legal Defense Fund (n.d.). Animal fighting: State laws. https://aldf.org/article/animal-fighting-facts/animal-fighting-state-laws (accessed 7 August 2021).

Gardiner, J. (2018). CANINE CODIS. https://vgl.ucdavis.edu/forensics/canine-codis (accessed 7 August 2021).

Governor's Commission on the Humane Treatment of Animals (2020). Animal cruelty investigation and prosecution: A user manual for New Hampshire law enforcement. http://neacha.org/resources/animal-cruelty-manual-2020.pdf (accessed 8 June 2021).

Humane Society (n.d.). Dogfighting fact sheet. https://www.humanesociety.org/resources/dogfighting-fact-sheet (accessed 7 August 2021).

Merck, M.D. (2013). Animal fighting. In: *Veterinary Forensics: Animal Cruelty Investigations*, 2e (ed. M.D. Merck), 243–253. Hoboken, NJ: Wiley-Blackwell.

National Sheriff's Association (2019). *Sheriff & Deputy*: 2019 special issue animal cruelty. https://www.sheriffs.org/sites/default/files/2019_SD_AA.pdf (accessed 8 June 2021).

Phillips, A. and Lockwood, R. (2013). Investigating and prosecuting animal abuse. https://nationallinkcoalition.org/wp-content/uploads/2013/09/Investigating-Prosecuting-AA-Phillips-Lockwood.pdf (accessed 8 June 2021).

Rogers, E.R. (2021). Blood sports. In: *Veterinary Forensics: Investigation, Evidence Collection, and Expert Testimony* (eds. E. Rogers and A.W. Stern), 8–14. London: CRC Press.

Webb, K.M. (2021). DNA evidence collection and analysis. In: *Veterinary Forensics: Investigation, Evidence Collection, and Expert Testimony* (eds. E. Rogers and A.W. Stern), 295–312. London: CRC Press.

Appendix B: Forms and Checklists

Title: Minimum Care Checklist

Purpose: This checklist is helpful when recording conditions related to food, water, shelter, and other aspects of minimum care in animal cruelty investigations

Title: Multi-Animal Site Visit Report

Purpose: This form provides specific areas for investigators to record conditions in suspected hoarding and other types of cases involving many animals

Title: On Scene Habitat Evaluation

Purpose: In multi-animal investigations, such as puppy mills and substandard rescue operations, this form is to be completed for each unit during inspections or crime scene processing as a means to accurately record conditions inside each cage or enclosure

Title: Large Animal Premises Inspection Report

Purpose: This form provides a means for the investigator to record conditions in livestock and horse multi-animal cases

Title: Action Notice

Purpose: This form is helpful when documenting and communicating instructions for correction of deficient conditions

Title: Animal Cruelty Case Consent to Search Form

Purpose: Documentation of an individual voluntarily consenting to a search of their person, residence, outbuildings, vehicle(s), and/or animals

Title: Animal Cruelty Case Relinquishment Form

Purpose: Documents the clear transfer of custody and/or ownership of an animal related to a criminal investigation

Title: Medical Exam Equipment Checklist

Purpose: A checklist of basic equipment, forms, and items to include when preparing to conduct live animal forensic examinations

Title: Veterinary Forensic Exam Form

Purpose: Provides an outline for the forensic live animal exam process and notations

Title: Game Cock Physical Evaluation Form

Purpose: Physical examination form for cockfighting cases

Title: Necropsy Exam Notes Form

Purpose: Provides an outline for the forensic necropsy process and notations

Title: Animal Observation Chart (Appetite, Elimination, and Weight)

Purpose: Form for recording daily observations of animals held in Protective Custody

Title: Live Evidence Tracking Form

Purpose: This form acts as an evidence report, chain of custody, and disposition form for live animals held as evidence

Title: Live Animal Evidence Tracking Continuation Page

Purpose: This form is a supplement to the Live Evidence Tracking Form and allows for continuous chain of custody documentation for the duration of a live animal's status as evidence

Title: Nonliving Evidence Tracking Form

Purpose: This form acts as an evidence report, chain of custody, and disposition form for nonlive evidence, such as animal remains, medication, documents, and weapons

Animal Cruelty Investigations: A Collaborative Approach from Victim to Verdict™, First Edition.
Edited by Kris Otteman, Linda Fielder, and Emily Lewis.
© 2022 John Wiley & Sons, Inc. Published 2022 by John Wiley & Sons, Inc.
Companion website: www.wiley.com/go/otteman/victimtoverdict

Title: Nonliving Evidence Tracking Continuation Page

Purpose: This form is a supplement to the Nonliving Evidence Tracking Form and allows for continuous chain of custody documentation of evidence

Title: Crime Scene Access Log

Purpose: Allows for documentation of all individuals accessing a crime scene. Helps ensure there is no unauthorized access to the scene

Title: Crime Scene Processing Roles and Responsibilities

Purpose: Provides guidelines and role assignments for thorough crime scene documentation and processing

Title: Evidence Placard

Purpose: Template for basic evidence photo placard

Title: Evidence Transport Inventory and Tracker

Purpose: This form tracks the chain of custody of animals (or other evidence) during loading on to transport vehicles at the scene and unloading at the evidence intake location. Confirms which animals/evidence were transported on which vehicle

Title: Transport Vehicle Log

Purpose: During search warrant execution and animal seizure, this form resides with the logistics coordinator and logs all of the vehicles transporting the evidence

Title: Case Animal Intake Checklist

Purpose: Outlines the process for the intake of animals to ensure all necessary steps are completed

Title: Affidavit and Search Warrant Drafting Checklist

Purpose: This document is useful to ensure that search warrant drafts are accurate and include all required elements

Title: Crime Scene Processing Supply List

Purpose: Supplies needed for seizures and crime scene-processing operations

Title: Camera Log

Purpose: For authentication purposes, this form creates a record of all individuals collecting photographic evidence at the crime scene

Title: Property in Custody and Evidence Receipt

Purpose: Use of this form provides a complete inventory of every item of evidence seized from the scene of a crime and taken into protective custody. Acts as a receipt to be provided to the owner of the property

Title: Case Submission Checklist

Purpose: This checklist will help ensure that all necessary steps are taken to collect and provide all discoverable information related to an animal cruelty investigation

Title: Case Submission Inventory

Purpose: Clearly notifies recipients of what is included in the submitted case packet

Title: Case Timeline

Purpose: A quick reference for anyone reviewing a case file to understand the order in which relevant events occurred

Title: Witness List

Purpose: For use during search warrant execution, scene processing, and case packet preparation this form provides a single location for the names, contact information, and roles of every participant

Title: Costs-of-Care Lien Foreclosure Checklist

    Purpose: This checklist ensures all necessary steps are followed to foreclose on a costs-of-care lien related to animals from a cruelty case

Title: Example Forfeiture Hearing Checklist

    Purpose: Use this checklist, amended to reflect the laws in your state, to confirm all elements of your bond-or-forfeit statute have been satisfied such that you are prepared to move forward with a hearing on the issue

Minimum Care Checklist

Purpose: This checklist is helpful when recording conditions related to food, water, shelter, and other aspects of minimum care in animal cruelty investigations

MINIMUM CARE CHECKLIST

AGENCY NAME	CASE	DATE	COMPLETED BY

SITE VISIT DETAILS

LOCATION	DATE / TIME
WEATHER CONDITIONS	TEMPERATURE

☐ INITIAL VISIT   ☐ RECHECK

ANIMAL LOCATION(S)

☐ HOUSE   ☐ TRAILER   ☐ CAGE
☐ APARTMENT   ☐ CORRAL   ☐ OTHER

ANIMAL INFORMATION

TOTAL NUMBER	SPECIES

ENVIRONMENT

OVERALL IMPRESSION OF THE ENVIRONMENT	PRESENCE OF HAZARDS OR DEBRIS

EXCESS URINE	EXCESS FECES
☐ YES ☐ NO	☐ YES ☐ NO

FOOD

FOOD AVAILABLE	QUANTITY SUFFICIENT FOR THE # OF ANIMALS
☐ YES ☐ NO	☐ YES ☐ NO
NUMBER OF FOOD BOWLS / FEEDERS PRESENT	TYPE OF FOOD

WATER

WATER AVAILABLE	QUANTITY SUFFICIENT FOR THE # OF ANIMALS
☐ YES ☐ NO	☐ YES ☐ NO
NUMBER OF WATER BOWLS / TROUGHS PRESENT	OTHER WATER PRESENT

WATER SOURCE	FROZEN
☐ WELL ☐ POND	☐ YES ☐ NO
☐ UTILITY ☐ OTHER	
☐ CREEK	

VETERINARY CARE

PREVENTIVE CARE UP TO DATE?	MEDICAL RECORDS AVAILABLE?
NAME OF CURRENT VETERINARIAN	VISIBLY ILL OR INJURED?
ANY TREATMENTS BEING ADMINISTERED?	

FENCE / TETHER

SECURE?	HAZARDOUS?
IF TETHER, LENGTH AND TYPE OF TETHER?	

SHELTER

TYPE OF SHELTER	IS IT ENCLOSED? ☐ YES ☐ NO
DOES IT OFFER PROTECTION FROM WIND, RAIN, SNOW, SUN?	TYPE OF BEDDING

IS IT MADE OF MATERIALS THAT ARE EASILY DEGRADED BY THE ELEMENTS?

MATERIALS DESCRIPTION

FLOORING DESCRIPTION

DESCRIBE HAZARDS AROUND THE SHELTER

NEXT STEPS

IF CONDITIONS OF PREMISES ARE NOT SATISFACTORY, WHAT ARE THE RECOMMENDATIONS?

☐ VET CARE ORDERED   ☐ ANIMALS REMOVED
☐ NOTICE TO COMPLY ISSUED   ☐ DEADLINE TO COMPLY
☐ CITATION ISSUED   ☐ FOLLOW UP INSPECTION SCHEDULED

INVESTIGATOR SIGNATURE: DATE:

VICTIM TO VERDICT™

Multi-Animal Site Visit Report

Purpose: This form provides specific areas for investigators to record conditions in suspected hoarding and other types of cases involving many animals

MULTI-ANIMAL SITE VISIT REPORT
Hoarded, bred, collected animals

AGENCY NAME	CASE	DATE	COMPLETED BY

TYPE OF RESIDENCE

☐ HOUSE   ☐ APARTMENT / TRAILER
☐ CONDO   ☐ OTHER

STATUS OF UTILITIES

WATER
☐ YES   ☐ NO

ELECTRICITY
☐ YES   ☐ NO

GAS
☐ YES   ☐ NO

TRASH PICKUP
☐ YES   ☐ NO

OTHER PEOPLE LIVING ONSITE (NUMBER)

CHILDREN (NUMBER & AGES)	PARENT(S) (NUMBER)	SPOUSE
PARTNER	RELATIVE(S) (& RELATION)	ROOMMATE(S)

INDICATE WHETHER THE FOLLOWING AREAS ARE FUNCTIONAL:

KITCHEN
☐ YES   ☐ NO   COMMENTS:

BATHROOM
☐ YES   ☐ NO   COMMENTS:

BEDROOM
☐ YES   ☐ NO   COMMENTS:

OTHER: _____
☐ YES   ☐ NO   COMMENTS:

EXTENT OF SQUALOR

AMMONIA ODOR
☐ 1   ☐ 2   ☐ 3   ☐ 4   ☐ 5 UNBEARABLE

FECAL ODOR
☐ 1   ☐ 2   ☐ 3   ☐ 4   ☐ 5 UNBEARABLE

VERMIN
☐ 1   ☐ 2   ☐ 3   ☐ 4   ☐ 5 INFESTATION   TYPE:

DO YOU THINK THIS PERSON IS LIVING IN SQUALOR?
☐ NO   ☐ YES: ☐ MILD   ☐ SEVERE

EXTENT OF HOARDING
CHECK OTHER ITEMS THAT HAVE BEEN COLLECTED AND INDICATE THE EXTENT ON A 1 – 5 SCALE, 5 = SEVERE

ANIMALS
☐ 1 ☐ 2 ☐ 3 ☐ 4 ☐ 5

NEWSPAPERS / MAGAZINE
☐ 1 ☐ 2 ☐ 3 ☐ 4 ☐ 5

FOOD OR FOOD GARBAGE
☐ 1 ☐ 2 ☐ 3 ☐ 4 ☐ 5

CONTAINERS
☐ 1 ☐ 2 ☐ 3 ☐ 4 ☐ 5

CLOTHING
☐ 1 ☐ 2 ☐ 3 ☐ 4 ☐ 5

CLUTTER OUTDOORS
☐ 1 ☐ 2 ☐ 3 ☐ 4 ☐ 5

OTHER
☐ 1 ☐ 2 ☐ 3 ☐ 4 ☐ 5

ANIMAL EVALUATION

TYPE OF ANIMAL	# IN ADEQUATE CONDITION	# IN POOR CONDITION (NOT IMMEDIATE RISK OF DEATH)	# ALIVE BUT SEVERELY INJURED OR SICK	# DEAD	TOTAL
DOGS					
PUPPIES (<1 YR)					
CATS					
KITTENS (<1 YR)					
BIRDS					
REPTILES					
SMALL MAMMALS					
HORSES					
CATTLE / SHEEP / GOATS					
OTHER					

HOW WERE THE MAJORITY OF THE ANIMALS ACQUIRED?

☐ ANIMALS BRED DELIBERATELY IN THE HOME
☐ ANIMALS BRED ACCIDENTALLY IN THE HOME
☐ OWNER ACTIVELY SOLICITED NEW ANIMALS BY ADVERTISEMENT, PICKING UP STRAYS

☐ PEOPLE BROUGHT ANIMALS TO THE HOME
☐ OWNER PURCHASED OR ADOPTED NEW ANIMALS
☐ OTHER:
_____

VICTIM TO VERDICT™

SUBJECT EVALUATION

HOW LONG HAS THIS INDIVIDUAL BEEN MONITORED / INVESTIGATED:

☐ LESS THAN 1 YEAR   ☐ 4 – 5 YEARS
☐ 1 – 3 YEARS   ☐ MORE THAN 5 YEARS

MARITAL STATUS OF THE OWNER:

☐ SINGLE   ☐ MARRIED
☐ DIVORCED   ☐ WIDOWED
☐ PARTNER / SIGNIFICANT OTHER   ☐ UNKNOWN

IS ANYONE CONNECTED WITH THE OWNER HELPING TO REMEDY THE SITUATION:

ADDITIONAL INFORMATION ON THE SITUATION:

VICTIM TO VERDICT™

On Scene Habitat Evaluation

Purpose: In multi-animal investigations, such as puppy mills and substandard rescue operations, this form is to be completed for each unit during inspections or crime scene processing as a means to accurately record conditions inside each cage or enclosure

ON SCENE HABITAT / ENCLOSURE EVALUATION

AGENCY NAME	CASE	DATE	COMPLETED BY

SITE ID

☐ STALL ☐ RUN ☐ CAGE ☐ YARD

☐ PEN ☐ ROOM ☐ OTHER _____

UNIT ID	DIMENSIONS (APPROXIMATE)

# OF ANIMALS	FLOORING MATERIAL	TEMPERATURE

FOOD ☐ YES ☐ NO NOTES:	WATER ☐ YES ☐ NO NOTES:
BEDDING ☐ YES ☐ NO NOTES:	SHELTER #: NOTES:
FECES ☐ YES ☐ NO NOTES:	INITIALS

VICTIM TO VERDICT™

Large Animal Premises Inspection Report

Purpose: This form provides a means for the investigator to record conditions in livestock and horse multi-animal cases

LARGE ANIMAL PREMISES INSPECTION REPORT

AGENCY NAME	CASE	DATE	COMPLETED BY

NAME OF BUSINESS	TELEPHONE
OWNER	TELEPHONE
MANAGER / FOREMAN	TELEPHONE
MAILING ADDRESS	
PHYSICAL ADDRESS	

GENERAL CONDITION OF THE PREMISES

ARE PREMISES CLEAN?	OFFENSIVE ODORS
EXCESSIVE FLIES / RODENTS?	EXCESSIVE MUD?
CURRENT WEATHER CONDITIONS	CONDITION OF FENCING
DEBRIS OR HAZARDS NOTED	

GENERAL CONDITION OF ANIMAL STALL OR ENCLOSURE

TYPE OF STALL BEDDING	CLEANLINESS OF ENCLOSURE OR BEDDING
FREQUENCY OF CLEANING	EXCESSIVE MANURE?
MANURE DISPOSAL METHOD	SHELTER TYPE
SHELTER COMMENTS	
SPECIFIC STALL COMMENTS	

VICTIM TO VERDICT™

GENERAL CONDITION OF FOOD AND WATER

WATER AVAILABLE / TYPES OF CONTAINERS / CONDITION

FOOD AVAILABLE AND TYPE OF FEED

ADEQUATE?	HOW OFTEN?

HOW FED

☐ GROUND ☐ FEEDERS ☐ MINERALS

HOW OFTEN?	ACCESS TO PASTURE ☐ YES ☐ NO

PASTURE SIZE, TYPE, GRAZING CONDITION

GENERAL CONDITION OF ANIMALS

SIGNS OF ILLNESS	SORES / WOUNDS
BODY CONDITION OBSERVATIONS	LAMENESS / CONDITION OF HOOVES

ARE ANIMALS INDIVIDUALLY IDENTIFIED? IF YES, HOW?

DOES ANYONE LIVE ON THE PROPERTY? NAME?

VETERINARIAN	TELEPHONE
FARRIER	TELEPHONE

IF CONDITIONS OF PREMISES OR ANIMALS ARE NOT SATISFACTORY, WHAT ARE THE RECOMMENDATIONS?

NEXT STEPS

☐ VET CARE ORDERED   ☐ FARRIER VISIT NEEDED?
☐ NOTICE TO COMPLY ISSUED   ☐ ANIMAL(S) SEIZED?
☐ CITATION ISSUED

TIME ALLOWED TO COMPLY WITH NOTICE	INVESTIGATING OFFICER

Action Notice

Purpose: This form is helpful when documenting and communicating instructions for correction of deficient conditions

ACTION NOTICE

AGENCY NAME	CASE	DATE	COMPLETED BY

CASE INFORMATION

INVESTIGATOR ASSIGNED	INVESTIGATOR CONTACT INFORMATION
SUBJECT NAME	SUBJECT PHONE NUMBER
SUBJECT ADDRESS	

NOTICE: A REPORT HAS BEEN FILED WITH OUR AGENCY FOR ALLEGED VIOLATION(S) OF STATE STATUTE(S).

DESCRIPTION OF ANIMAL(S):

INVESTIGATOR'S FINDINGS

PHYSICAL CONDITION	SHELTER	WATER
☐ THIN	☐ NONE	☐ NONE
☐ SICK	☐ INADEQUATE	☐ INADEQUATE
☐ LAME	☐ DANGEROUS	☐ LARGER CONTAINER
☐ INJURED	☐ OTHER: _____	☐ SECURE CONTAINER
☐ HAIR LOSS		☐ CONTAMINATED
☐ DECEASED		☐ OTHER: _____
☐ OTHER: _____		

SANITATION	CONFINEMENT	ANIMAL POSSIBLY ABANDONED
☐ POOR	☐ TIED SHORT	☐ YES
☐ TRASH	☐ ENTANGLED	☐ NO
☐ FECES	☐ DANGEROUS	
☐ URINE	☐ OTHER: _____	
☐ OTHER: _____		

VICTIM TO VERDICT™

FINDINGS IN NEED OF IMMEDIATE ACTION

PHYSICAL CONDITION	SHELTER
☐ HAVE VET EXAMINE / TREAT ☐ SUBMIT VETERINARY RECORDS TO: NAME: _____ CONTACT INFO: _____	
SANITATION	CONFINEMENT

OTHER CORRECTIONS / REMARKS

ACKNOWLEDGEMENT

FAILURE TO COMPLY WITH ANY OF THESE ITEMS CAN RESULT IN CRIMINAL PROSECUTION. I UNDERSTAND THE REQUIREMENTS AND WILL MAKE THE NECESSARY CORRECTIONS INDICATED.

OWNER / AGENT SIGNATURE: _____

OWNER / AGENT NAME PRINTED: _____

STATUS OF ACTION NOTICE

☐ CONTACTED
☐ POSTED NOTICE:
    TIME: _____ LOCATION: _____

INVESTIGATOR SIGNATURE: _____ DATE:

VICTIM TO VERDICT™

Animal Cruelty Case Consent to Search Form

Purpose: Documentation of an individual voluntarily consenting to a search of their person, residence, outbuildings, vehicle(s), and/or animals

ANIMAL CRUELTY CASE CONSENT TO SEARCH FORM

AGENCY NAME	CASE	DATE	COMPLETED BY

I, _____ [NAME] have been informed that officer(s) or agent(s) of the _____
[AGENCY NAME] wish to search my:

- ☐ PERSON
- ☐ PERSONAL BELONGINGS IN MY POSSESSION
- ☐ VEHICLE
    - MAKE _____ MODEL _____ PLATE # _____
- ☐ ANIMAL
    - SPECIES _____ BREED _____
    - COLOR _____ NAME _____
    - OTHER IDENTIFIERS _____
- ☐ ANIMAL REMAINS
    - SPECIES _____ BREED _____
    - COLOR _____ NAME _____
    - OTHER IDENTIFIERS _____
- ☐ RESIDENCE
    - ☐ OUTBUILDING / SHEDS
    - ☐ GARAGE
    - ☐ OTHER _____

For evidence of a crime, including but not limited to: living animals, animal remains, veterinary records, kennels/cages, animal food, medications, radiographs, photographs, tissue samples, blood samples, urine/fecal samples, and/or other items which they may consider pertinent to this or any other criminal investigations.

I understand that my animal(s) may be part of a criminal investigation, and could be held as evidence until the conclusion of the case.

I understand that performing a necropsy can alter the state and condition of my animal's remains.

I have been informed that I have a constitutional right to deny consent to search and require that the officers obtain a search warrant prior to any search being conducted.

I have been informed that I have a right to stop the search at any time and require that the officers obtain a search warrant.

By signing below, I am providing written consent / permission for officer(s) or agent(s) of the _____
[AGENCY NAME] to conduct the search without obtaining a warrant and seize any evidence outlined above. I give consent / permission freely and voluntarily without threats or promises of any kind, either express or implied, made to me or someone close to me to convince me to grant consent / permission to search the property described above.

CONSENTING PARTY

SIGNATURE:	DATE:

WITNESSING OFFICER

SIGNATURE:	DATE:

DATE	TIME	LOCATION	RIGHTS EXPLAINED BY (PRINT)

VICTIM TO VERDICT™

Animal Cruelty Case Relinquishment Form

Purpose: Documents the clear transfer of custody and/or ownership of an animal related to a criminal investigation

ANIMAL CRUELTY CASE RELINQUISHMENT FORM

AGENCY NAME	CASE	DATE	COMPLETED BY

ANIMAL OWNER INFORMATION

NAME	LICENSE / ID NUMBER
PHONE NUMBER	EMAIL ADDRESS
PHYSICAL ADDRESS	

ANIMAL INFORMATION (TYPE AND NUMBER)

CAT	DOG	KITTEN	PUPPY
OTHER			
NAME(S)			

SEX

☐ UNALTERED MALE(S) _____   ☐ UNALTERED FEMALE(S) _____
☐ ALTERED MALE(S) _____   ☐ ALTERED FEMALE(S) _____
☐ UNKNOWN _____

PHYSICAL DESCRIPTION (BREED, COLOR, MARKINGS, ETC)

TYPE OF RELINQUISHMENT

☐ FULL RELINQUISHMENT OF OWNERSHIP TO _____ [AGENCY NAME]

_____[INITIAL] I CERTIFY THAT I AM THE OWNER/AGENT FOR THE ANIMAL(S) DESCRIBED ABOVE. I UNCONDITIONALLY RELINQUISH ALL RIGHTS OF OWNERSHIP TO SAID ANIMAL(S). I UNDERSTAND THAT THE ANIMAL MAY BE PLACED INTO AN ADOPTIVE HOME OR HUMANELY EUTHANIZED IF FOUND TO BE IN POOR HEALTH OR OF DANGEROUS OR UNSOCIAL TEMPERAMENT. IN CONNECTION WITH THIS VOLUNTARY RELINQUISHMENT I HEREBY FOREVER RELEASE, ACQUIT, AND DISCHARGE THE _____ [AGENCY NAME] AND THEIR OFFICERS, AGENTS, EMPLOYEES, SUCCESSORS, AND ASSIGNS FROM ANY CLAIM, DEMAND, PROCEEDING, LIEN, OR OTHER THEORY OF RECOVERY OR REDRESS IN CONNECTION WITH THE ANIMAL(S) AND THE CIRCUMSTANCES THAT GAVE RISE TO MY DECISION TO RELINQUISH. I UNDERSTAND THAT BY SIGNING THIS FORM I GIVE UP ALL CLAIMS TO THE RELINQUISHED ANIMAL(S) OR TO ANY MONEY OR OTHER CONSIDERATION FROM _____ [AGENCY NAME]. I ALSO AGREE TO HOLD HARMLESS, INDEMNIFY, AND DEFEND _____ [AGENCY NAME] FROM ANY AND ALL LIABILIRY, ACTIONS, CLAIMS, LOSSES, DAMAGES, OR OTHER COSTS THAT MAY BE ASSERTED BY ANY PERSON OR ENTITY ARISING FROM ANY DISPUTE AS TO THE OWNERSHIP OF THE ANIMAL(S) SUBJECT TO THIS RELINQUISHMENT.

☐ TEMPORARY RELINQUISHMENT OF CUSTODY FOR MEDICAL EXAM / TREATMENT / PROCEDURE

_____[INITIAL] I CERTIFY THAT I AM THE OWNER/AGENT FOR THE ANIMAL(S) DESCRIBED ABOVE. I HEREBY AUTHORIZE _____ [AGENCY NAME] TO PROVIDE MEDICAL TREATMENT / SERVICES TO THE ANIMAL(S). I UNDERSTAND THAT THERE ARE INHERENT RISKS INVOLVED WITH ANESTHETIC USE, SURGICAL PROCEDURES, AND MEDICAL CARE. IN RECOGNITION OF SUCH RISKS I AGREE TO NOT HOLD THE [AGENCY NAME] LIABLE FOR DEATH OR INJURY SUSTAINED BY MY ANIMAL RESULTING FROM ANESTHETIC REACTION OR PROCEDURAL COMPLICATION. I UNDERSTAND THAT I MAINTAIN OWNERSHIP OF THE ANIMAL(S) AND THAT I MAY INCUR CHARGES FOR TREATMENT OR SERVICES PROVIDED TO MY ANIMAL(S) BY _____ [AGENCY NAME] AND THAT CONTINUED AND FUTURE MEDICAL CARE AND TREATMENT IS MY FULL RESPONSIBILITY IN ORDER TO MAINTAIN THE HEALTH AND WELFARE OF MY ANIMAL(S).

☐ TO THE BEST OF MY KNOWLEDGE AND BELIEF, SAID ANIMAL(S) HAS NOT BITTEN ANY PERSON IN THE PAST 10 DAYS.

NOTES

SIGNATURE:	DATE:

VICTIM TO VERDICT™

Medical Exam Equipment Checklist

Purpose: A checklist of basic equipment, forms, and items to include when preparing to conduct live animal forensic examinations

MEDICAL EXAM EQUIPMENT CHECKLIST

EVIDENCE

- ☐ CAMERA
- ☐ FORMS
- ☐ PLACARD
- ☐ EVIDENCE MARKER
- ☐ EVIDENCE LOG (FOR SAMPLES REMOVED)
- ☐ PHOTO SCALES
- ☐ COTTON SWABS

- ☐ SAMPLE COLLECTION SUPPLIES
  - ☐ BLOOD – COLLECTION TUBES
  - ☐ FECES – FECAL LOOP
  - ☐ URINE
- ☐ LABELS & PACKAGING MATERIALS (PAPER/PLASTIC)
- ☐ DRY ERASE MARKER
- ☐ PERMANENT MARKER

EXAMINATION

- ☐ PHYSICAL EXAM FORM
- ☐ CLIPBOARD
- ☐ OTOSCOPE
- ☐ THERMOMETER
- ☐ WEIGH SCALE
- ☐ STETHOSCOPE
- ☐ OPHTHALMOSCOPE
- ☐ MICROCHIP READER
- ☐ FECAL LOOP

- ☐ ALTERNATIVE LIGHT SOURCE
- ☐ NAIL TRIMMER
- ☐ PEN LIGHT
- ☐ SLIDES / SLIDE PROTECTORS
- ☐ SWAB PROTECTORS
- ☐ STERILE COTTON SWABS
- ☐ STERILE POLYESTER SWABS
- ☐ PORTABLE CLIPPERS
- ☐ SMALL SCISSORS

FORMS

- ☐ PHYSICAL EXAM FORM
- ☐ CHAIN OF CUSTODY FORMS
- ☐ EVIDENCE PLACARD

- ☐ LAB SAMPLE SUBMISSION FORM
- ☐ LAB SAMPLE CHAIN OF CUSTODY FORM

Veterinary Forensic Exam Form

Purpose: Provides an outline for the forensic live animal exam process and notations

VETERINARY FORENSIC EXAM FORM

AGENCY NAME	CASE	DATE	COMPLETED BY

ANIMAL IDENTIFICATION AND SIGNALMENT

ID # / EVIDENCE ID	SPECIES / BREED
AGE	COLOR
MARKINGS	SEX
MICROCHIP / TATTOO / BRAND / TAGS / ID BANDS	OTHER

ANIMAL VITAL SIGNS

TEMPERATURE	WEIGHT
RESPIRATION	PULSE
BODY CONDITION SCORE	

PHYSICAL EXAM FINDINGS

	N	ABN	NE		N	ABN	NE
GENERAL APPEARANCE				CARDIOVASCULAR			
EARS				GASTROINTESTINAL			
EYES				NERVOUS SYSTEM			
NOSE				MUSCULAR / SKELETAL			
MOUTH / TEETH				HYDRATION			
RESPIRATORY				GENITOURINARY			

COAT / SKIN
☐ MATTED   ☐ HAIR LOSS   ☐ ODOR   ☐ PARASITES   ☐ URINE / FECAL STAINING

MEDICAL NOTES | OVERALL ASSESSMENT AND SPECIFIC DIAGNOSIS:

BEHAVIOR ASSESSMENT

☐ UNHANDLEABLE ☐ FEARFUL ☐ COMPLIANT ☐ FRIENDLY

BEHAVIORAL OBSERVATIONS AND ASSESSMENT:

PLAN

RADIOLOGY SERVICES REQUESTED

MEDICATIONS AND PRESCRIPTIONS RECOMMENDED / ORDERED

LABORATORY SERVICES
☐ CBC PANEL ☐ FECAL ☐ OTHER: _____

VETERINARIAN SIGNATURE: DATE:

CONTACT INFORMATION:

VICTIM TO VERDICT™

Game Cock Physical Evaluation Form

Purpose: Physical examination form for cockfighting cases

GAME COCK PHYSICAL EVALUATION FORM

AGENCY NAME	CASE	DATE	COMPLETED BY

ANIMAL IDENTIFICATION AND SIGNALMENT

ID # / EVIDENCE ID	SPECIES / BREED

AGE RANGE ☐ ADULT ☐ JUVENILE	COLOR

MARKINGS	SEX

MICROCHIP / TATTOO / BRAND / TAGS / ID BANDS	OTHER

PHYSICAL ALTERATIONS

☐ SPURS _____

☐ COMB _____

☐ EARLOBES _____

☐ WATTLES _____

☐ FEATHER REMOVAL OBSERVATIONS: _____

_____

☐ OTHER: _____

_____

MEDICAL NOTES | OVERALL ASSESSMENT AND SPECIFIC DIAGNOSIS:

PLAN

LABORATORY SERVICES – DIAGNOSTIC TESTS ORDERED:

RADIOLOGY SERVICES REQUESTED:

MEDICATIONS AND PRESCRIPTIONS NEEDED:

OTHER:

SIGNATURE: DATE:

Necropsy Exam Notes Form

Purpose: Provides an outline for the forensic necropsy process and notations

NECROPSY EXAM NOTES

AGENCY NAME	CASE	DATE	COMPLETED BY

☐ 5 VIEW INTAKE PHOTOS TAKEN   ☐ FULL BODY IMAGING
☐ CHAIN OF CUSTODY IN PLACE   ☐ ANCILLARY ITEMS LOGGED/STORED

IN ATTENDANCE

VET (PERFORM EXAM)	CONTACT INFORMATION
SCRIBE (DOCUMENT FINDINGS AS DIRECTED)	CONTACT INFORMATION
PHOTOGRAPHER (5 VIEW PHOTOS AND SPECIFIC CONDITIONS OR INJURIES)	CONTACT INFORMATION

ANIMAL IDENTIFICATION

ID # / EVIDENCE ID	SPECIES
AGE	WEIGHT
BREED / COLOR	SEX
MICROCHIP / TATTOO / ID	OTHER

CASE PRESENTATION

AGENCY INVOLVED	TIME / DATE OF DEATH IF KNOWN
STORAGE HISTORY	DIAGNOSTIC IMAGING COMPLETED ☐ YES ☐ NO
OTHER DIAGNOSTIC TESTS COMPLETED	
OTHER DOCUMENTATION PROVIDED WITH REMAINS	
OTHER INFORMATION OR ACCOMPANYING EVIDENCE RELATED TO REMAINS	

VICTIM TO VERDICT™

EXAMINATION FINDINGS | EXTERNAL EXAM

RIGOR	LIVIDITY
BODY CONDITION SCORE	TEMPERATURE
DECOMPOSITION	COAT CONDITION

ENTOMOLOGICAL FINDINGS

HEAD

EYES / EARS / NOSE

THORAX / ABDOMEN

PERINEUM / EXTERNAL GENITALIA

LEGS

FEET / NAILS

TAIL

EVIDENCE OF MEDICAL OR SURGICAL INTERVENTION

FULL BODY IMAGING COMPLETED / INTERPRETATION

☐ YES   ☐ NO

EXAMINATION FINDINGS | INTERNAL EXAM

SKIN REFLECTION FINDINGS

HEAD

NECK

MUSCULOSKELETAL SYSTEM – NOTE ALL INJURIES AND FRACTURES

THORACIC CAVITY

RESPIRATORY TRACT:

CARDIOVASCULAR SYSTEM:

ABDOMINAL CAVITY

STOMACH:

GASTROINTESTINAL TRACT:

LIVER:

GALLBLADDER:

PANCREAS:

SPLEEN:

KIDNEYS:

ADRENAL GLANDS:

URINARY TRACT:

REPRODUCTIVE TRACT:

SUMMARY OF FINDINGS

LIST OF SAMPLES COLLECTED

SIGNATURE: DATE:

VICTIM TO VERDICT™

Animal Observation Chart (Appetite, Elimination, and Weight)

Purpose: Form for recording daily observations of animals held in Protective Custody

ANIMAL OBSERVATION CHART
Appetite, Elimination, and Attitude

AGENCY NAME	CASE	DATE	COMPLETED BY

ANIMAL INFORMATION

NAME		ID #	
SPECIES / BREED		SEX	
COLOR		INTAKE WEIGHT	
LOCATION			

APPETITE

	SUNDAY	MONDAY	TUESDAY	WEDNESDAY	THURSDAY	FRIDAY	SATURDAY
INITIALS	/	/	/	/	/	/	/
AM							
PM							

1 = NOTHING | 2 = SOME | 3 = MOST | 4 = EATING EVERYTHING THAT WAS OFFERED

ELIMINATION

	SUNDAY	MONDAY	TUESDAY	WEDNESDAY	THURSDAY	FRIDAY	SATURDAY
INITIALS	/	/	/	/	/	/	/
AM							
PM							

1 = NOTHING | 2 = NORMAL | 3 = LOOSE | 4 = DIARRHEA

ATTITUDE

	SUNDAY	MONDAY	TUESDAY	WEDNESDAY	THURSDAY	FRIDAY	SATURDAY
INITIALS	/	/	/	/	/	/	/
AM							
PM							

1 = FROZEN / CATATONIC | 2 = FEARFUL | 3 = QUIET | 4 = BAR (BRIGHT, ALERT, RESPONSIVE)

REPORT TO SUPERVISOR OR MEDICAL STAFF IF ANY OF THE FOLLOWING IS OBSERVED

- ☐ DIARRHEA
- ☐ BLOOD IN FECES OR ENCLOSURE
- ☐ VOMITING
- ☐ EXTREME LETHARGY

VICTIM TO VERDICT™

Live Evidence Tracking Form

Purpose: This form acts as an evidence report, chain of custody, and disposition form for live animals held as evidence

LIVE EVIDENCE TRACKING FORM

AGENCY NAME	CASE	DATE	COMPLETED BY

SUSPECT		DATE / TIME SEIZED	
LOCATION OF SEIZURE		OBTAINED BY	
RECEIVED BY (PRINT)	RECEIVED BY (SIGN)	DATE	TIME

DESCRIPTION OF EVIDENCE

PROPERTY ITEM #	ANIMAL ID	ANIMAL NAME	PHYSICAL DESCRIPTION OF ITEM (SEX, COLOR, SPECIES, DISTINCT MARKINGS, ETC.)

TRANSFER OF CUSTODY (USE WHEN EVIDENCE CHANGES LOCATION OR CUSTODY)

PROPERTY ITEM #	DATE / TIME	RELEASED BY (PRINT / SIGNATURE)	RECEIVED BY (PRINT / SIGNATURE)	REASON

DESCRIPTION OF EVIDENCE		
PROPERTY ITEM #	ANIMAL ID	ANIMAL NAME

CHAIN OF CUSTODY – SIGN OUT / IN (USE WHEN EVIDENCE IS BEING INTERACTED WITH WHILE IN CUSTODY)				
DATE	TIME IN	REASON	TIME OUT	PRINTED INITIALS

VICTIM TO VERDICT™

DESCRIPTION OF EVIDENCE

PROPERTY ITEM #	ANIMAL ID	ANIMAL NAME

LIVE EVIDENCE DISPOSITION (USE WHEN EVIDENCE IS BEING RELEASED FROM EVIDENCE STATUS)

AUTHORIZATION FOR DISPOSITION

ITEM #: _____ ON THIS DOCUMENT PERTAINING TO (CASE # / SUSPECT): _____ / _____
IS NO LONGER NEEDED AS EVIDENCE AND IS AUTHORIZED FOR DISPOSITION BY (CHECK APPROPRIATE DISPOSITION METHOD)

☐ RELEASE ITEM TO: _____

☐ SEND LETTER TO OWNER: _____

☐ CONTACT OTHER AGENCY: _____

☐ DISPOSE OF EVIDENCE

NAME OF AUTHORIZING INDIVIDUAL: _____

SIGNATURE: _____ DATE: _____

RELEASE TO LAWFUL OWNER

ITEM #: _____ ON THIS DOCUMENT WAS RELEASED BY:

PRINT	SIGN
TITLE	ON DATE / TIME

RELEASED TO NAME	ADDRESS	
CITY	STATE	ZIP	TELEPHONE

UNDER PENALTY OF LAW, I CERTIFY THAT I AM THE LAWFUL OWNER OF THE ABOVE ITEM.

SIGNATURE	DATE

COPY OF GOVERNMENT-ISSUED PHOTO IDENTIFICATION IS ATTACHED.

☐ YES   ☐ NO

RELEASE TO THIRD PARTY (NOT OWNER)

ITEM #: _____ ON THIS DOCUMENT WAS RELEASED BY:

PRINT	SIGN
TITLE	ON DATE / TIME

RELEASED TO NAME	ADDRESS	
CITY	STATE	ZIP	TELEPHONE

UNDER PENALTY OF LAW, I CERTIFY THAT I AM THE INDIVIDUAL AUTHORIZED FOR DISPOSITION OF THE ABOVE NAMED ITEM.

SIGNATURE	DATE

COPY OF GOVERNMENT-ISSUED PHOTO IDENTIFICATION IS ATTACHED.

☐ YES   ☐ NO

VICTIM TO VERDICT™

Live Animal Evidence Tracking Continuation Page

Purpose: This form is a supplement to the Live Evidence Tracking Form and allows for continuous chain of custody documentation for the duration of a live animal's status as evidence

LIVE EVIDENCE TRACKING CONTINUATION PAGE
CHAIN OF CUSTODY – SIGN OUT / IN

AGENCY NAME	CASE	DATE

DESCRIPTION OF EVIDENCE

PROPERTY ITEM #	ANIMAL ID	ANIMAL NAME	PHYSICAL DESCRIPTION OF ITEM (SEX, COLOR, SPECIES, DISTINCT MARKINGS, ETC.)

CHAIN OF CUSTODY – SIGN OUT / IN

DATE	TIME IN	REASON	TIME OUT	PRINTED INITIALS

VICTIM TO VERDICT™

Nonliving Evidence Tracking Form

Purpose: This form acts as an evidence report, chain of custody, and disposition form for nonlive evidence, such as animal remains, medication, documents, and weapons.

NON-LIVING EVIDENCE TRACKING FORM

AGENCY NAME	CASE	DATE	COMPLETED BY

SUSPECT		DATE / TIME SEIZED	
LOCATION OF SEIZURE		OBTAINED BY	
RECEIVED BY (PRINT)	RECEIVED BY (SIGN)	DATE	TIME

DESCRIPTION OF EVIDENCE

PROPERTY ITEM #	PHYSICAL DESCRIPTION OF ITEM (IF ANIMAL REMAINS, INCLUDE IF POSSIBLE: SEX, COLOR, SPECIES, DISTINCT MARKINGS, NAME, MICROCHIP NUMBER, ETC.)

TRANSFER OF CUSTODY (USE WHEN EVIDENCE CHANGES LOCATION OR CUSTODY)

PROPERTY ITEM #	DATE / TIME	RELEASED BY (PRINT / SIGNATURE)	RECEIVED BY (PRINT / SIGNATURE)	REASON

CHAIN OF CUSTODY – SIGN OUT / IN (USE WHEN EVIDENCE IS BEING INTERACTED WITH WHILE IN CUSTODY)

DATE	TIME IN	REASON	TIME OUT	PRINTED INITIALS

VICTIM TO VERDICT™

DESCRIPTION OF EVIDENCE

PROPERTY ITEM #	PHYSICAL DESCRIPTION OF ITEM (IF ANIMAL REMAINS, INCLUDE IF POSSIBLE: SEX, COLOR, SPECIES, DISTINCT MARKINGS, NAME, MICROCHIP NUMBER, ETC.)

NON-LIVING EVIDENCE DISPOSITION (USE WHEN EVIDENCE IS BEING RELEASED FROM EVIDENCE STATUS)

AUTHORIZATION FOR DISPOSITION

ITEM #: _____ ON THIS DOCUMENT PERTAINING TO (CASE # / SUSPECT): _____ / _____
IS NO LONGER NEEDED AS EVIDENCE AND IS AUTHORIZED FOR DISPOSITION BY (CHECK APPROPRIATE DISPOSITION METHOD)

☐ RELEASE ITEM TO: _____

☐ SEND LETTER TO OWNER: _____

☐ CONTACT OTHER AGENCY: _____

☐ DISPOSE OF EVIDENCE

NAME OF AUTHORIZING INDIVIDUAL: _____

SIGNATURE: _____ DATE: _____

WITNESS TO DISPOSITION OF EVIDENCE

ITEM #: _____ ON THIS DOCUMENT WAS RELEASED BY (PRINT / SIGN): _____ /

TITLE	IN MY PRESENCE ON (DATE)	
NAME OF WITNESS TO DISPOSITION	SIGNATURE	DATE

RELEASE TO LAWFUL OWNER

ITEM #: _____ ON THIS DOCUMENT WAS RELEASED BY (PRINT / SIGN): _____ /

TITLE	ON DATE / TIME	
RELEASED TO NAME	ADDRESS	
CITY	STATE	ZIP	TELEPHONE

UNDER PENALTY OF LAW, I CERTIFY THAT I AM THE LAWFUL OWNER OF THE ABOVE ITEM.

SIGNATURE	DATE

COPY OF GOVERNMENT-ISSUED PHOTO IDENTIFICATION IS ATTACHED.

☐ YES   ☐ NO

RELEASE TO THIRD PARTY (NOT OWNER)

ITEM #: _____ ON THIS DOCUMENT WAS RELEASED BY (PRINT / SIGN): _____ /

TITLE	ON DATE / TIME	
RELEASED TO NAME	ADDRESS	
CITY	STATE	ZIP	TELEPHONE

UNDER PENALTY OF LAW, I CERTIFY THAT I AM THE INDIVIDUAL AUTHORIZED FOR DISPOSITION OF THE ABOVE NAMED ITEM.

SIGNATURE	DATE

COPY OF GOVERNMENT-ISSUED PHOTO IDENTIFICATION IS ATTACHED.

☐ YES   ☐ NO

Nonliving Evidence Tracking Continuation Page

Purpose: This form is a supplement to the Nonliving Evidence Tracking Form and allows for continuous chain of custody documentation of evidence

NON-LIVING EVIDENCE CONTINUATION PAGE
CHAIN OF CUSTODY – SIGN OUT / IN

AGENCY NAME	CASE	DATE

DESCRIPTION OF EVIDENCE

PROPERTY ITEM #	PHYSICAL DESCRIPTION OF ITEM (IF ANIMAL REMAINS, INCLUDE IF POSSIBLE: SEX, COLOR, SPECIES, DISTINCT MARKINGS, NAME, MICROCHIP NUMBER, ETC.)

CHAIN OF CUSTODY – SIGN OUT / IN

DATE	TIME IN	REASON	TIME OUT	PRINTED INITIALS

VICTIM TO VERDICT™

Crime Scene Access Log

Purpose: Allows for documentation of all individuals accessing a crime scene. Helps ensure there is no unauthorized access to the scene

CRIME SCENE ACCESS LOG

AGENCY NAME		CASE		DATE

LOCATION ADDRESS	LOCATION CITY

ACCESS LOG

NAME / PHONE		AGENCY	
TIME IN	TIME OUT	REASON FOR ACCESS	
NAME / PHONE		AGENCY	
TIME IN	TIME OUT	REASON FOR ACCESS	
NAME / PHONE		AGENCY	
TIME IN	TIME OUT	REASON FOR ACCESS	
NAME / PHONE		AGENCY	
TIME IN	TIME OUT	REASON FOR ACCESS	
NAME / PHONE		AGENCY	
TIME IN	TIME OUT	REASON FOR ACCESS	
NAME / PHONE		AGENCY	
TIME IN	TIME OUT	REASON FOR ACCESS	
NAME / PHONE		AGENCY	
TIME IN	TIME OUT	REASON FOR ACCESS	

VICTIM TO VERDICT™

Crime Scene Processing Roles and Responsibilities

Purpose: Provides guidelines and role assignments for thorough crime scene documentation and processing

CRIME SCENE PROCESSING ROLES AND RESPONSIBILITIES

AGENCY NAME	CASE	DATE	COMPLETED BY

CASE INFORMATION

DATE	CASE #
COUNTY	LEAD INVESTIGATOR
LEAD VETERINARIAN	ASSISTING AGENCIES
WARRANT READER	

SCENE PROCESSING

INITIAL WALK THROUGH TEAM
ROLE: LOOK FOR EMERGENCIES, IDENTIFY NUMBER OF CRIME SCENES, ESTABLISH PLAN FOR EVIDENCE PROCESSING.

NAME: _____

PHOTO / VIDEO EVIDENCE
ROLE: DOCUMENT THE SITE BY VIDEO. ADDITIONAL PHOTOGRAPHS OF THE OUTDOOR ASPECTS OF THE PROPERTY MAY BE NECESSARY.

NAME: _____

SITE MAPPING
ROLE: DRAW A MAP OF THE PROPERTY LAYOUT, IDENTIFYING EACH STRUCTURE ON THE PROPERTY.

NAME: _____

NON-LIVE EVIDENCE
ROLE: DOCUMENT ENVIRONMENTAL CONDITIONS INCLUDING TEMPERATURE AND ODOR. COLLECT ALL VETERINARY MEDICINE RECORDS, MEDICATIONS, FECAL SAMPLES, AND ANIMAL HUSBANDRY MATERIALS.

NAME: _____

ANIMAL INVENTORY AND ID
ROLE: DOCUMENT NUMBER OF LIVE AND DECEASED ANIMALS, PHOTOGRAPH, ASSIGN A UNIQUE IDENTIFIER, AND AFFIX THE ID TO THE INDIVIDUAL ANIMAL.

NAME: _____

VICTIM TO VERDICT™

ANIMAL TRANSPORT
ROLE: COMMUNICATE WITH INTAKE FACILITY, COORDINATE HUMANE TRANSPORT OF ANIMALS FROM THE SCENE TO THE INTAKE FACILITY, MAINTAIN CHAIN OF CUSTODY.

NAME: _____

PUBLIC INFORMATION OFFICER
ROLE: CONTACT FOR MEDIA.

NAME: _____

PROPERTY IN CUSTODY EVIDENCE LOG
ROLE: INVENTORY AND LOG ALL EVIDENCE COLLECTED, NON-LIVE AND/OR LIVE ANIMAL.

NAME: _____

WITNESS LOG
ROLE: DOCUMENT ALL WITNESSES ON SCENE, INCLUDE CONTACT INFORMATION.

NAME: _____

FINAL WALK THROUGH
ROLE: CONFIRM ALL AREAS HAVE BEEN PROCESSED AND LEGAL PAPERWORK IS COMPLETE.

NAME: _____

INTAKE-SHELTER ARRIVAL (WITHIN 24 HOURS)

PUBLIC INFORMATION OFFICER CONTACT
ROLE: MEDIA AT THE SHELTER, PRESS RELEASE.

NAME: _____

ADMISSIONS INTAKE
ROLE: RECEIVE ANIMALS INTO FACILITY DATABASE.

NAME: _____

VETERINARIAN
ROLE: OVERSEE PHYSICAL EXAMS, DEVELOP A PLAN FOR CARE.

NAME: _____

ANIMAL CARE / MEDICAL TEAM
ROLE: COLLECT WEIGHT, FECAL, TEMPERATURE, PULSE, RESPIRATION, ADMINISTER PREVENTIVE CARE, AND COLLECT SAMPLES AS DIRECTED.

NAME: _____

EVIDENCE PHOTOS
PHOTOGRAPH EVERY ANIMAL TAKING 5 OVERALL VIEWS OF THE ANIMAL(S) WITH A PLACARD AND DOCUMENTING SPECIFIC CONDITIONS.

NAME: _____

Evidence Placard

Purpose: Template for basic evidence photo placard

EVIDENCE PLACARD

DATE:	CASE NUMBER:
IDENTIFICATION / EVIDENCE ID:	NAME:
COLOR:	SEX:
SPECIES / BREED:	
PHOTOGRAPHER / HANDLER:	

Evidence Transport Inventory and Tracker

Purpose: This form tracks the chain of custody of animals (or other evidence) during loading onto transport vehicles at the scene and unloading at the evidence intake location. Confirms which animals/evidence were transported on which vehicle

EVIDENCE TRANSPORT INVENTORY AND TRACKER

AGENCY NAME	CASE	DATE	COMPLETED BY

VEHICLE NAME / # / IDENTIFIER		DRIVER	
DESTINATION		DEPARTURE TIME FROM SITE	ARRIVE TIME AT DESTINATION

#	EVIDENCE ID	TYPE / SPECIES	COLOR	OTHER COMMENTS	LOADED (INITIALS)	UNLOADED (INITIALS)
1						
2						
3						
4						
5						
6						
7						
8						
9						
10						
11						
12						
13						
14						
15						
16						

VICTIM TO VERDICT™

Transport Vehicle Log

Purpose: During search warrant execution and animal seizure, this form resides with the logistics coordinator and logs all of the vehicles transporting the evidence

TRANSPORT VEHICLE LOG

AGENCY NAME	CASE	DATE	COMPLETED BY

	VEHICLE NAME / # / IDENTIFIER	DRIVER	DESTINATION
TRIP 1			
	DESCRIPTION OF EVIDENCE TRANSPORTED		

	VEHICLE NAME / # / IDENTIFIER	DRIVER	DESTINATION
TRIP 2			
	DESCRIPTION OF EVIDENCE TRANSPORTED		

	VEHICLE NAME / # / IDENTIFIER	DRIVER	DESTINATION
TRIP 3			
	DESCRIPTION OF EVIDENCE TRANSPORTED		

	VEHICLE NAME / # / IDENTIFIER	DRIVER	DESTINATION
TRIP 4			
	DESCRIPTION OF EVIDENCE TRANSPORTED		

	VEHICLE NAME / # / IDENTIFIER	DRIVER	DESTINATION
TRIP 5			
	DESCRIPTION OF EVIDENCE TRANSPORTED		

	VEHICLE NAME / # / IDENTIFIER	DRIVER	DESTINATION
TRIP 6			
	DESCRIPTION OF EVIDENCE TRANSPORTED		

	VEHICLE NAME / # / IDENTIFIER	DRIVER	DESTINATION
TRIP 7			
	DESCRIPTION OF EVIDENCE TRANSPORTED		

Case Animal Intake Checklist

Purpose: Outlines the process for the intake of animals to ensure all necessary steps are completed

CASE ANIMAL INTAKE CHECKLIST

AGENCY NAME	CASE	DATE	COMPLETED BY

DATE OF INTAKE		ANIMAL NAME	
ANIMAL ID		LOCATION	
VET ASSIGNED		STATUS ☐ LIVE ☐ DEAD	

LIVE ANIMALS

☐ ENTERED INTO FACILITY DATABASE
☐ CHAIN OF CUSTODY IN PLACE
☐ OBSERVATION DOCUMENTATION IN PLACE
☐ 5-VIEW PHOTOS
☐ VETERINARY EXAM REQUESTED
☐ INITIAL WEIGHT RECORDED
☐ MICROCHIP SCAN
☐ IDENTIFICATION COLLAR (OR OTHER)
☐ DATABASE PHOTO
☐ NAIL TRIM / BATH / GROOMING REQUESTED
INSURE NECESSARY EVIDENCE HAS BEEN COLLECTED BEFORE GROOMING
☐ FLEA / MITE TREATMENT

VACCINES AND PREVENTIVE CARE
☐ RABIES
☐ FVRCP
☐ DHLPP
DA2PP
☐ BORDATELLA
☐ FeLV TEST
☐ HEART WORM TEST
☐ PARVO/PANLEUK TEST (IF ILL)
☐ DEWORMER
INSURE NECESSARY EVIDENCE HAS BEEN COLLECTED BEFORE DEWORMING
☐ FLEA-TICK TREATMENT
☐ OTHER: _____

DECEASED ANIMAL

☐ ENTERED INTO FACILITY DATABASE
☐ SECURE AREA FOR REMAINS
☐ CHAIN OF CUSTODY IN PLACE
☐ 5-VIEW PHOTOS TAKEN
☐ NECROPSY REQUESTED

NOTES:

SIGNATURE: DATE:

Affidavit and Search Warrant Drafting Checklist

Purpose: This document is useful to ensure that search warrant drafts are accurate and include all required elements

AFFIDAVIT AND SEARCH WARRANT DRAFTING CHECKLIST

AGENCY NAME	CASE	DATE	COMPLETED BY

AFFIDAVIT

- ☐ TRAINING AND EXPERIENCE IS OUTLINED IN A WAY THAT IS RELEVANT TO THE CRIMES BEING INVESTIGATED
- ☐ AFFIANT'S BASIS OF KNOWLEDGE IS ESTABLISHED (I.E. FIRSTHAND, PASSED ON FROM SOMEONE ELSE, ETC.)
- ☐ CRIMES ARE IDENTIFIED
- ☐ PLACES TO BE SEARCHED ARE DESCRIBED WITH PARTICULARITY
- ☐ REQUEST TO "SEARCH" AND "SEIZE" IS INCLUDED
- ☐ STATEMENTS OF PROBABLE CAUSE RELATE THE EVIDENCE SOUGHT TO THE CRIME (I.E. COULD THE MAGISTRATE REASONABLY CONCLUDE THAT THE FACTS (WITH REASONABLE INFERENCES) ESTABLISH THAT SEIZABLE THINGS WILL PROBABLY BE FOUND AT THIS LOCATION?)
- ☐ EVIDENCE TO BE SEIZED IS DESCRIBED WITH PARTICULARITY
- ☐ WITNESS / INFORMANTS ARE NAMED AND THE BASIS OF THEIR KNOWLEDGE IS IDENTIFIED
- ☐ INFORMATION IS "FRESH" AND JUSTIFIES THE ASSERTION THAT SEIZABLE EVIDENCE WILL BE PRESENT AT THE TIME OF THE WARRANT EXECUTION
- ☐ IF NIGHTTIME SERVICE IS REQUESTED, EXPLANATION IS INCLUDED

WARRANT

- ☐ CRIME IS IDENTIFIED
- ☐ LANGUAGE MATCHES AFFIDAVIT **EXACTLY:**
  - ☐ DESCRIPTION OF THE LOCATION / PERSON
  - ☐ DESCRIPTION OF THE EVIDENCE TO BE SEARCHED FOR AND SEIZED
- ☐ DIRECTS TO "SEARCH AND SEIZE" (USING THOSE WORDS)
- ☐ PERIOD OF TIME TO EXECUTE IS SPECIFIED
- ☐ PERIOD OF TIME TO RETURN THE WARRANT IS SPECIFIED
- ☐ AUTHORITY TO BRING NON-SWORN PEOPLE TO ASSIST WITH PROCESSING THE SCENE IS STATED

SPECIFIC LANGUAGE TO INCLUDE

1. Probable Cause
   a. Based on the stated facts, I have probable cause to believe that the crime of [insert crime] has been committed and that evidence of this crime will be located at [insert location] in "all structures to include primary residence, outbuildings, as well as curtilage".

2. Premises
   a. The premises located at [insert location] is described as follows [describe in detail]
      i. House number
      ii. Tax lot number
      iii. Distinguishing features of the property and / or buildings

iv. Signage

v. Property layout

vi. Owners

vii. **Include a photo if possible**

3. Evidence

    a. To search, seize, and the analysis thereof: [list evidence to be seized]

    b. You are further commanded to open closed containers.

    c. You are further commanded to subject substances seized to analysis.

    d. I respectfully request that the court specifically authorizes [insert lead agency's name] to impound all abused and neglected animals located on the premises under [insert statute authorizing animal seizure in criminal case], with the understanding that [insert lead agency's name] may/will use other animal care providers as their agents to help fulfill their obligations under [list statute requiring minimum care for animals].

PROCESS

☐ THE AFFIDAVIT AND WARRANT HAVE BEEN REVIEWED BY A PROSECUTOR FOR THE JURISDICTION.

☐ COPIES OF THE AFFIDAVIT AND WARRANT MADE AND ORIGINALS PRESERVED FOR MAGISTRATE.

NOTES:

SIGNATURE: DATE:

Crime Scene Processing Supply List

Purpose: Supplies needed for seizures and crime scene-processing operations

CRIME SCENE PROCESSING SUPPLY LIST

IDENTIFICATION, EVIDENCE COLLECTION, AND PACKAGING SUPPLIES			
	AMOUNT NEEDED	PACKED BY (INITIALS)	WHERE PACKED
SMALL PAPER BAG			
LARGE PAPER BAG			
SMALL PAPER ENVELOPE			
SMALL PLASTIC BAG			
MEDIUM PLASTIC BAG			
LARGE PLASTIC BAG			
EVIDENCE TAGS			
ALTERNATE LIGHT SOURCE			
RUBBER BANDS			
ZIP TIES			
EVIDENCE TAPE			
EXTRA SD CARDS			
USB			
CAMERAS			
VIDEO CAMERA			
CHARGERS			
SHOVELS			
AXE			
BOLT CUTTERS			
TARPS			

PRUNERS			
ROPE			
DUCT TAPE			
MULTI-TOOL			
THERMOMETER			
BIOHAZARD BAGS / STICKERS			
SPECIMEN JARS FOR ENTEMOLOGICAL EVIDENCE			
COOLER			
EVIDENCE MARKERS / TENTS			
CRIME SCENE TAPE			
HAY SAMPLE CORING TOOL			
PENS: BALL POINT, PERMANENT, HIGHLIGHTER			
SHARPIES / PERMANENT MARKERS			
CLIPBOARDS			
PAPER – GRAPH, BLANK, LINED			
GLOVES – VINYL			
SCISSORS			
TRASH BAGS – DIFFERENT SIZES, RED HAZMAT			
FLASHLIGHT			
INDEX CARDS FOR PHOTO PLACARDS			
PHOTO PLACARDS			

FORMS

	AMOUNT NEEDED	PACKED BY (INITIALS)	WHERE PACKED
WARRANT			
MAPS			
ON-SITE ANIMAL ID / INVENTORY			
SCENE SIGN-IN / OUT LOG			
CAMERA SIGN IN / OUT LOG			
PROPERTY IN CUSTODY FORMS			
HARDCOPY STATUTORY LANGUAGE RE FORFEITURE AND/OR COSTS OF CARE			
CONSENT TO SEARCH			
OWNER RELEASE FORM			
INVENTORY OF VEHICLES TRANSPORTING EVIDENCE			
TRANSPORT INVENTORY (FOR EACH VEHICLE)			
CLIPBOARDS			
ACCIDENT / INJURY PACKET			
CONFIDENTIALITY AGREEMENT / ONE-DAY VOLUNTEER			
ON-SCENE HABITAT EVALUATION SHEETS			

MAPPING SUPPLIES

	AMOUNT NEEDED	PACKED BY (INITIALS)	WHERE PACKED
CLIPBOARD			
GRAPH PAPER			
PENCILS / MARKERS			
TAPE MEASURE			
RULER			

VICTIM TO VERDICT™

PPE & RESPONDER SUPPLIES	AMOUNT NEEDED	PACKED BY (INITIALS)	WHERE PACKED
POP UP CANOPY			
PROCESSING TABLES			
SCENE LIGHTING			
FLASHLIGHTS / HEADLAMPS			
TOWELS			
FIRST AID KIT			
HAND SANITIZER			
RUBBER GLOVES			
PROTECTIVE GLOVES			
TYVEK SUITS			
BOOT COVERS			
RESPIRATORS			
SNACKS / FOOD			
POTABLE WATER			
TRASH BAGS			
SHARPS CONTAINER			
EXTENSION CORD			

VETERINARY FIELD SUPPLIES	AMOUNT NEEDED	PACKED BY (INITIALS)	WHERE PACKED
LRS FLUIDS			
NUTRICAL / KARO SYRUP			
FLUID LINES			
NEEDLES (18G, 20G, 22G, 25G)			
SYRINGES (1CC, 3CC, 6CC, 20CC, 60CC)			
THERMOMETER			
LUBRICANT			
SHOCK KIT			
SALINE			
SCISSORS			
ISOPROPYL ALCOHOL			
GAUZE PADS / GAUZE WRAP			
VET WRAP			
STERILE COTTON SWABS			
CULTURE SWAB KITS			
SUTURE KIT			
FECAL COLLECTION CUP			
FECAL LOOP			
FIELD NECROPSY KIT			
EVIDENCE BAGS			
EMPTY SAMPLE CONTAINERS			

FIELD EUTHANASIA KIT			
TOE TAGS			
LAVENDER TOP BLOOD COLLECTION TUBE			
RED TOP BLOOD COLLECTION TUBE			
NON-ADDITIVE COLLECTION TUBE			
MICROSCOPE SLIDES			
SLIDE HOLDING CONTAINER			
CLEAR TAPE			
GLOVES			
NAIL TRIMMERS			
KWIK STOP			
DEXTROSE			

CATS	AMOUNT NEEDED	PACKED BY (INITIALS)	WHERE PACKED
CRATES			
CAT FOOD (WET / DRY)			
FOOD / WATER BOWLS / PAPER TRAYS			
GLOVES – HEAVY DUTY / BITE PROOF / LEATHER			
LEATHER BITE GUARDS			
CLAM CAT TRAPPER NET			
ZIPPERED CAT TRAPPING NET			
MEDICAL: KARO SYRUP, LRS SETUP			
PAPER COLLARS			
CARDBOARD CAT CARRIERS			
FERAL CAT TRAP(S)			
MICROCHIP SCANNER			
TOWELS			

BIRDS	AMOUNT NEEDED	PACKED BY (INITIALS)	WHERE PACKED
CRATES			
CARDBOARD CARRIERS			
NET(S)			
GLOVES – HEAVY DUTY / BITE PROOF / LEATHER			
LEATHER BITE GUARDS			
LEG BANDS (OR OTHER ID PLAN)			

DOGS			
	AMOUNT NEEDED	PACKED BY (INITIALS)	WHERE PACKED
CRATES			
LEASHES			
CONTROL STICK(S)			
SNAPPY SNARE(S)			
GLOVES – HEAVY DUTY / BITE PROOF / LEATHER			
LEATHER BITE GUARDS			
FOOD / WATER BOWLS			
DOG FOOD (WET / DRY)			
DOG TREATS			
WEARABLE TREAT POUCH			
MICROCHIP SCANNER			
PAPER COLLARS			
MEDICAL: PARVO SNAP TEST			

HORSES & LIVESTOCK			
	AMOUNT NEEDED	PACKED BY (INITIALS)	WHERE PACKED
PLACARD EXTENSION POLE			
HALTERS / LEAD ROPES			
LIVESTOCK TAGGING MARKERS			
TALLY COUNTER			
HOG SORTING PANELS			
FEED / GRAIN			
WATER BUCKETS			
BODY CONDITION CHARTS			
WEIGHT / HEIGHT TAPE			
SQUEEZE CHUTE			
SORTING FLAGS			

REPTILES & SMALL ANIMALS			
	AMOUNT NEEDED	PACKED BY (INITIALS)	WHERE PACKED
RUBBERMAID CONTAINERS WITH VENTILATION			
TRAVEL HABITATS / SECURE TANKS			
PILLOW CASES			
SNAKE HOOK			
INSULATED CONTAINERS			
ZIP TIES			
PROTECTIVE GLOVES / BITE GLOVES			
DISPOSABLE HAND WARMER PACKS			
SMALL ANIMAL BEDDING			
DUCT TAPE			
STYROFOAM COOLERS			
ID MARKING PLAN			
THERMOMETER			

Camera Log

Purpose: For authentication purposes, this form creates a record of all individuals collecting photographic evidence at the crime scene

CAMERA LOG

AGENCY NAME	CASE	DATE	COMPLETED BY

CAMERA NAME OR IDENTIFIER
PHOTOGRAPHER'S NAME

SIGN OUT TIME (INITIAL)	SIGN IN TIME (INITIAL)

CAMERA NAME OR IDENTIFIER
PHOTOGRAPHER'S NAME

SIGN OUT TIME (INITIAL)	SIGN IN TIME (INITIAL)

CAMERA NAME OR IDENTIFIER
PHOTOGRAPHER'S NAME

SIGN OUT TIME (INITIAL)	SIGN IN TIME (INITIAL)

CAMERA NAME OR IDENTIFIER
PHOTOGRAPHER'S NAME

SIGN OUT TIME (INITIAL)	SIGN IN TIME (INITIAL)

CAMERA NAME OR IDENTIFIER
PHOTOGRAPHER'S NAME

SIGN OUT TIME (INITIAL)	SIGN IN TIME (INITIAL)

Property in Custody and Evidence Receipt

Purpose: Use of this form provides a complete inventory of every item of evidence seized from the scene of a crime and taken into protective custody. Acts as a receipt to be provided to the owner of the property

PROPERTY IN CUSTODY & EVIDENCE RECEIPT

AGENCY NAME	CASE	DATE
COMPLETED BY	RECEIPT #	PAGE # OF

LOCATION INFORMATION

OWNER	SUSPECT? (YES OR NO)	SEX
D.O.B.	PHONE	OTHER
STREET ADDRESS		CITY
COUNTY	STATE	ZIP

PROPERTY TYPE CODES

F = FOUND	S = SEIZED	LE = LIVE EVIDENCE	NLE = NON-LIVE EVIDENCE
P = PRISONER PROPERTY	S = SAFEKEEPING	DOA = DECEASED	O = OTHER

INVENTORY

PROPERTY TYPE (CHECK ALL THAT APPLY)

☐ F   ☐ S   ☐ LE   ☐ NLE   ☐ P   ☐ S   ☐ DOA   ☐ O

QUANTITY	ITEM OR SPECIES	BRAND OR BREED	UNIQUE IDENTIFIERS (MARKINGS, MICROCHIP, MODEL #, SERIAL #)	
COLOR		EVIDENCE IDENTIFIER	LOCATION ON SCENE	OTHER NOTES

PROPERTY TYPE (CHECK ALL THAT APPLY)

☐ F   ☐ S   ☐ LE   ☐ NLE   ☐ P   ☐ S   ☐ DOA   ☐ O

QUANTITY	ITEM OR SPECIES	BRAND OR BREED	UNIQUE IDENTIFIERS (MARKINGS, MICROCHIP, MODEL #, SERIAL #)	
COLOR		EVIDENCE IDENTIFIER	LOCATION ON SCENE	OTHER NOTES

PROPERTY TYPE (CHECK ALL THAT APPLY)

☐ F   ☐ S   ☐ LE   ☐ NLE   ☐ P   ☐ S   ☐ DOA   ☐ O

QUANTITY	ITEM OR SPECIES	BRAND OR BREED	UNIQUE IDENTIFIERS (MARKINGS, MICROCHIP, MODEL #, SERIAL #)	
COLOR		EVIDENCE IDENTIFIER	LOCATION ON SCENE	OTHER NOTES

APPROVED BY (PRINT)	SIGNATURE	BADGE / CERTIFICATION #	DATE

VICTIM TO VERDICT™

AGENCY NAME	CASE	RECEIPT #	PAGE # OF

INVENTORY

PROPERTY TYPE (CHECK ALL THAT APPLY)

☐ F ☐ S ☐ LE ☐ NLE ☐ P ☐ S ☐ DOA ☐ O

QUANTITY	ITEM OR SPECIES	BRAND OR BREED	UNIQUE IDENTIFIERS (MARKINGS, MICROCHIP, MODEL #, SERIAL #)	
COLOR		EVIDENCE IDENTIFIER	LOCATION ON SCENE	OTHER NOTES

PROPERTY TYPE (CHECK ALL THAT APPLY)

☐ F ☐ S ☐ LE ☐ NLE ☐ P ☐ S ☐ DOA ☐ O

QUANTITY	ITEM OR SPECIES	BRAND OR BREED	UNIQUE IDENTIFIERS (MARKINGS, MICROCHIP, MODEL #, SERIAL #)	
COLOR		EVIDENCE IDENTIFIER	LOCATION ON SCENE	OTHER NOTES

PROPERTY TYPE (CHECK ALL THAT APPLY)

☐ F ☐ S ☐ LE ☐ NLE ☐ P ☐ S ☐ DOA ☐ O

QUANTITY	ITEM OR SPECIES	BRAND OR BREED	UNIQUE IDENTIFIERS (MARKINGS, MICROCHIP, MODEL #, SERIAL #)	
COLOR		EVIDENCE IDENTIFIER	LOCATION ON SCENE	OTHER NOTES

PROPERTY TYPE (CHECK ALL THAT APPLY)

☐ F ☐ S ☐ LE ☐ NLE ☐ P ☐ S ☐ DOA ☐ O

QUANTITY	ITEM OR SPECIES	BRAND OR BREED	UNIQUE IDENTIFIERS (MARKINGS, MICROCHIP, MODEL #, SERIAL #)	
COLOR		EVIDENCE IDENTIFIER	LOCATION ON SCENE	OTHER NOTES

PROPERTY TYPE (CHECK ALL THAT APPLY)

☐ F ☐ S ☐ LE ☐ NLE ☐ P ☐ S ☐ DOA ☐ O

QUANTITY	ITEM OR SPECIES	BRAND OR BREED	UNIQUE IDENTIFIERS (MARKINGS, MICROCHIP, MODEL #, SERIAL #)	
COLOR		EVIDENCE IDENTIFIER	LOCATION ON SCENE	OTHER NOTES

PROPERTY TYPE (CHECK ALL THAT APPLY)

☐ F ☐ S ☐ LE ☐ NLE ☐ P ☐ S ☐ DOA ☐ O

QUANTITY	ITEM OR SPECIES	BRAND OR BREED	UNIQUE IDENTIFIERS (MARKINGS, MICROCHIP, MODEL #, SERIAL #)	
COLOR		EVIDENCE IDENTIFIER	LOCATION ON SCENE	OTHER NOTES

APPROVED BY (PRINT)	SIGNATURE	BADGE / CERTIFICATION #	DATE

VICTIM TO VERDICT™

Case Submission Checklist

Purpose: This checklist will help ensure that all necessary steps are taken to collect and provide all discoverable information related to an animal cruelty investigation

CASE SUBMISSION CHECKLIST

AGENCY NAME	CASE	DATE	COMPLETED BY

COLLECT

- ☐ CRIME REPORTS
- ☐ VETERINARY REPORTS
- ☐ RECORDS
  - ☐ RADIOGRAPHS
  - ☐ LAB RESULTS
  - ☐ SPREADSHEETS
  - ☐ EXAM FORMS
- ☐ BODY CONDITION SCORING CHART
- ☐ ANY OTHER DOCUMENTS COLLECTED OR CREATED IN THE COURSE OF THE INVESTIGATION (I.E. ACTION NOTICES)
- ☐ PHOTOS AND VIDEOS
- ☐ CHAIN OF CUSTODY FORMS
- ☐ CURRICULUM VITAE (CV) OF EXPERTS INCLUDED IN CASE SUBMISSION
- ☐ ALL NOTES FROM ANIMAL CARE DATABASE REGARDING VICTIM ANIMALS

CREATE

- ☐ LETTER TO PROSECUTOR PROVIDING RELEVANT INFORMATION ON THE JURSIDICTION'S ANIMAL PROTECTION LAWS AND BOND-OR-FORFEIT STATUTES
- ☐ CASE SUBMISSION INVENTORY (NOTING EVERYTHING THAT IS INCLUDED IN THE CASE SUBMISSION)
- ☐ WITNESS LIST
- ☐ SUCCINCT TIMELINE OF THE INVESTIGATION AND ASSOCIATED EVENTS (I.E. VETERINARY VISITS, WITNESS INTERACTIONS, ETC.)
- ☐ REQUEST FOR RESTITUTION
  - ☐ ACCOUNTING FOR EACH INDIVIDUAL ANIMAL
  - ☐ SUMMARY WITH TOTAL COST
  - ☐ NOTICE GIVEN IF RESTITUTION AMOUNT IS EXPECTED TO CONTINUE TO ACCRUE
- ☐ NOTICE DOCUMENT REGARDING CONTINUING VETERINARY MEDICAL DISCOVERY IF TREATMENT IS ONGOING AT TIME OF CASE SUBMISSION

COMPLETE

- ☐ UPDATE AGENCY DATABASE WITH CURRENT STATUS / INFORMATION ON THE CASE AND SUSPECT(S)
- ☐ UPDATE INTERNAL RESTITUTION TRACKING SYSTEM WITH AMOUNT REQUESTED
- ☐ DOUBLE CHECK ACCURACY OF DATES LISTED IN REPORTS (INQUIRE WITH AUTHOR IF NECESSARY)
- ☐ EMAIL THE PROSECUTOR TO ALERT THEM TO THE CASE SUBMISSION AND ARRAIGNMENT DATE
- ☐ DOCUMENT ARRAIGNMENT DATE ON INTERNAL CALENDAR(S)
- ☐ FILL OUT AND SUBMIT NIBRS FORM TO APPROPRIATE RECIPIENT

NOTES

Case Submission Inventory

Purpose: Clearly notifies recipients of what is included in the submitted case packet

CASE SUBMISSION INVENTORY

AGENCY NAME	CASE	DATE	COMPLETED BY

DOCUMENTS

SUPPLEMENTAL (FLASHDRIVES, CITATION(S), BUSINESS CARDS, ETC.)

NOTES

VICTIM TO VERDICT™

Case Timeline

Purpose: A quick reference for anyone reviewing a case file to understand the order in which relevant events occurred

CASE TIMELINE

AGENCY NAME	CASE	DATE	COMPLETED BY

DATE	TIME AND LOCATION	NAME / WITNESSES ASSOCIATED WITH EVENT
	SUMMARY OF EVENT	
	LIST OF RELATED RECORDS / DOCUMENTATION ENCLOSED	

DATE	TIME AND LOCATION	NAME / WITNESSES ASSOCIATED WITH EVENT
	SUMMARY OF EVENT	
	LIST OF RELATED RECORDS / DOCUMENTATION ENCLOSED	

DATE	TIME AND LOCATION	NAME / WITNESSES ASSOCIATED WITH EVENT
	SUMMARY OF EVENT	
	LIST OF RELATED RECORDS / DOCUMENTATION ENCLOSED	

DATE	TIME AND LOCATION	NAME / WITNESSES ASSOCIATED WITH EVENT
	SUMMARY OF EVENT	
	LIST OF RELATED RECORDS / DOCUMENTATION ENCLOSED	

DATE	TIME AND LOCATION	NAME / WITNESSES ASSOCIATED WITH EVENT
	SUMMARY OF EVENT	
	LIST OF RELATED RECORDS / DOCUMENTATION ENCLOSED	

DATE	TIME AND LOCATION	NAME / WITNESSES ASSOCIATED WITH EVENT
	SUMMARY OF EVENT	
	LIST OF RELATED RECORDS / DOCUMENTATION ENCLOSED	

DATE	TIME AND LOCATION	NAME / WITNESSES ASSOCIATED WITH EVENT
	SUMMARY OF EVENT	
	LIST OF RELATED RECORDS / DOCUMENTATION ENCLOSED	

VICTIM TO VERDICT™

Witness List

Purpose: For use during search warrant execution, scene processing, and case packet preparation this form provides a single location for the names, contact information, and roles of every participant

WITNESS LIST

AGENCY NAME	CASE	DATE	COMPLETED BY	

NAME	CONTACT INFORMATION	ORGANIZATION AFFILIATION AND TITLE	ROLE

VICTIM TO VERDICT™

Costs-of-Care Lien Foreclosure Checklist

Purpose: This checklist ensures all necessary steps are followed to foreclose on a costs-of-care lien related to animals from a cruelty case

COSTS-OF-CARE LIEN FORECLOSURE CHECKLIST

DISCLAIMER: THE REQUIREMENTS AND TIME PARAMETERS ASSOCIATED WITH A COSTS-OF-CARE LIEN MAY DIFFER STATE TO STATE. THIS CHECKLIST SHOULD BE UPDATED TO REFLECT THE PROCEDURAL REQUIREMENTS OF YOUR JURISDICTION.

AGENCY NAME	CASE	DATE	COMPLETED BY

CHECKLIST

- ☐ CALCULATE COST OF LIEN
- ☐ PICK A DATE FOR THE FORECLOSURE SALE
- ☐ PICK A DATE TO PROVIDE NOTICE (USUALLY 30 DAYS BEFORE FORECLOSURE SALE)
- ☐ SEARCH UCC FOR OTHER PEOPLE WITH SECURITY INTEREST AND INCLUDE DOCUMENTATION OF THIS SEARCH IN YOUR FILES
- ☐ DRAFT THE NOTICE DOCUMENT
- ☐ GET THE NOTICE DOCUMENT NOTARIZED
- ☐ GIVE NOTICE:
  - ☐ AT THE COURTHOUSE ON THE PUBLIC FORECLOSURE BOARD (TAKE A PICTURE AND SAVE IT IN THE FILE)
  - ☐ AT THE PLACE OF SEIZURE (TAKE A PICTURE AND SAVE IT IN THE FILE)
  - ☐ SEND NOTICE THROUGH CERTIFIED MAIL TO THE LIEN DEBTOR'S LAST KNOWN ADDRESS
  - ☐ SEND COPY OF NOTICE TO:
    - ☐ LIEN DEBTOR'S ATTORNEY(S)
    - ☐ PROSECUTOR ASSIGNED TO THE CRIMINAL CASE
  - ☐ PURCHASE AN AD IN THE PROMINENT NEWSPAPER TO RUN ON THE TWO SUNDAYS BEFORE THE SALE
- ☐ PUT FORECLOSURE SALE DATE ON THE CALENDAR

NOTES

Example Forfeiture Hearing Checklist

Purpose: Use this checklist, amended to reflect the laws in your state, to confirm all elements of your bond-or-forfeit statute have been satisfied such that you are prepared to move forward with a hearing on the issue

Example Forfeiture Hearing Checklist (Oregon)

☐ The animal was impounded pursuant to ORS 167.345.
- ○ A "peace officer" (definition at ORS 161.015 (4)) had PC to believe that the animal was being subjected to treatment in violation of [specific animal cruelty law] and impounded the animal.

☐ The animal is being held by a county animal shelter or an animal care agency.

☐ There is a pending criminal action charging a violation of the animal cruelty laws.
- ○ Have judge take judicial notice of charging document or citation.
- ○ Note: As of 2017, each individual animal does not need its own separate criminal charge to be forfeited.

☐ There is probable cause to believe that the animal was subjected to a violation of [specific animal cruelty law].
- ○ Note: Not a requirement to prove which specific person subjected the animal to the violation.

☐ (**If necessary**) Proper notice for the hearing was given, either in person or by publication, to all potential claimants.

☐ Establish an amount sufficient to repay all reasonable costs incurred, and anticipated to be incurred, in caring for the animals from the date of initial impoundment to the date of trial.

Credit: Jake Kamins

Appendix C: Templates and Agreements

Title: Memorandum of Understanding Template

Purpose: Sample language for agreements to assist between law enforcement agency and animal care/rescue entities

Title: Communications–Media Policy Template

Purpose: Outlines the communication channels between the media and the organization, and provides guidelines on releasable information in criminal cases that protects both the individuals involved and the community

Title: Confidentiality Agreement

Purpose: This document ensures all volunteers assisting with a criminal investigation and the animals related to criminal investigations understand the importance of and agree to maintain confidentiality

Title: Protective Custody Foster Care Agreement

Purpose: This adaptable agreement provides clear parameters around the requirements of fostering an animal in protective custody status. This allows the victim animal to be housed in the most humane way while not creating a vulnerability in the criminal case

Title: Sample Veterinary Clinic Reporting Policy/Protocol

Purpose: This document serves as an adaptable policy and protocol template for veterinary clinics to implement regarding the process for reporting suspected animal cruelty

Title: Summary Vet Report

Purpose: This form may be used to summarize veterinary examination findings and connect the findings with circumstances of the case where relevant

Title: Scene Processing Witness Report

Purpose: Provides a template for participants in a search warrant execution or crime scene processing to document their role and what they observed

Title: Animal Cruelty Affidavit Template

Purpose: This template provides the structure for an affidavit in an animal cruelty case that will prompt officers to provide the necessary information about training, probable cause, and evidence

Title: Animal Cruelty Search Warrant Template

Purpose: This template pairs with the Animal Cruelty Affidavit Template to ensure that the information included in the warrant is clear, thorough, and mirrors that of the affidavit where necessary

Title: Animal Cruelty Warrant Return Template

Purpose: This template completes the Animal Cruelty Affidavit and Search Warrant package by providing guidance on language for generating thorough search warrant return documentation

Title: Bill of Sale and Relinquishment of Animal Ownership Template

Purpose: Use this template when an agreement with a suspect animal owner is made to relinquish ownership of some or all of their animals who are being held in protective custody in relation to a criminal animal cruelty investigation

Animal Cruelty Investigations: A Collaborative Approach from Victim to Verdict™, First Edition.
Edited by Kris Otteman, Linda Fielder, and Emily Lewis.
© 2022 John Wiley & Sons, Inc. Published 2022 by John Wiley & Sons, Inc.
Companion website: www.wiley.com/go/otteman/victimtoverdict

Title: Forfeiture Petition Template

Purpose: This template gives guidance on the petition filed with the court to request a hearing that initiates the bond-or-forfeit process where state law allows

Title: Forfeiture Order Template

Purpose: Where state law allows, use this template to generate the order made at the conclusion of the bond-or-forfeit process

Title: Lien Foreclosure Notice Document Template

Purpose: Provides a template (to be adapted to comply with your state guidelines) for creating the document that gives the required legal notice of a lien foreclosure

Title: Sample Newspaper Notice Ad Template for Lien Foreclosure

Purpose: Provides sample language for posting notice of foreclosure hearing as required by law

Title: Script Template for Lien Foreclosure Sale

Purpose: This script ensures that all the necessary components of a lien foreclosure sale are met when conducting the sale, but should be reviewed and adapted to comport with state laws in the jurisdiction

Title: Notice Letter of Future Discovery Template

Purpose: This letter, to be included with the discovery materials in a case, puts the prosecutor and other parties on notice that animals are still being cared for in connection with the case and additional discovery should be expected/requested

Title: Restitution Cover Letter Template

Purpose: Include this restitution cover letter in the discovery provided to the prosecutor's office to summarize the costs associated with the case up to the point of submission and provide notice of expected future costs

Title: Restitution Waiver Template

Purpose: If you will not be seeking restitution in a case, use this template to notify the prosecutor's office

Title: Request for Live Animal Evidence Disposition Template

Purpose: This request can accompany the submission of the Live Evidence Tracking Form, and may be used to inform law enforcement and prosecutor contacts about the importance of a timely release of live animal evidence

Memorandum of Understanding Template

Purpose: Sample language for agreements to assist between law enforcement agency and animal care/rescue entities

Template: Memorandum of Understanding
BETWEEN
[insert organization providing care]
AND
[insert agency name]

This MEMORANDUM OF UNDERSTANDING, hereafter referred to as MOU, is by and between [**insert agency name**], hereinafter referred to as [**insert abbreviation**], and the [**insert organization**], [**insert description of organization**] located in [**insert city and state**], hereinafter referred to as [**insert abbreviation**].

A) **PURPOSE**

The purpose of this MOU is to establish a partnership between [**insert agency**] and [**insert organization**] with respect to [**insert case number**]. The MOU will clearly identify the roles and responsibilities of each party. The purpose of the partnership is to ensure the successful enforcement of [**insert state**]'s animal welfare laws and to streamline cooperation between the agencies in order to expedite the criminal justice process.

B) **ROLES AND RESPONSIBILITIES**

[**Insert agency**] agrees to:

a) [**List terms the agency needs to meet in order to collaborate with the organization, the following are examples. . .**]

- Seize animals by warrant only.
- Reference authority under [**insert statute**] in the warrant.
- Submit warrant affidavit to [**insert organization**] for review prior to warrant service (days prior when possible).
- Ensure adequate communication with [**insert organization**] on all correspondence regarding the progress of the case.
- Provide notice of forfeiture and foreclosure remedies to animal owner(s) on the day of the seizure.
- Notify animal owner(s) of costs that will accrue in connection with the animal(s) care on the day of the seizure.
- Defer to [**insert organization**] choice of veterinarian for on-site care.
- Defer to [**insert organization**] veterinary recommendations for continued care of the animals.
- Collaborate with [**insert organization**] in a timely manner with regard to press releases and media involvement.
- Provide finalized reports related to the case to [**insert organization**].

- Submit case to the prosecutor's office for consideration of charges in a timely manner after animal seizure.
- Adhere to the following stipulations regarding expenses incurred in connection with caring for and medically treating all seized animals:
  - **[Outline the terms of the agreement with respect to who is responsible for paying these costs and the method by which those costs will be invoiced and paid.]**

[**Insert organization**] agrees to:

a) [**List terms the organization needs to meet in order to collaborate with the agency. The following are examples. . .**]

- Review warrant affidavit prior to submission to prosecutor or judge.
- Take custody of animals that were procured by warrant only.
- Respond to all correspondence with [**insert agency**] in a timely manner.
- Adhere to scene safety protocols.
- Maintain confidentiality regarding the case and the victim animals.
- Provide all necessary daily care to all animals seized, including but not limited to proper nutrition and adequate shelter.
- Provide all veterinary care to all seized animals.
- Hold animals in "Protective Custody" until documentation is received indicating their release from this status.
- Maintain chain of custody for all seized animals.
- Provide behavior training and enrichment to all seized animals.
- Notify [**insert agency**] and the prosecutor's office if any animal from this population experiences a medical emergency, dies, or produces offspring.
- Adhere to the following stipulations regarding expenses incurred in connection with caring for and medically treating all seized animals:
  - **[Outline the terms of the agreement with respect to who is responsible for paying these costs and the method by which those costs will be invoiced and paid.]**

This MOU will be in effect until final resolution of the criminal case.

In the event of any dispute between the parties concerning the terms of this MOU, the prevailing party shall be entitled to collect from the other party all reasonable costs incurred, including attorneys' fees.

[**Insert organization**]

Authorized official: _____   _____
                                        Signature   Printed name and title

[**Insert agency**]

Authorized official: _____   _____
                                        Signature   Printed name and title

VICTIM TO VERDICT™

Communications–Media Policy Template

Purpose: Outlines the communication channels between the media and the organization, and provides guidelines on releasable information in criminal cases that protects both the individuals involved and the community

Purpose

The media has an important responsibility in helping the public understand our valuable role in the community and acts as an essential community partner in raising awareness around animal cruelty. It is imperative that the media is provided lawful, timely, and accurate information on animal cruelty cases to relay to the public, particularly given the substantiated link between animal crime and human violence.

To mitigate potential conflicts in the freedom to report the news and the right of an accused to a fair trial, [**insert agency/organization name**] has adopted the [**insert state/local guidelines on permissible information to release**]. These guidelines are intended to keep the public informed without violating the rights of any individual. It is the intent of [**insert agency/organization name**] to adhere to those guidelines as addressed below.

The [**insert agency/organization name**] will supplement the [**insert state/local guidelines on permissible information to release**] with additional standards that address the unique circumstance of living evidence.

These guidelines are intended to assist those assigned the task of releasing information to the media and public. They do not prohibit release of, or publication of, information needed to identify or aid in the capture of a suspect and protect animals, or information appropriate for disclosure after arrest in the public interest. Neither do they proscribe publication of information already in the public domain.

Policy

[**Insert agency/organization name**] must balance promoting public understanding of the seriousness of animal crimes through media coverage, the constitutional rights of a suspect or a defendant, the integrity of the criminal investigation, including evidence, and the safety of all involved.

It is the policy of [**insert agency/organization name**] to furnish to members of the media such timely information as may properly be published, broadcast, or televised. The purpose of this policy is to provide a reference to assist the employees of [**insert agency/organization name**] in this endeavor by providing an outline of releasable information.

[**Insert agency/organization name**] shall designate an employee as the Public Information Officer (PIO). Only the PIO is authorized to release sanctioned case information to the media. The PIO is available to answer communications-related questions, prepare news releases, and help coordinate [**insert agency/organization name**]'s response during and following major events. The PIO coordinates all direct media inquiries.

The PIO is expected to be familiar with all guidelines outlined in this policy. [**Insert agency/organization name**] employees are expected to seek assistance or information from the PIO in high-profile matters or cases where the employee is unsure of the proper way to proceed with respect to communication issues.

Guidelines

According to [**insert state/local guidelines on permissible information to release**], it is generally appropriate to disclose or report the following:

- [**Include a list of the information approved for release as per the guidelines in your jurisdiction.**]

Procedure

Procedure for Interdepartmental Exchange of Information

The following guidelines consist of principles outlined in the [**insert state/local guidelines on permissible information to release**] as well as internal [**insert agency/organization name**] principles regarding disclosure and reporting of information associated with criminal investigations:

- In all criminal cases, the PIO will generate a "Case Summary" to be distributed to internal departments/programs as needed. The production of the Case Summary will be a component of the internal case finalization process and is provided to aid [**insert agency/organization name**] in coordinating the organization's response to a case.
- The "Case Summary" will include:
  - Name of suspect, only after arraignment or grand jury proceedings
  - Location of the incident: street and city
  - Other agencies involved
  - Current status of the case
    - If citation has been issued, then charges listed on the cite
  - Facts establishing the nature of the incident
  - Status of any victim animals in the case
  - Any photos or video footage approved for release as per this policy.

- The PIO will not make available to the media primary witnesses in any case unless the case is closed or adjudicated.
  - "Adjudicated" is defined as the legal process of judicially deciding a case. As it is used in this policy, a criminal case will be considered "closed" or "adjudicated" when a judgment has been entered by the circuit court with jurisdiction.
- Any and all photos or video taken of an animal involved in a criminal case, regardless of ownership status, while it is in the custody or control of [**insert agency/organization name**] shall be turned over as discovery in the case.
- Photographs and information regarding a wanted suspect may be released by [**insert agency/ organization name**] as necessary to enlist the public's help in apprehending the individual, provided the release does not interfere with enforcement of the law. Such disclosure may include photographs as well as records of prior arrests and convictions to the extent the information helps inform the public of the danger posed by the wanted suspect.
- The PIO is responsible for informing relevant [**insert agency/organization name**] departments in a timely manner of any court proceedings or status changes with the animals in every animal cruelty criminal case.
- Once a case has been adjudicated, the PIO will send a follow-up report to relevant [**insert agency/organization name**] departments with the following information:
  - Case outcome
  - Sentence (if applicable)

VICTIM TO VERDICT™

- Name of the judge who sentenced or acquitted the defendant(s)
- Digital copies of any photos or video that were used as exhibits in the case (if applicable)
- "Adjudicated" is defined as the legal process of judicially deciding a case. As it is used in this policy, a criminal case will be considered "closed" or "adjudicated" when a judgment has been entered by the circuit court with jurisdiction.

Procedure When Live Evidence Is Seized
Photos and video
The PIO (or designee) may take photo and video footage of the evidence animals postseizure and this footage may be made available to the media.

- All photos and video taken shall be provided in the discovery materials for the case.
- The PIO (or designee) must adhere to chain of custody protocols while photographing or videotaping seized animals.
- The PIO (or designee) shall not take any photos or video footage of the forensic exam or any other evidentiary process taking place.
- There will be no private media events to view or photograph seized animals.
- No photos taken on scene will be released by [**insert agency/organization name**] unless there is written consent by the owner (animal and property owner if not the same).

Procedure in Cases Involving a Search Warrant

- If circumstances require it, the PIO may respond to the location of the search warrant execution for the sole purpose of being the point of contact for any media interactions that take place at the scene.
- After the warrant has been executed and the property has been cleared, the following information will be provided to the PIO as soon as the warrant return has been submitted:
  - A copy of the signed affidavit/search warrant/search warrant return
  - Digital copies of any photos and/or exhibits to the affidavit or warrant return.
- The PIO shall not provide copies of the affidavit, the search warrant, or the search warrant return to any outside media contacts.

Procedure for Disseminating Information

[**Insert agency/organization name**] will disseminate information to the news media primarily through two methods:

1) A written media release for email delivery that is prepared by the PIO based on the Case Summary materials, any publicly available documents and/or photos and video footage, and any photo and/or video footage taken by [**insert agency/organization name**] in compliance with this policy.
2) Invitations to the media to attend a press conference with the PIO as the spokesperson for [**insert agency/organization name**].

  - Any statements made by the PIO should not include opinions about the evidence and should not include any information that could deprive the suspect or defendant of a fair trial. Thus, comments made by the PIO should be consistent with the guidelines noted above.

Confidentiality Agreement

Purpose: This document ensures all volunteers assisting with a criminal investigation and the animals related to criminal investigations understand the importance of and agree to maintain confidentiality

Statement of Confidentiality

I, _____, have successfully applied for a position as a volunteer

with _____.

[Institution of volunteer placement]

I acknowledge my participation as a volunteer may give me the opportunity to see or hear information of a sensitive or confidential nature. With this in mind, I will not take photographs, videos, or audio recordings during my volunteer hours. I will also not divulge sensitive or confidential information learned directly or indirectly during the course of my volunteering to anyone, in any manner, without the permission of an agency representative. Such information includes, but is not limited to:

- Personal information of victims (human and animal), paid staff, volunteers, trainees, police officers, veterinarians, suspects, witnesses, or any other individuals present or learned about during the course of my volunteering. Personal information includes names, addresses, phone numbers, and any identifying descriptors.
- The subject matter or nature of any and all completed, current, or potential criminal investigations, including but not limited to charges filed or to be filed, locations of investigations, and parties involved.
- Operational strategies involving deployment of police, security resources, and support staff.

In the event of my withdrawal or termination, I will not disclose any confidential information that I received during my involvement with _____ [institution of volunteer placement].

Additionally, I understand that during the course of my volunteering, I may observe activity that could be of evidentiary value. I may be utilized as a witness to an incident and my testimony may be needed during a civil or criminal proceeding.

If I violate this agreement, I will be subject to termination and possible criminal prosecution.

My signature below affirms that I have read and understand the contents of this confidentiality agreement. My signature below also indicates that I agree to comply with the policies laid out in this agreement at all times. If I have any questions regarding confidentiality, I will ask an agency representative.

Volunteer print name: _____

Volunteer signature: _____ Date: _____

Agency representative: _____ Date: _____

Protective Custody Foster Care Agreement

Purpose: This adaptable agreement provides clear parameters around the requirements of fostering an animal in protective custody status. This allows the victim animal to be housed in the most humane way while not creating a vulnerability in the criminal case

PROTECTIVE CUSTODY FOSTER CARE AGREEMENT

AGENCY NAME	CASE	DATE	COMPLETED BY

PROTECTIVE CUSTODY FOSTER CARE INTRODUCTORY STATEMENT

There are several unique aspects we must consider when placing animals in protective custody foster care. Please read and consider all these factors and your family's ability to adhere to them before making the final commitment to bring one of these animals into your home. Please share this information with anyone who will be residing with your foster animal.

THESE ANIMALS ARE EVIDENCE and are the responsibility of the agency in charge of the case. In an animal cruelty case, the evidence is alive. It must be fed, watered, walked (in some cases), and cleaned up after. It is, however, still highly confidential and must be kept safe. Therefore, in fostering animals held as evidence, these special and critical rules apply:

- Information about your foster animal is confidential. That means you will not be allowed to post comments or photographs of him/her on Facebook, Twitter, Instagram, Craigslist, blogs or any other social media. You must not discuss information about the case, or your foster animal's condition or progress with the media or any outside parties. The information posted by _____ or reported to the media is likely all you will learn about the investigation, but remember, even reports from the media may be inaccurate or speculative. This rule of confidentiality extends to your family, roommates, coworkers, and anyone who comes in contact with your foster animal.
- By agreeing to foster a protective custody animal you are a representative of _____ and therefore statements you make about the condition or progress of your foster animal could potentially be attributed to _____ and be used in court to damage the integrity of the investigation. If you feel that you or anyone in your family is unable to uphold strict confidentiality, you are ineligible to foster a protective custody animal.
- Protective Custody foster animals must be kept safe and in a secure place at all times.
- All veterinary care and treatments must be facilitated through _____. If the animal you are fostering is underweight or emaciated it is imperative that you follow a strict feeding plan that will be provided to you.
- With protective custody animals, the length of time an animal needs foster is often an unknown. While we will explore all avenues available to us to receive custody of the animals, they are sometimes held in evidence status for several months. Your commitment to these animals even for a short duration of time is extremely helpful.

Thank you for your generosity and desire to help these animals in their recovery. Thank you also for understanding the importance of the information above.

ANIMAL INFORMATION

NAME	UNIQUE IDENTIFIER	
SPECIES	BREED	SEX

AGE

- ☐ NEONATE (ORPHAN OR WITH MOTHER)   ☐ JUNIOR
- ☐ ADULT   ☐ SENIOR

NOTES _____

ANIMAL INFORMATION

NAME	CELL PHONE
ADDRESS	CITY, STATE, ZIP
ALTERNATE CONTACT NAME & PHONE	EMAIL ADDRESS

ANIMAL INFORMATION

VETERINARY EMERGENCY

NAME	PHONE	EMAIL

GENERAL INQUIRIES

NAME	PHONE	EMAIL

TERMS OF THE AGREEMENT

1. I agree to foster the above described animal(s), ID(s) _____, _____ (*initial*)
2. I understand that this animal(s) does not belong to me and the pending court process will dictate the ultimate disposition of this animal(s). I understand this process could result in returning this animal(s) to the original owner. _____ (*initial*)
3. I have been informed of any circumstances or diagnosis related to this animal(s) that are relevant to the care and documentation that I may be required to provide. _____ (*initial*)
4. I understand that I have been entrusted to ensure the safety of this animal(s). _____ (*initial*)
5. I understand that a _____ representative may visit my home for a home inspection before my foster application is approved. _____ (*initial*)
6. I understand that this animal(s) must not be surgically altered without express authorization. _____ (*initial*)
7. I understand that any medical concerns must be brought to the immediate attention of _____ and that all instructions are to be followed. _____ (*initial*)
8. I understand that this animal(s) should not be routinely taken to public places, animal shows, events, dog parks, day care, boarding facility, or anywhere that the identity of the animal(s) could be made known. _____ (*initial*)
9. I understand that the details of the investigation or any information about the case, including my observations of the animal(s)'s condition or behavior, must not be released to any individual. _____ (*initial*)
10. I understand that any and all paragraphs, recordings, or other media made or taken of the animal(s) may be evidence. I understand that I may not delete any forms of media taken and agree to send all photos, recordings, and other media of the animal(s) to _____ within 24 hours of taking the photos or making the recording. _____ (*initial*)
11. I understand that this animal(s) must be kept safe and in a secure place at all times. Birds and cats must not be allowed outdoors and dogs must remain under strict supervision when outside and only in an escape-proof yard or on a leash. _____ (*initial*)
12. I understand that the animal(s) must reside only at the address provided in this agreement and I must report any changes in my location or contact information as they occur. _____ (*initial*)
13. I understand if this animal(s) is lost or stolen I must notify _____ immediately. _____ (*initial*)
14. I understand that I am prohibited from transferring care of this animal(s) to any location or interested party without express authorization of _____. If I can no longer keep or safely house this animal(s) I must immediately notify _____. _____ (*initial*)
15. I understand that I have temporary custody of this animal(s) as a custodial agent of _____ and must return the animal(s) upon request. _____ retains legal possession and control of the animal(s) while it is in my custody and this agreement does not release or waive any lien _____ may have in this animal(s). _____ (*initial*)
16. I understand that I am not authorized to incur any expense or other obligation on behalf of _____ unless previously arranged, and I am solely responsible for any damage, injury, or harm resulting from my negligence or actions inconsistent with this agreement. _____ (*initial*)

NOTES

FOSTER CONTACT

PRINT:	SIGNATURE:	DATE:

WITNESS TO AGREEMENT

PRINT:	SIGNATURE:	DATE:

VICTIM TO VERDICT™

Sample Veterinary Clinic Reporting Policy/Protocol

Purpose: This document serves as an adaptable policy and protocol template for veterinary clinics to implement regarding the process for reporting suspected animal cruelty

Sample Veterinary Clinic Reporting Policy/Protocol

The American Veterinary Medical Association (AVMA) encourages veterinarians to educate clients, recognize the signs of animal abuse and neglect, and familiarize themselves with relevant laws and the appropriate authorities to whom they should report suspected cases of animal abuse or neglect within their jurisdiction.

The law does not require absolute assurance of cruelty, abuse, and/or neglect to provoke a report to animal care and control authorities who will, under their responsibilities, investigate further and determine appropriate action.

It is the policy of this hospital that veterinarians, technicians, and support staff who suspect animal cruelty, abuse, or neglect in the context of a veterinarian–client–patient relationship observe the following clinic procedures to report concerns to the proper authorities.

NOTE: ***If, at any time you perceive the situation to be an emergency and are concerned for the immediate safety of staff, clients, or patients, dial 911.***

1) At the time staff is made aware of the possibility of abuse or neglect, suspicions must be reported to the manager or lead veterinarian on duty.
2) Provide the manager/lead veterinarian with details regarding the suspicion, notes from calls or conversations, and any other information relevant to the concern.
3) The manager/lead veterinarian will determine next steps based on the facts presented, whether the client and patient are present in the hospital, level of risk to patient, clients, and staff, and severity of injuries to patient.
4) The manager/lead veterinarian will report the concern to the appropriate agency (animal control, humane agent, law enforcement, human services, etc.) and follow all instructions provided.
5) Clinic staff will provide a written witness statement of the incident/suspicion if requested by clinic management or investigating agency.
6) The veterinary team will provide necessary treatment to the animal and produce a detailed record of exam findings, collect photographs/video of relevant findings, and save any and all items of evidence such as collars, bedding, mats, nail clippings, etc.
7) Clinic staff will provide investigating agencies with records, evidence, notes, and reports as requested.
8) Clinic staff will not share details, images, or other information about the incident/case outside of the clinic and as requested by investigating authorities.
9) It is beyond the clinic's authority to hold animals without the client's consent. If animals must be discharged before investigating agencies arrive, investigators will be expected to pursue the investigation at the home of the client/suspect.

[Consider listing relevant state statutes]
[Consider listing contact information for relevant agencies]

VICTIM TO VERDICT™

Summary Vet Report

Purpose: This form may be used to summarize veterinary examination findings and connect the findings with circumstances of the case where relevant

SUMMARY VET REPORT

AGENCY NAME	CASE	DATE	COMPLETED BY

ACCOMPANYING ATTACHMENTS

☐ PHOTOS / VIDEOS _____

☐ DIAGNOSTICS _____

☐ RADIOGRAPHS _____

☐ PHYSICAL EXAM NOTES _____

☐ OTHER _____

INTRODUCTION (PRESENTATION OF CASE, DESCRIPTION OF ANIMAL(S))

NARRATIVE

FINDINGS

VICTIM TO VERDICT™

SUMMARY

CONCLUSION

SIGNATURE: DATE:

Scene Processing Witness Report

Purpose: Provides a template for participants in a search warrant execution or crime scene processing to document their role and what they observed

SCENE PROCESSING WITNESS REPORT

AGENCY NAME	CASE	DATE	COMPLETED BY

NAME	DATE OF REPORT
AGENCY / ORGANIZATION AFFILIATION	TITLE
PHONE	EMAIL

ADDRESS
DATE AND LOCATION OF RESPONSE
CASE ROLE / DUTIES

OBSERVATIONS MADE

DISCUSS IN NARRATIVE OR BULLET POINT FORMAT WHAT YOU PERSONALLY OBSERVED / WITNESSED WHILE YOU WERE CARRYING OUT YOUR DUTIES DURING THIS CASE.

SIGNATURE: DATE:

VICTIM TO VERDICT™

Animal Cruelty Affidavit Template

Purpose: This template provides the structure for an affidavit in an animal cruelty case that will prompt officers to provide the necessary information about training, probable cause, and evidence

In The State of [Insert State]
for The County of [Insert County]

State of [**insert state**]   )

County of [**insert county**]   )   ss: AFFIDAVIT FOR SEARCH WARRANT

I, the undersigned, upon my oath, do hereby depose and say that, I, [**insert title and name**], am a sworn [**insert title**] employed by [**insert agency name**] and that I am investigating [**insert agency name**] case number [**insert case number**]. The victim in this case is/are [**insert description of animal(s)**] and the crime that has been committed is [**insert statute**]. The elements of [**insert statute**] in this case are: [**insert applicable elements of the offense**].

A) TRAINING AND QUALIFICATIONS OF [**insert title and name**]

I, [**insert name**], being duly sworn, depose and say that I have been employed by [**insert agency name**] for [**insert number**] years. [**Insert all trainings and experience with criminal case work, animal cruelty investigations, animal forensics, and animal behavior/care.**]

B) INVESTIGATION/PROBABLE CAUSE

[**Give the narrative and timeline of the investigation. Include any relevant photos taken.**]

APPLICATION FOR SEARCH WARRANT

Based upon the stated facts I have probable cause to believe that the crime of [**insert statute**] has been committed. That the crime has been committed at [**insert location**]. That [**insert suspect's name**] [**describe the aspects of the crime committed and the victim animal**] on [**insert date**]. And that based on my training and experience [**Connect the evidence you want to search/seize with the crime alleged. For example:**

Based on my training and experience, animals that are victims of abuse and neglect often have a history of abuse and neglect and that evidence of this abuse and neglect can be found in the radiographs of the animal's body and by performing an exam (or necropsy) of the body. And that the evidence may be in the form of broken bones in various stages of repair, internal injuries not visible from the exterior of the body, and foreign objects that may have been injected or impregnated into the body such as BBs, pellets, darts, arrows or other projectiles, and any other signs of abuse or neglect or cause of death.

OR, FOR EXAMPLE:

Based on my training and experience animals that are victims of neglect often have a history of neglect and that evidence of this can be found by performing thorough examinations of the animals. The evidence of neglect may be in the form of injuries or abnormal

results seen on radiographs, bloodwork, necropsies, urinalysis, and/or fecal tests, and not visible from the exterior of the body. Based on my training and experience, I know that bloodwork done can confirm dehydration, anemia, and muscle wasting in an animal. I know that fecal testing can detect the existence of parasites in an animal and determine whether that parasite load was impacting the animal's body condition or overall health.

AND:

Based on my training and experience I know that evidence of animal neglect and/or abuse can be found on the premise where the pet is housed, within the pet owner's dwelling, curtilage, and transportation vehicles.]

And that the evidence will be, but is not limited to: [**list all evidence to search for and seize**]

Which are located at [**insert location**], [**describe with specificity (i.e. tax lot #, physical description, etc. Include a photo if possible)**].

[insert location]	[insert photo]

That based on the above information the undersigned respectfully requests a search warrant for the described location to search and seize and evaluate and analyze the listed evidence for the aforementioned crime.

Further, pursuant to the court's authority under [**insert statute authorizing seizure of animals**], I respectfully request that the court specifically authorize [**insert agency name**] to impound all abused and/or neglected animals located on the premises, with the understanding that [**insert agency name**] may/will use other animal care providers as their agents to help fulfill their obligations under [**list statute requiring minimum care for animals**].

_____
Signature of Affiant

SUBSCRIBED AND SWORN before me this _____ day of _____, 20____

_____
CIRCUIT COURT JUDGE

Animal Cruelty Search Warrant Template

Purpose: This template pairs with the Animal Cruelty Affidavit Template to ensure that the information included in the warrant is clear, thorough, and mirrors that of the affidavit where necessary

IN THE STATE OF [**insert state**]   )

)   SEARCH WARRANT

FOR THE COUNTY OF [**insert county**]   )

TO ANY POLICE OFFICER IN THE STATE OF [**insert state**], GREETINGS:

Upon information given under oath to me by an affidavit signed and sworn to by [**insert title and name**], this Court finds good reason and probable cause to believe that the following crime has been committed in [**insert county**] and that evidence of the following crime is currently located in [**insert county**]: [**insert statute**].

You are hereby commanded to search and seize and test, evaluate, analyze, and photograph evidence from the below-described property: search all structures to include primary residence, outbuildings as well as curtilage of the following location.

The premises located at [**insert location**]. Described as follows: [**give an in depth physical description of the property, include specifics like tax lot #, color of the buildings, any signage or landmarks that can be seen, etc. (THIS MUST MATCH THE AFFIDAVIT)**].

[**insert location**]	[**Insert photo of location**]

For the following described evidence: [**list all evidence to search for and seize (THIS MUST MATCH THE AFFIDAVIT)**].

The court specifically authorizes [**insert agency name**] to impound all abused and/or neglected animals located on the premises, with the understanding that [**insert agency name**] may/will use other animal care providers as their agents to help fulfill their obligations under [**insert statute requiring minimum care for animals**].

___This warrant may be executed any time of the day or night.

___This warrant may be executed more than five (5) days but not more than ten (10) days from the date of issuance.

_____   _____

Title of Magistrate   Signature of Magistrate

VICTIM TO VERDICT™

Animal Cruelty Warrant Return Template

Purpose: This template completes the Animal Cruelty Affidavit and Search Warrant package by providing guidance on language for generating thorough search warrant return documentation

In The Circuit Court of the State of [insert state]
for The County of [insert county]

STATE OF [**insert state**]   )

)   **RETURN OF SEARCH WARRANT**

County of [**insert county**]   )   For [**insert agency name**] Case [**insert #**]

I, [**insert name**], the undersigned [**insert title**], executed the attached search warrant on [**insert date**] at [**insert time**] a.m., and state that the following is a true list of items seized by me pursuant to the warrant:

_____ The property listed on the inventory attached hereto and incorporated herein.

_____ The following property, to wit: [**list seized property**]

1) [**Insert total number**] Living [**insert species**]
2) [**Insert total number**] DOA [**insert species**]
3) [**List other inanimate property like care supplies, food samples, blood samples, leashes, medications, etc.**]
4) Records (see attached Property in Custody inventory)
5) Two (2) SD cards of photos taken on scene (representative sample attached and incorporated herein) [**create a separate document with a sample of the photos taken on scene that are representative of the conditions you found and support the probable cause described in the affidavit**]
6) One (1) SD card of video taken on scene

_____

Signature of [**insert title**]
[**insert name**]

Received by [**insert county**] Circuit Court Office

On ____ day of _____, 20___

Received by: _____

             Printed name and signature

Bill of Sale and Relinquishment of Animal Ownership Template

Purpose: Use this template when an agreement with a suspect animal owner is made to relinquish ownership of some or all of their animals who are being held in protective custody in relation to a criminal animal cruelty investigation

Bill of Sale and Relinquishment of Animal Ownership Template (in lieu of foreclosure under [insert statute if applicable])

The undersigned [**insert animal owner**] (herein after referred to as the Transferor), does hereby relinquish any claim, right, title, and interest in the animals seized during the execution of a search warrant on [**insert date**], at [**insert address**], by the [**insert seizing agency**] _____(#) [**insert species**] and _____ (#) [**insert species**] that are **specifically identified in the attached pages** from Appendix A, which is incorporated herein by this reference and includes any and all offspring of those animals – hereinafter referred to as the Animals), and hereby transfer ownership of the Animals to [**insert seizing agency**]. The consideration for this transfer of ownership is the agreement by the [**insert seizing agency**] (herein after, the Transferee) to waive Transferee's claim for all costs of care that accrue going forward from the date of this agreement in connection with the Animals, and the Transferee's promise to refrain from filing civil suit (including, without limitation, a civil foreclosure of Transferee's possessory chattel lien attaching by operation of [**insert statute if applicable**]) against the Transferor.

Transferor expressly acknowledges that this transfer of ownership in the Animals noted herein shall not be construed as an offer or an agreement to civilly compromise the criminal charge or charges that may be prosecuted against Transferor as a result of this incident. This transfer of ownership does not waive the Transferee's right to seek restitution in the criminal case for the costs of care of the Animals accrued up to the date of this agreement.

Transferor further represents and warrants that s/he has clear and marketable title to the Animals and that s/he has actual authority to transfer ownership of the Animals. Transferor shall hold harmless, indemnify, and defend the Transferees, their officers, agents, and employees from any and all liability, actions, claims, losses, damages, or other costs including attorney's fees and witness costs (at both trial and appeal level, whether or not a trial or appeal ever takes place) that is asserted by any person or entity arising from any dispute as to the ownership of the Animals subject to the Bill of Sale and Relinquishment of Animal Ownership.

Transferor further expressly represents and warrants that s/he is making this decision of his own free will, after ample opportunity to confer with counsel, without duress. Transferor further warrants that s/he has good and marketable title to the Animals, free of all liens and encumbrances (other than the lien(s) attaching to Transferees by operation of [**insert statute if applicable**]).

This Bill of Sale and Relinquishment of Animal Ownership embodies the entire agreement that Transferor has with the Transferees.

_____
Name   (printed)

_____
Signature/date

VICTIM TO VERDICT™

Forfeiture Petition Template

Purpose: This template gives guidance on the petition filed with the court to request a hearing that initiates the bond-or-forfeit process where state law allows

In The Circuit Court of the State of [insert state]
for the County of [insert county]

STATE OF [**insert state**],)	
)	Case no. [**insert number**]
Plaintiff,)	
)	DA no. [**insert number**]
vs.)	
)	PETITION FOR FORFEITURE OF
[**Insert defendant name**])	SEIZED ANIMALS PURSUANT
)	TO [**insert statute**]
Defendant,)	
)	
_____)	
[**Insert county**], a political subdivision of)	
the State of [**insert state**],)	
)	(HEARING REQUESTED (within [**number**]
Petitioner,)	days), estimated time four hours)
)	
vs.)	
)	
[**Insert defendant name**])	
)	
Respondent.)	

Comes now [**insert county**], by and through [**insert prosecutor name**], pursuant to [**insert statute**], and moves this Court for a pretrial order of forfeiture for an animal seized and impounded in the above-entitled case.

1) Deputy _____, a peace officer with [**insert agency name**], seized and impounded the animal listed below on or about [**insert date**].
2) The impounded animal was placed in care at the [**insert animal care provider**].
3) The impounded animal is described as follows:
4) [**Insert description of animal(s)**].
5) There is probable cause to believe that the impounded animal has been subjected to treatment in violation of [**insert statute**].
6) The Defendant-Respondent has been charged by information with [**insert charges**] in [**insert county**] Circuit Court case [**insert number**].
7) [**Insert county**] has incurred expenses related to the feed, care, and medical treatment of the impounded animal, and those costs are expected to be ongoing as the criminal case continues.

WHEREFORE, the Petitioner requests this Court set a hearing, and upon determination that the impounded animal was subjected to a violation of [**insert statute**], the Petitioner prays for judgment against the Defendant-Respondent as follows:

1) For the immediate forfeiture of the impounded animal and for such other relief as may be just and equitable; or
2) In the alternative, requiring the Defendant-Respondent (or any other claimant) to post a security deposit or bond, within [**insert number**] hours of the hearing of this matter, in an amount sufficient to repay all reasonable costs incurred, and anticipated to be incurred, by the Petitioner in caring for the impounded animal from the date of the initial impoundment to the date of the trial in the underlying criminal matter.

Respectfully submitted this [**insert date**],

_____

[**Insert prosecutor name and bar #**]

Forfeiture Order Template

Purpose: Where state law allows, use this template to generate the order made at the conclusion of the bond-or-forfeit process

In The Circuit Court of the State of [insert state]
for the County of [insert county]

STATE OF [**insert state**],	)	
	)	Case no. [**insert number**]
Plaintiff,	)	
	)	DA no. [**insert number**]
vs.	)	
	)	
[**Insert defendant name**]	)	
	)	
Defendant,	)	
	)	ORDER FORFEITING
_____)		SEIZED ANIMALS PURSUANT
[**Insert county**], a political subdivision of	)	TO [**insert statute**]
the State of [**insert state**],	)	
	)	
Petitioner,	)	
	)	
vs.	)	
	)	
[**Insert defendant name**]	)	
	)	
Respondent.	)	

This matter came before the Court on [**insert date**], for a hearing on Plaintiff-Petitioner's Petition for Forfeiture of Seized Animals Pursuant to [**insert statute**], filed on [**insert date**]. Judge [**insert name**] presided. The Plaintiff-Petitioner was represented by [**insert prosecutor name**]; the Defendant-Respondent was represented by [**insert attorney name**].

The animal the Plaintiff-Petitioner sought forfeited (hereinafter referred to as "the animal") is a [**insert species**], further described as:

1) [**Insert description of animal(s)**]
   The Court, having reviewed the petition, and having heard the testimony of witnesses, makes the following findings:
   a) The animal was lawfully impounded by a peace officer pursuant to [**insert statute**] and is currently being held by [**insert animal care provider**] pending outcome of criminal action charging violations of [**insert statute**].
   b) There is probable cause to believe that the animal was subjected to a violation of [**insert statute**].

c) [**Insert county**] has incurred costs in caring for the animals, and those costs are expected to be ongoing to the date of trial (currently set for [**insert trial date**]).

d) The costs in caring for the animal through the date of trial will be [**insert amount**].

IT IS HEREBY ORDERED that all right, title, and interest in the animal, currently in the legal custody of [**insert county**], shall be and is FORFEITED by Defendant-Respondent, and lawful ownership in the animals is now hereby vested in [**insert county**], pursuant to [**insert statute**].

This order is effective as of [**insert time/date**], unless, prior to said date and time, the Defendant-Respondent or any other claimant posts with the clerk of this court a full cash security bond in the amount of [**insert amount**], to repay all reasonable costs incurred, and anticipated to be incurred, by the Plaintiff-Petitioner in caring for the animals from the date of initial impoundment to the date of trial. If Defendant-Respondent or any other claimant posts the security bond specified above, the forfeiture and transfer of ownership in the animals as ordered herein is stayed pending the outcome of the underlying criminal matter.

If the above-mentioned security bond is paid, [**insert county**] is entitled to withdraw funds from the security bond in order to repay the costs (both incurred and anticipated) related to its care of the animals.

If a bond is posted, and the trial in the underlying criminal action is not commenced on [**insert trial date**], the Court shall require the Defendant-Respondent or any other claimant to post an additional security deposit or bond in an amount determined by the Court that shall be sufficient to repay all additional reasonable costs anticipated to be incurred by the Plaintiff-Petitioner in caring for the animal until the anticipated date of trial.

Dated this [**insert date**],

_____

[**Insert Judge's name/title**]

Lien Foreclosure Notice Document Template

Purpose: Provides a template (to be adapted to comply with your state guidelines) for creating the document that gives the required legal notice of a lien foreclosure

CLAIM OF POSSESSORY LIEN
_____

[**Insert animal care provider**]
Lien Claimant,

vs.

[**Insert name of animal owner(s)**],
Lien Debtor(s)

NOTICE OF FORECLOSURE SALE

(Applicable for Food, Vet Care, Labor, Materials, and Related Services – Animal Seized Pursuant to [**insert statute**] *with the lien attaching pursuant to* [**insert lien statute**]*)*

Notice is hereby given that:

1) The undersigned, [**insert animal care provider**], hereinafter referred to as the Claimant, pursuant to the provisions of [**insert lien statute(s)**] inclusively, continues to claim and intends to foreclose a possessory lien upon the Animal(s) noted below (which is, under [**insert state**] law, considered personal property) particularly described as follows:

   a) [**Insert description of animal(s): evidence ID, species, breed, age, color, name, etc.**]

   (hereinafter collectively referred to as the Animal(s)), for the following charges for services provided, materials supplied, and/or labor performed for the Lien Debtor in transporting, caring for, sheltering, feeding, grooming, and treating the Animal(s), said Animal(s) having been seized pursuant to a criminal investigation of animal neglect pursuant to [**insert statute(s)**] resulting in criminal charges filed and pending in [**insert county**] Circuit Case Number [**insert criminal case number(s)**].

2) The actual or reputed owners of the Animal(s), hereinafter referred to as the Lien Debtor(s), are [**insert name of animal owner(s)**], whose last known address is [**insert address**].

3) The total charges are:

   a) The reasonable charges for Claimant's services noted above, including labor and materials at a *daily rate of $*[**insert amount**] *per animal ($*[**insert amount**] *per day total) over* [**insert number**] *days (measured from* [**insert date range**]*) is*. . . . . $ _____

   b) Claimant has incurred expenses in providing medical treatment and care to the Animal(s) and a reasonable fee for the medical care, beyond the day-to-day care noted above is the sum of . . . . $ _____

   c) No part of the charges has been paid except for the sum of. . . . . . $ _____

   d) The **TOTAL** amount of claimant's lien is (a + b − c). . . . . $ _____

4) Claimant obtained possession of the Animal(s) in [**insert county**], [**insert state**].

5) The date the lien was attached to the Animal(s) is [**insert date lien attached**], and the Lien Debtor either knew or should reasonably have known that the sum noted above was beginning to accrue and due. Since that date, legal possession of the Animal(s) has been and is now retained by the claimant.

NOTICE IS HEREBY GIVEN to Lien Debtor and to any whom it may concern that on [**insert date of foreclosure sale**], Claimant will sell the Animal(s) at public auction to the highest bidder for cash, in [**insert county where seizure occurred**], [**insert state**], where Claimant obtained possession thereof, at the following place in that county, **the front steps of the** [**insert county**] **Courthouse, [insert address], City of [insert city]**, State of [**insert state**], at [**insert time**]. The name of the person foreclosing the lien is the [**insert animal care provider**]. All of the above information is incorporated into the Notice of Sale by reference.

6) At the conclusion of the foreclosure sale, the proceeds of the sale will be applied as follows: first, to the payment of the reasonable and necessary expenses of the sale; second, to satisfy the indebtedness secured by the lien under which the sale was made; third (if one or more written requests satisfying [**insert statute**] are submitted to the person foreclosing the lien), to satisfy the indebtedness secured by any subordinate lien(s), in order of priority, in the Animal(s); and fourth, to the treasurer of the county in which the sale is made, accompanied by a copy of the statement of account described in [**insert statute**].

7) On or before [**insert date**], and more than 30 days prior to the day so fixed for the foreclosure sale, Claimant gave this notice by registered or certified mail to the following persons:

   a) To the Lien Debtor at Lien Debtor's last known address, or if the Lien Debtor is a corporation, to its registered agent at the agent's registered office.

   b) To all persons with a security interest in the Animal(s) who have filed a financing statement perfecting that interest in the office of the Secretary of the State of [**insert state**], or in the office of the appropriate county officer of the county in which the foreclosure sale is to be held.

   c) If the chattel to be sold is one for which a certificate of title is required by the laws of this state, to all those persons whom the certificate of title indicates have a security interest in or lien upon the chattels.

8) On or before the date mentioned in paragraph 7, this notice was posted in a public place at or near the front door of the county courthouse of the county in which the sale is to be held and in a public place where Claimant obtained possession of the Animal(s) from the Lien Debtor in [**insert county**], [**insert state**].

9) Claimant has also purchased ads in [**insert name of publication**] and will publish notice in compliance with [**insert statute**].

In construing this instrument, where the context so requires, the singular includes the plural, and all grammatical changes shall be made or implied so that this instrument shall apply equally to corporations and to individuals.

DATE: _____

By _____
[**Insert Attorney name and bar #**]
Attorney for Lien Claimant
[**Insert contact information**]

STATE OF [**insert state**],   )
) ss.
County of [**insert county**]   )

I, [**insert name**], the Attorney for Claimant named in the foregoing instrument, being first duly sworn, depose and say that I know the contents thereof. The statements and claims made therein are true and correct as I verily believe.

_____

[**Insert Attorney name and bar #**]
Attorney for Lien Claimant
[**Insert contact information**]

Signed and sworn to before me on

_____

Notary Public for [**insert state**].
My commission expires _____

Sample Newspaper Notice Ad Template for Lien Foreclosure

Purpose: Provides sample language for posting notice of foreclosure hearing as required by law

Sample Newspaper Notice Ad Template for Lien Foreclosure Sale

NOTICE OF FORECLOSURE SALE [**insert statute**]

Lien claimant, the [**insert animal care provider**] hereby gives notices that it will hold a foreclosure sale on [**insert date**] at [**insert time**] on the front steps of the [**insert county**] Courthouse, [**insert location address**], to foreclose its possessory chattel lien held pursuant to [**insert statute**] for the cost of caring for [**insert number**] [**insert species**] seized as part of a criminal investigation by the [**insert seizing agency**] on or about [**insert date**], said animals being further described as (1) [**insert specific description of each animal (sex, name, ID, color, etc.)**]. The amount owed by the lien debtor(s) ([**insert animal owner(s) name(s)**] whose last known address [**insert address**]), to [**insert lien claimant name**] is $[**insert amount of the lien**] as of the foreclosure sale date. For further information, contact [**insert attorney name**], Attorney for [**insert lien claimant name**] at [**insert phone number**].

Script Template for Lien Foreclosure Sale

Purpose: This script ensures that all the necessary components of a lien foreclosure sale are met when conducting the sale, but should be reviewed and adapted to comport with state laws in the jurisdiction

Script Template for Lien Foreclosure Sale

Introduction

We are here today to complete the nonjudicial lien foreclosure process under [**insert applicable statute**] – via public sale – of the possessory chattel lien attached to a total of [**insert number and species of animal(s)**] that were seized by [**insert seizing agency**] on or about [**insert date of seizure**] [**insert seizing agency's case number**] under the care of Lien Claimants [**insert lien claimant's name**].

All [**insert number of animals**] are being sold "as is," in one lot, for cash to the highest bidder in one sale. It should be noted that these [**insert number of animals**] remain subject to a continuing evidence hold in the underlying criminal cases, meaning that transfer of possession of the [**insert species**] to the highest cash bidder will not be completed unless and until the evidence hold is released or modified by the State of [**insert state**] through the [**insert prosecutor office**] to reflect the results of today's sales (or for some other lawful reason). The successful bidder will be solely responsible for dealing with the State's evidence hold and supplying written proof to the Lien Claimants that the State's evidence hold has been lifted or modified to allow for transfer of possession of the [**insert species of animal(s)**] in completion of the sale or sales conducted this morning.

The lien amount at issue under [**insert statute**] is [**insert amount of lien**].

The successful bidder must make payment this morning, at the close of bidding, in cash or by cashier's check/money order made payable to the Lien Claimant. In addition, the successful bidder must provide proof of identity in the form of a current valid driver's license or State-issued DMV ID card.

Conduct the Sale

I will now read the lien claim and notice of foreclosure sale – this lien is in favor of [**insert lien claimant's name**].

[**Now read out loud the claim of possessory chattel lien/notice of foreclosure sale documents.**]

I will now open the bidding for these [**insert number and species of animal(s)**] at [**insert amount of lien**]. I have a bid from [**insert lien claimant's name**] in the lien amount of [**insert amount of lien**] for the [**insert number and species of animal(s)**] at issue in this case.

FIRST CALL:
Are there any other bids higher than the current bid amount? (pause for five seconds)

SECOND CALL:
Are there any other bids higher than the current bid amount? (pause for five seconds)

THIRD CALL:
Are there any other bids higher than the current bid amount? (pause for five seconds)

    The animal(s) identified in the lien claim and notice of foreclosure sale are SOLD to [**insert lien claimant's name**] for [**insert amount of lien or highest bid**]. I hereby declare this sale closed and the [**insert number and species of animal(s)**] at issue are sold to [**insert lien claimant's name**] subject to the evidence hold previously noted.

Conclusion

Lien Claimant's Attorney will file the formal statement of account of foreclosure sale for this sale as is required under [**insert applicable statute**]. Thank you for coming out today.

END

Notice Letter of Future Discovery Template

Purpose: This letter, to be included with the discovery materials in a case, puts the prosecutor and other parties on notice that animals are still being cared for in connection with the case and additional discovery should be expected/requested

Template: Notice Letter of Future Discovery

[**Insert prosecutor name**]
[**Insert address**]
[**Insert address**]

[**Insert date**]

Dear [**insert prosecutor office**],

As this case proceeds, there will be subsequent documentation produced in connection with the care of the animals associated with this case. Consequently, you should expect to receive additional discovery within three or four weeks. It is our hope that this letter provides you with sufficient notice of such future discovery.

Please do not hesitate to contact our department with any further questions.

Respectfully,

Restitution Cover Letter Template

Purpose: Include this restitution cover letter in the discovery provided to the prosecutor's office to summarize the costs associated with the case up to the point of submission and provide notice of expected future costs

Template: Restitution Cover Letter

[Insert date]

[Insert prosecutor name]
[Insert address]
[Insert address]

RE: **[Insert case # and defendant(s) name(s)]**

To Whom It May Concern:

Thank you for prosecuting this case. Attached please find an itemized list of the costs the **[insert animal care provider]** has incurred thus far in caring for and rehabilitating the **[insert type of animal(s)]** associated with this case; this is provided to you for purposes of restitution.

The total cost of caring for **[insert animal name]**, animal ID **[insert animal identifier]**, as of **[insert date]**, is $ **[insert amount]**.

Please do not hesitate to contact **[insert contact name at animal care provider]** at **[insert contact information]** with any questions you have regarding this submission.

Sincerely,

Restitution Waiver Template

Purpose: If you will not be seeking restitution in a case, use this template to notify the prosecutor's office

Template: Restitution Waiver

[**Insert date**]

[**Insert prosecutor name**]
[**Insert address**]
[**Insert address**]

RE: [**insert case # and defendant(s) name(s)**]

To Whom It May Concern:

Thank you for reviewing this case. Should you decide to file on this case we are not seeking any amount of restitution and do not expect to accrue any costs associated with restitution in the future for this case.

Please do not hesitate to contact me with any questions you have regarding this submission.

Sincerely,

Request for Live Animal Evidence Disposition Template

Purpose: This request can accompany the submission of the Live Evidence Tracking Form, and may be used to inform law enforcement and prosecutor contacts about the importance of a timely release of live animal evidence

Template: Request for Live Animal Evidence Disposition

[**Insert address**]

[**Insert date**]

Re: [**insert agency case number**], [**insert suspect/defendant name**]

Dear [**insert agency name**]:

Please see the attached disposition paperwork for the live animal(s) we have in our custody related to a criminal investigation conducted by your agency. Live animal evidence is unique and requires customized evidence collection, care, and disposition procedures. Using the enclosed form, it is our request and recommendation that you release the animal(s) from their evidence hold so they can move on to their next chapter in life.

The evidentiary value of an animal usually declines rapidly after intake. Initial documentation of the physical condition of the animal(s) and any injuries or illnesses sustained will take place while our agency retains custody of the animal(s). Continued documentation is likely to occur as the animal(s) are rehabilitated and treated; occasionally in a constructive custody situation such as "Protective Custody Foster." This documentation will be retained and turned over as part of discovery in your case. At a certain point, the animal(s) may be mostly or completely rehabilitated and animal ownership issues resolved, **which is the current status of the animal(s) listed on the attached disposition form**. We have documented the improvement and **any additional documentation would have little relevance to the initial condition of the animal(s)**.

Additionally, unlike all other evidence seized by law enforcement, living animals require active and regular care. Any individual or organization that takes in a seized animal is held to the same standards of care required under the law that every other citizen must meet. This correlates to a direct cost to the individual/organization caring for that evidence. The state has an interest in mitigating these costs of care for those individuals/organizations.

Finally, our facility is specially designed for the ***temporary*** holding of animals. It is in the animals' best interest to have their evidence hold lifted as soon as practicable. We will document the disposition of the animal and make adopters aware of the animals' involvement in an ongoing criminal matter. With ample documentation of the animal(s)' condition and status, it is unlikely that rehoming a rehabilitated animal would impinge on a defendant's due process rights, or their ability to have a fair trial.

Please contact us with any questions or concerns you have regarding this disposition request.

Appendix D: Resources

Title: Investigations Triage Matrix (Example)

Purpose: An example of agency response priority to help organize site visits and rechecks based on risk and severity

Title: Guidance for Compliance/Recheck Planning

Purpose: This form provides a template for outlining improvement plans and ongoing rechecks

Title: Animal Cruelty Case Field Operations Structure

Purpose: This diagram represents the key responder roles and chain of command structure for large-scale animal cruelty-related incidents

Title: Animal Crime Scene Processing Roles

Purpose: Outline of responder roles for search warrant and animal seizure operations

Title: Animal Cruelty Case Probable Cause Examples

Purpose: These examples demonstrate how an officer can connect their training and experience with the probable cause in a case and the related evidence

Title: Outline for Conducting Search Warrant Briefing

Purpose: Provides guidance on leading a prewarrant service briefing in an animal cruelty seizure

Title: Evidence in Animal Cruelty Cases

Purpose: This list provides examples of evidence to include in search warrant application language. It can also serve as a guide to searchers when collecting and/or documenting evidence at the crime scene

Title: Examples of On Scene Veterinary Assessments

Purpose: To provide the veterinarian with model language for reporting on observations and findings at a crime scene

Title: Language Options for Adoption Contracts

Purpose: This document lists special considerations when placing animals from cruelty cases for adoption. Special considerations should be customized to the case or your agency's needs

Title: State Evidence Retention and Disposition Rules

Purpose: A reference for state specific laws or regulations on the retention and disposition of evidence in criminal cases

Title: Resource List: Grants for Animal Cruelty Case Work

Purpose: A list of organizations that may provide funding to support animal cruelty investigation and case work

Animal Cruelty Investigations: A Collaborative Approach from Victim to Verdict™, First Edition.
Edited by Kris Otteman, Linda Fielder, and Emily Lewis.
© 2022 John Wiley & Sons, Inc. Published 2022 by John Wiley & Sons, Inc.
Companion website: www.wiley.com/go/otteman/victimtoverdict

Investigations Triage Matrix (Example)

Purpose: An example of agency response priority to help organize site visits and recheck based on risk and severity

Investigations Triage Matrix (Example)

Response time is dependent on resources and geography.
Agencies may find a triage matrix helpful in determining response prioritization.

Minor incident | Target response time: 3 days or less

Witnessed rough handling/no injuries noted

Chronic pet shop complaints

Sanitation issues

Report of abuse/neglect concerning animal in custody

Secondary incident | Target response time: 2 days or less

Shelter/food/water-related neglect in mild weather

Thin or confined animals

Abandoned animal not in immediate danger

Non-life-threatening abuse or neglect report with or without injury

Unlawful tethering

Major incident | Target response time: within 24 hours

Hoarding/crowding with ill or injured animals

Animal sexual abuse

Animal cruelty in conjunction with child abuse or domestic violence

Inadequate shelter in severe weather

Critical incident | Target response time: same day

Abandoned or confined with imminent risk of death (hot vehicle, weather-related)

Downed horses or livestock

Ill, Emaciated, Injured, unable to stand or walk, probable pain

Dead, mutilated, or intentionally killed

Animal fighting with injuries

Request from government agency or veterinarian for onsite assistance

---

VICTIM TO VERDICT™

Guidance for Compliance/Recheck Planning

Purpose: This form provides a template for outlining improvement plans and ongoing rechecks

Guidance for Compliance/Recheck Planning

No human contact made		
Incident	**Step 1: recheck**	**Step 2: if noncompliance or no contact**
Critical	Later same shift or first thing next morning	Return each shift until contact made
Major	1 day	Return each shift until contact made
Secondary	1–2 day or next shift	Return each shift until contact made
Minor	1–3 day or next shift	Return each shift until contact made

Emergency		
Instructions	**Step 1: recheck**	**Step 2: if noncompliance or no contact**
Animal unable to walk/stand	Remain on scene until veterinarian responds	Same day
Provide water	Remain on scene while owner provides water or 1 day if no one home	Return each shift until contact made
Provide food	1 day or if given a supply of food by investigator, 5–7 day	Return each shift until contact made
Provide adequate shelter or bedding in extreme temperatures	1 day	Return each shift until compliance met

Urgent		
Instructions	**Step 1: recheck**	**Step 2: if noncompliance or no contact**
Provide adequate shelter or bedding in mild temperatures	5–7 day	Return every 1–2 day until compliance met
Remove excess feces/urine	2 day	Return each shift until compliance met
Remove hazards	7–14 day	Return every 2–3 day until compliance met
Address unlawful tethering	7–14 day	Return every 2–3 day until compliance met
Address overcrowding/confinement	2 day or next shift	Return each shift until compliance met
Other care to preserve health and well-being	3 day	Return every 1–2 day until compliance met

Animal Cruelty Case Field Operations Structure

Purpose: This diagram represents the key responder roles and chain of command structure for large-scale animal cruelty-related incidents

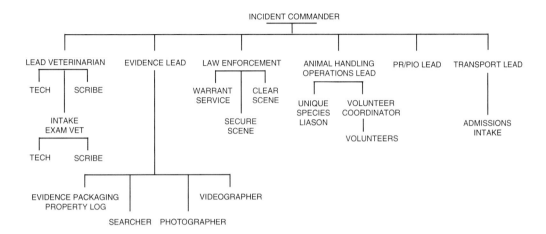

Animal Crime Scene Processing Roles

Purpose: Outline of responder roles for search warrant and animal seizure operations

Animal Crime Scene Processing Roles

Understanding and assigning roles supports an organized and effective effort when processing a crime scene. While not all roles will be essential to every case, search warrant execution and cases involving multiple animals will most certainly benefit from clearly defined roles. Many agencies are familiar with incident command structure, and the following roles fit well into that type of organized response. Each lead individual may have one or more responders assigned to them and their coordination, training, and oversight will be included in their duties.

Law Enforcement: The agency that has jurisdiction over the case is responsible for all law enforcement duties, including: citations, search warrant application, service, and return. These agencies should perform a risk assessment for all locations prior to warrant service and create an emergency or traumatic incident plan. They will serve the warrant, detain the suspect if necessary, declare the scene safe for processing teams to enter, and secure the scene for the duration of processing. Law enforcement should be alerted to any firearms, drugs, or other dangerous contraband found in the search. The agency may oversee evidence collection and packaging as well as property in custody form completion in cooperation with the Evidence Chief. The law enforcement agency will issue any criminal citations.

Incident Commander: The Incident Commander oversees all aspects of planning, preparation, execution, and follow-up of a crime scene response. They will work with law enforcement and animal sheltering teams to assign roles and train responders in their duties. The Incident Commander acts as a point of communication for all assigned roles and is responsible for adjusting plans as needed.

Medical Lead: The individual assigned this role is responsible for on scene medical duties. This is ideally a veterinarian who will conduct an initial walk-through of the scene to assess the animals and their conditions, identify and triage animal emergencies, and perform any medical exams or treatment on scene as required. They are a critical partner in identifying relevant evidence at a crime scene and can offer guidance to searchers in what is important to document and/or collect. The Medical Lead can consult on the capture, handling, and transport of animals based on their species, temperament, age, and condition and may liaise with the Intake Exams Veterinarian on exam procedures and treatment plans for animals upon intake to the sheltering facility.

Unique Species Liaison: If the case includes animal species that the primary sheltering agency is not trained or equipped to capture, handle, transport, or house, an individual from an organization skilled in these areas is required. A Unique Species Liaison will assist with and consult in the plan for the seizure, and coordinate the acquisition of skilled handlers and the appropriate handling, capture, and transport equipment. This individual may possess expertise that also proves valuable when assessing the scene, identifying relevant evidence, and responding to unforeseen circumstances.

Evidence Lead: The Evidence Lead will coordinate the search for and seizure of evidence including photo and video documentation. They will oversee the search and evidence collection, property in custody logs, evidence packaging, and the assignment of evidence identification letters or numbers. This individual will monitor and assign still and video cameras for use in documenting the scene and collect equipment and SD cards prior to clearing the scene. When the search is concluded, the Evidence Lead oversees the processing and storage of physical evidence, videos, and photographs.

Inventory and Transport Lead: Working closely with the Evidence Lead, the Inventory and Transport Lead is responsible for the safe loading and transport of animals from the scene to the medical or sheltering facility. They will create and maintain accurate vehicle inventory forms for each vehicle and monitor the health and safety of the animals during staging and loading for transport, en route, and unloading at the destination.

Animal Shelter Intake Lead: The Animal Shelter Intake Lead remains in communication with the Incident Commander and Transport Lead to facilitate the receipt of animals removed from the scene. Their duties include oversight of animal unloading and kenneling, verifying accuracy of transport logs on arrival, facilitating the entry of shelter or clinic admissions data and creation of daily care logs, cage or stall identification forms or placards, and the application of any additional identification collars, tags, bands, or markings needed to identify each animal.

Public Information Lead: This individual works closely with the primary agency as well as all other organizations involved in the response as a point of contact for all media inquiries. They may be posted outside the crime scene to intercept media representatives that may show up during a search. The Public Information Officer is rarely allowed on private property unless directly involved in the search and seizure operation, and may not take photos or videos on scene for publication. They will often produce press releases and may provide interviews for media outlets and therefore must be trained in what information is appropriate to share with the public.

Outline for Conducting Search Warrant Briefing

Purpose: Provides guidance on leading a prewarrant service briefing in an animal cruelty seizure

Outline for Conducting Search Warrant Briefing

Search warrant briefings should always be conducted on the day of the warrant service prior to arriving on scene with all responding agencies and individuals present. This is a time to instruct all responders, including volunteers, in the procedural plan, expectations, and safety protocols. This briefing must include the reading of the warrant and review of the incident command structure and assigned roles.

Outline
1) Introduction of command staff
2) Collect names/contact info for all responders and sign confidentiality agreements, waivers, emergency contact forms (pass around clipboard/forms)
3) Review incident command structure, roles, and lead assignments
4) Review emergency/critical incident protocol/procedure
5) Other safety instructions (personal protective equipment, handling safety, required equipment, etc.)
6) Discuss warrant execution timeline and procedural plan
7) Discuss confidentiality and expectations for conduct on scene
8) Read the warrant
9) Questions

Evidence in Animal Cruelty Cases

Purpose: This list provides examples of evidence to include in search warrant application language. It can also serve as a guide to searchers when collecting and/or documenting evidence at the crime scene

Evidence in Animal Cruelty Cases

Specific language for use in warrant drafting

Animals	
Name of specific animal(s) or ID Number/ear tag, etc.	
Types of animals (species, breed, etc.)	Living and deceased
Above and below ground	Born and unborn

Records	
Veterinary records	Vaccination records
Care and treatment logs/notebooks	Ownership documents
Animal transfer/transport documents	Animal sale records
Animal purchase records	Medication receipts
Animal care contracts/agreements	Staff/caretaker payroll records, schedules
Feed store/supply receipts	Rendering and other animal disposal receipts
Birth/death records	

Medical/animal care	
Medication (over-the-counter)	Medication containers
Prescriptions	Veterinary supplies
Vaccines/antiparasiticides	Food and feed packaging
Feed and water containers	Blood samples
Stool/fecal samples	Refrigerated or frozen medical supplies
Tissue samples	Evaluations and lab testing of all samples
Radiographs	DNA
Weapons or objects used as weapons	Halters
Blood spatter/blood-soiled items	Leashes
Tethers	Other restraints
Collars	Camera/camera SD cards
Photographs	Computers/tablets/cell phones
Video	Garbage/trash containers
First aid supplies	

VICTIM TO VERDICT™

Animal habitats	
Bedding	Light fixtures
Heat sources	Nest boxes, whelping boxes
Water bowl/containers/bottles	Containers
Aquariums/tanks	Cages
Kennels	Other instruments of confinement/restraint
Gates	

Animal fighting (or other cases as relevant)	
Gaffs/knives/boots/muffs	Training supplies/treadmills/jenny mills
Steroids/home remedies/shears/scales	First aid supplies/bandages/chalk
Trophies/plaques/memorabilia	Game/match announcements/derby cards
Sport/game magazines, books, videos	Contact lists/shipping labels/order forms
Vehicle search	Credit card receipts

Bestiality (or other cases as relevant)	
Social media profiles and history	DNA (human and animal)
Chat room history/transcripts	Cell phones
Pornographic media	
Restraints – collars, leashes, muzzles, harnesses, stockades	
Computers, hard drives, electronic storage devices	

Examples of On Scene Veterinary Assessments

Purpose: To provide the veterinarian with model language for reporting on observations and findings at a crime scene

Examples of on Scene Veterinary Assessments

Example 1

As I walked around the kennels that were set up in the warehouse, it became evident to me that this group of dogs was in dire condition. I observed that most of the dogs were very, very thin. Many were emaciated to the point of skeletal, with their entire boney structures visible under their skin. They all appeared very anxious, vocalizing and pacing or jumping up on the sides of the kennels. Most approached me as I went from pen to pen looking at them. The majority of the dogs appeared friendly and social to the point that I felt comfortable reaching through the wire kennels to touch them. I also observed about 20 dogs with both fresh and old bite wounds on their ears, tails, paws, nose, head and forelimbs. About a dozen dogs appeared to be severely ill and/or injured. These dogs did not react when I approached or called to them, and instead remained curled tightly in the corners of their enclosures. Many of the dogs had significant generalized hair loss of the paws, face and body consistent with external parasites. Most of the large breed dogs were housed individually and occasionally with one or two kennel mates.
 	
   Along the left side of the warehouse I observed a series of round wire exercise pens and plastic pens, some with empty wading pools inside of the pens. These pens housed between two and six dogs each. Many of the pens had an accumulation of fecal material present among the wood chip bedding.
 	
   Along the back wall of the warehouse I saw a stack of small, cat-sized plastic travel crates in which three, four, or five small dogs were literally crammed together with no room to move around and no food or water. More crates along this wall contained single small breed dogs. The dogs in these stacked crates were standing in feces and urine with no place to get away from it. The stench from these animals and crates was awful. The overcrowding of the animals in the crates was one of the worst environments I had ever seen humans put dogs in. The inability to turn around, lie down and get away from their own feces and urine was terrible for them. If the intent was to move these dogs in these crates even a short distance (15–30 minutes) the crowding of this many animals into tight confinement is inappropriate, unsafe, and unsanitary.
 	
   There was a large stack of 20 or more garbage bags near the front of the warehouse that were full of wood chip kennel bedding, dog feces, and debris.
 	
   After my initial visual examination of the dogs and the conditions, I could visually assess and diagnose issues that appeared to be chronic in nature and would have taken weeks or months to develop. Examples of these observations include:
 	
• Feces and urine staining of the coat and paws of many of the dogs.
• Very strong ammonia odor in the warehouse.
• Skin disease with hair loss and skin damage that had been present for long periods of time (months).

- Bite wounds of various durations and scarring consistent with old bite wounds. Some bite wounds appeared to be very recent (within days) and others were very old (weeks to months).
- The degree of emaciation (weight loss and loss of body fat and muscle due to starvation) was severe in the vast majority of the dogs.
- Severe illness or injury/extremely depressed or catatonic state.
- Dangerous overcrowding.
- No access to food/water.

Example 2

Overall, the pasture at that property was overgrazed and offered very little to no nutritive value to the animals. A few empty protein tubs were found and a limited water source – consisting of two automatic watering troughs holding approximately 35 gallons each – was available to the animals in the pastures, but not to those in the alleyway. About 80% of the cattle had a marginal health status as evidenced by the low (1–2) BCS, poor hair coat and lower than expected overall body weight, condition and size. Approximately 10% had the body condition score of a solid 3 and 10% at a solid 4. Some of the cattle were suffering from unattended medical conditions such as cancer eye and pink eye that had caused permanent damage to their eyes. Polled Hereford cattle, because of the typically white skin around their eyes, have a predisposition to "cancer eye" which is squamous cell carcinoma (skin cancer). Good husbandry includes monitoring cattle for this condition and intervening with removal or cryotherapy before the cancer becomes significant. If the cancer cannot be reduced, the tissue around the eye, and many times the eye, is removed. Pink eye is an infectious kerato-conjunctivitis that causes a very painful infection of the eye globe (ball). The incidence of this disease is significantly reduced or prevented through vaccination which is considered part of good husbandry for beef cattle. In the event cattle contract pink eye the treatment includes antibiotics in order to limit and cure the infection. Permanent damage to the eye can be avoided with vaccination and treatment in most cases.

We sorted and removed 14 of the cattle that were in the worst condition. This included the 6 cattle in the east pasture that were in emaciated condition, two calves in very poor condition and 6 other very thin adult cattle that we sorted out of the group from the south pasture.

Example 3

I entered the building at 10:02 AM through a door at the front of the building and immediately saw that a small (approx. 6 feet by 6 feet) entry area housed three cages and that the walls and ceiling were covered in fly droppings. The odor inside the building was very, very strong and smelled of feces and decomposition. The temperature in the building felt approximately 10 degrees warmer than outside.

The investigations team had already been through the site, numbering all of the cages and assigning letters to the birds, which are the designations I will use as references in this report. Video and photos had already been taken and as I walked through I used yellow evidence tents to mark areas I felt were relevant for photos or notes related to the care of the birds.

In the entry area the three cages that I observed labeled "1," "2," and "3," were representative of the cages in the other areas of the building. No water, no perches, very small and inadequate habitat, no food or food contaminated with feces, large piles of feces and cage debris (bedding, seed) were piled up under the cages or below the wire floors of cages. Many of the piles had been present long enough to grow mold and for bird seed to sprout and grow in some cases 3–6 inches in height.

Under cage "2," immediately in the front door, the debris measured just over 2 inches deep and was packed down indicating that it had settled for weeks or more.

In cage "3," just inside the door, I saw a kinkajou hiding under a blanket. The cage for this animal was 20 inches by 36 inches approximately which is many, many times too small for this species. The cage lacked food, water, enrichment (activity space or toys) or an enclosed area within the cage that is concealed for comfort and security or a space sufficient for exercise.

Cage "1" in the entry area contained two pigeons with no water, debris that was so deep in the bottom of the cage that it was up against the wire floor and lack of sufficient space for the birds to move around without feather damage. (See photos please.)

After the entry way I entered a large room (approx. 20 by 40 feet) that was filled with birds of many, many types in cages. Over 12 fly tapes that were covered in flies hung from the ceiling, and the walls and ceiling were covered in fly feces.

My immediate observations of the birds and the environment indicated to me that they were in very, very poor conditions and needed immediate assistance.

Example 4

A large, red colored barn on the property was vacant on the bottom floor and had several stalls made of pallets that were tied together. In one stall I saw some small bales of straw material that looked suitable for stall bedding and a domestic short haired black and white cat that ran away when approached. The second stall was empty.

In the third stall I observed a chestnut colored horse with a body condition score of one, meaning emaciated. That mare had a very long, knotted mane and tail, was emaciated and had a deep wound visible on her left rear leg just below the fetlock. The limb was swollen with edema (fluid accumulation). There was a small amount of granulation tissue forming around the wound indicating the wound was over 7–10 days old. I saw a 50 gallon garbage can tied to the inside of the stall with some water in it. The water level was at about 50% and I saw the horse was having difficulty reaching it. There was no hay in the stall at the time of my visit.

A fourth stall had a black and white paint pony type horse inside it. The horse's body condition score was a one, meaning emaciated. I could clearly see the horse's ribs and tail pins. The watering system in this stall was set up the same way. The horse was about 11–12 hands tall and the water remaining in the garbage can was 6 inches deep and could not be reached by the horse. There was no food in the stall with the horse.

Behind the red barn in an area with an overhang another horse was standing on a deep pile (4 feet plus) of manure and straw and looking out at us. That was also a smaller paint pony-type horse with a body condition score of three. There was no water receptacle available to the horse in this area.

Language Options for Adoption Contracts

Purpose: This document lists special considerations when placing animals from cruelty cases for adoption. Special considerations should be customized to the case or your agency's needs

Options for Adoption Contract Clauses for Animal from Criminal Cases

- I agree to provide food, water, shelter, exercise, socialization, and veterinary treatment as my companion animal may require throughout its lifetime at levels equal to or greater than the minimum care standards codified in [**insert statute**].
- I affirm that I will be the sole caretaker and owner of [**insert animal identifier**]. I further affirm that I am not adopting [**insert animal identifier**] on behalf of any third person or entity.
- I understand that [**insert animal identifier**] is part of a criminal case filed by [**insert prosecutor office**]. I understand that, due to the pending criminal case in [**insert county**], I must make [**insert animal identifier**] available at the request of [**insert agency/organization name**] or [**insert prosecutor office**] for any evidentiary purpose until the case is resolved.
- Until this criminal case is resolved I will keep [**insert agency/organization name**] apprised of [**insert animal identifier**]'s location. If I relocate with [**insert animal identifier**], I will provide an updated address for [**insert animal identifier**]'s location within 48 hours to [**insert agency/organization name**].
- I understand that the transfer of ownership of [**insert animal identifier**] to me has been approved on the condition that I do not rehome, sell, or otherwise permanently transfer the physical custody of [**insert animal identifier**] to any other person, agency, corporation, or entity without adequate notice to [**insert agency/organization name**].
- I understand that [**insert state**] law prohibits an animal forfeited in a criminal case from being returned to the person or persons it was originally forfeited from. Under [**insert statute**] this crime of [**insert name of the offense**] is a [**insert offense level**].
  (*This is state specific. Check your state laws to determine if a stipulation like this would be relevant in your jurisdiction.*)

State Evidence Retention and Disposition Rules

Purpose: A reference for state specific laws or regulations on the retention and disposition of evidence in criminal cases

State Evidence Retention and Disposition Rules

Resources
1) Alaska   a) Alaska Stat. § 12.36.200
2) Arizona   a) Ariz. Rev. Stat. Ann. § 13-4221
3) Arkansas   a) A.C.A. § 12-12-104
4) California   a) Cal Pen Code § 1417.9
5) District of Columbia   a) D.C. Code § 22-4134
6) Georgia   a) Ga. Code Ann. § 17-5-56
7) Kentucky   a) Ky. Rev. Stat. Ann. § 524.140
8) Louisiana   a) La. Rev. Stat. Ann. § 15:621
9) Massachusetts   a) Mass. Gen. Laws. Ch. 278A § 16
10) Michigan   a) Mich. Comp. Laws. Ann. § 770.16
11) Minnesota   a) Minn. Stat. Ann. § 590.10
12) Mississippi   a) Miss. Code Ann. § 99-49-1
13) Montana   a) Mont. Code Ann. 46-21-111
14) Nebraska   a) Neb. Rev. Stat. Ann. § 29-4125
15) Nevada   a) Nev. Rev. Stat. Ann. § 176.0912
16) New Hampshire   a) N.H. Rev. Stat. Ann. § 651-D:3
17) North Carolina   a) N.C. Gen. Stat. Ann. § 15A-268
18) Ohio   a) Ohio Rev. Code Ann. § 2933.82
19) Oklahoma   a) Okla. Stat. Ann. Tit. 22 § 1372
20) Rhode Island   a) R.I. Gen. Laws Ann. § 10-9.1-11
21) Texas   a) Tex. Code Crim. Proc. art. 38.43
22) Wisconsin   a) Wis. Stat. Ann. § 978.08

Resource List: Grants for Animal Cruelty Case Work

Purpose: A list of organizations that may provide funding to support animal cruelty investigation and case work

Resource List: Grants for Animal Cruelty Case Work

- Animal Legal Defense Fund
  - https://aldf.org/how_we_work/criminal-justice
- The Association of Prosecuting Attorneys
  - https://www.sheriffs.org/programs/national-law-enforcement-center-animal-abuse
- The American Society for the Prevention of Cruelty to Animals (ASPCA)
  - https://www.aspca.org/about-us/aspca-grants
- National District Attorneys Association
  - https://ndaa.org/programs/animal-abuse
- American Humane
  - https://www.americanhumane.org/initiative/second-chance-grants
- The Humane Society of the United States
  - https://humanepro.org/grant-listings
- The Glaser Progress Foundation
  - http://www.glaserprogress.org/grants/index.asp
- Red Rover Relief
  - https://redrover.org/relief
- The Association for Animal Welfare Advancement
  - https://theaawa.org/page/GrantSources
- California Department of Food and Agriculture
  - https://www.cdfa.ca.gov/SpayNeuter
- Kenneth A. Scott Charitable Trust
  - https://kennethscottcharitabletrust.org/mission-and-grant-guidelines
- Forensic Veterinary Investigations, LLC
  - http://www.vetinvestigator.com/animaldoeproject
- The William and Charlotte Parks Foundation for Animal Welfare
  - https://www.parksfoundation.org/types-of-grants
- Oklahoma Alliance for Animals
  - https://animalallianceok.org/programs/fighting-cruelty
- Bikers Against Animal Cruelty
  - https://www.bikersagainstanimalcruelty.org/about-us
- Banfield Foundation
  - https://vet.banfield.com/banfield-foundation/programs
- Hugs and Kisses Animal Fund
  - https://hugsandkissesanimalfund.org/grant-application
- Ian Somerhalder Foundation
  - https://www.isfoundation.com/ISFEmergencyMedicalGrant
- Second Chance Fund
  - https://thesecondchancefund.org
- Napa Valley Community Foundation
  - https://www.napavalleycf.org/wp-content/uploads/2020/11/FY21-NVCF-Gotelli-Fund-RFP.pdf

VICTIM TO VERDICT™

Index

Page numbers in *italics* refer to illustrations; those in **bold** refer to tables

Animal Cruelty Investigations: A Collaborative Approach from Victim to Verdict™, First Edition.
Edited by Kris Otteman, Linda Fielder, and Emily Lewis.
© 2022 John Wiley & Sons, Inc. Published 2022 by John Wiley & Sons, Inc.
Companion website: www.wiley.com/go/otteman/victimtoverdict